T0187163

David Miles has two decades of experience as a scientist and educator in the field of infectious disease immunology. He began his scientific career as a zoologist before moving to The Gambia to study the infant immune response to vaccines against infectious diseases, and spent the next ten years leading research projects there, in Malawi and in South Africa. After his research career was ended by lymphoma, David moved into education. He is now a tutor on the London School of Hygiene and Tropical Medicine's distance learning MSc in infectious diseases.

HOW VACCINES WORK

The Science and History Behind Every
Question You've Wanted to Ask

DAVID MILES

PIATKUS

PIATKUS

First published in Great Britain in 2023 by Piatkus

1 3 5 7 9 10 8 6 4 2

Copyright © David Miles 2023

The moral right of the author has been asserted.

All rights reserved.
No part of this publication may be reproduced, stored in a
retrieval system, or transmitted, in any form, or by any means, without
the prior permission in writing of the publisher, nor be otherwise circulated
in any form of binding or cover other than that in which it is published
and without a similar condition including this condition being
imposed on the subsequent purchaser.

A CIP catalogue record for this book
is available from the British Library.

ISBN: 978-0-3494-2890-1

Typeset in Sabon by M Rules
Printed and bound in Great Britain by
Clays Ltd, Elcograf S.p.A.

Papers used by Piatkus are from well-managed forests
and other responsible sources.

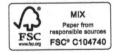

Piatkus
An imprint of
Little, Brown Book Group
Carmelite House
50 Victoria Embankment
London EC4Y 0DZ

An Hachette UK Company
www.hachette.co.uk

www.littlebrown.co.uk

To every under-appreciated postgrad, field worker, laboratory technician, postdoc, research nurse, medical officer and data manager whose efforts have enabled countless millions of people to live long and healthy lives.

Never forget what you achieved.

Contents

III: The myths and mysteries of vaccination

Introduction

The seed for this book was planted by an MMR vaccination.

Not in the way you're probably thinking. It was nothing to do with the two-decades-and-counting row over the evidence-free assertion that the MMR causes autism. It was a mundane appointment to receive the MMR at my GP's surgery.

The GP's nurse delivered the 'slight scratch', as they call it, and asked if she could pick my brains about her adult son.

It happens. Like most medical researchers, I am often asked medical questions. More often than not, they're in areas I know nothing about and I have to explain that I'm a scientist, not a doctor; I may or may not be able to explain why a doctor told you to do something, but don't, whatever you do, mistake anything I say for medical advice. I usually end up falling back on my standard response: 'I think you should see a doctor about that.'

A nurse working in a GP's surgery didn't need medical advice from me. She wanted to understand why her son, who had recently recovered from a lymphoma, had been advised against being vaccinated against yellow fever before travelling to South America.

That was a question I was comfortable with. Most of my research has been on how our immune systems interact with the microbes they protect us against, and how vaccines stack the deck in our favour. I was happy to pontificate about how a lymphoma, being a cancer of the lymphocyte cells that are key to the immune response, would have left her son with a weakened immune system. That mattered, because the yellow fever vaccine is a type called 'live attenuated': a strain of the yellow fever virus modified to be much weaker than the 'wild-type' circulating in nature.

Challenging the immune system with an attenuated virus is a bit like sending a boxer into the ring with one hand tied behind his back. He'll be able to throw a couple of punches at the immune system, letting it know it's in a fight but leaving no doubt about the outcome. As long as the vaccine strain is reasonably similar to the wild-type, it triggers protection against the real thing.

The catch is that the mildness of the infection depends on the immune system stamping it out while it's still mild. If her son's immune system was still reeling from lymphoma and chemotherapy, it might not be able to handle even the mild vaccine strain. To stay with the boxing analogy, her son's immune system might be going into the ring with both hands tied behind its back, unable to protect him from the one-punch vaccine strain.

The nurse seemed happy with my explanation, and I was happy with my immunity to the three viruses in the MMR, but the nurse's question crystallised something I'd been thinking about for some time. I get asked a lot of questions about vaccines, mostly by people bamboozled by the accusations and counter-accusations that fly around whenever a vaccine finds its way into the media. It leaves many people struggling to sift evidence from rhetoric and unsure of what's best for themselves and their children.

The things that worry the people asking me questions are rarely the things that worry the researchers and public health professionals who work on vaccines. Diseases caused by viruses and bacteria shape our society in ways we barely notice, or so I mused in those halcyon days before COVID-19 reshaped our lives. Few of us give much thought to the microbial reason why there's a sink next to every toilet.

In Britain, as in most high-income countries, vaccinations against the most dangerous microbes nature throws at us are available for every child, and we have been so successful at banishing them that it's easy to forget why we need vaccines.

That's what led to my first encounter with serious infectious disease. The year I was born, a long-simmering debate over whooping cough vaccination burst out of academic conferences and medical journals and into *The Times* and television news. Some doctors and scientists believed the vaccine was causing permanent brain damage in some of the children it was given to. Others saw no evidence that it was dangerous and were more worried about putting parents off the vaccine. The latter side would ultimately be proved correct,[1] but that lay in the future.

My parents were intelligent people, but they weren't equipped to evaluate the accusations of peddling dangerous vaccines from one side and counter-accusations of scaremongering from the other. They were as bamboozled as the people who ask me about vaccines now. All they knew was that highly qualified people were saying that the whooping cough vaccine might cause brain damage.

Watching one's baby being jabbed with a steel needle is distressing enough without worrying that its contents might damage his developing brain, and by the 1970s, whooping cough was no longer the disease most likely to kill a child, as it had been when my parents were children.[2] My parents decided that protecting me against a disease that belonged to the era of steam locomotives and air-raid sirens wasn't worth any possible risk to my brain.

They weren't alone. Two thirds of British parents decided their children were better off not being vaccinated against whooping cough. What happened next was inevitable. Whooping cough returned with a vengeance. Between 1977 and 1979, nearly 115,000 British children caught it.[3]

I was one of them. Paroxysms of coughing left me gasping

for air with the 'whoop' that gives the disease its name, while my fevers kept both me and my parents up night after night. I recovered after a few months, as did most of the victims of the 1970s epidemic. Not all; thirty-eight children died,[4] which scared parents back to the vaccine clinics. By the 1990s, whooping cough was once again a rare disease in Britain.

I don't remember my brush with it, so I give whooping cough no credit for the career choice I made in my mid-twenties. With a newly minted doctorate in zoology and no job, I changed direction and applied for a post researching the infant immune system in The Gambia, a tiny West African country whose many mysteries include the definite article in its name.

In 2002, I left Britain in the throes of a new vaccine scare. The one you probably thought of when I mentioned the MMR. Researchers at London's Royal Free Hospital were asserting that another vaccine caused brain damage. This time, the vaccine was the MMR, combining live attenuated vaccine strains of the measles, mumps and rubella (aka German measles) viruses, and the feared brain damage was regressive autism.

At the time, my colleagues and I thought the Royal Free team had raised a legitimate point of concern. If there was any chance that the MMR might cause autism, the researchers had been right to raise it so that it could be properly investigated.

We didn't know that the whole thing was based on falsified data,[5] and backed up by research practices so unethical that they would get the lead researcher struck off the medical register[6] – although not until those practices had put a child in intensive care.[7]

The whole story didn't come to light until years later, but we did know that the original research had only involved twelve children, and that subsequent studies, looking at hundreds of thousands of children, found no link between the MMR and autism.

But that wasn't how it had been reported. As a rather green researcher, I remember chuckling at a headline in one of the more reputable broadsheets: 'Research puts MMR autism link in doubt.'[8] I didn't think the link was in *doubt*; it was never proved in the first place, and had since been shown not to exist.

I didn't fully appreciate that for parents, it was nothing to chuckle about. Like my parents a generation earlier, they were trying to make sense of media coverage that gave more space to strident opinion than to calm evaluation of evidence. Many parents of the 2000s made the same judgement that my parents had made in the 1970s: that erring on the side of caution meant not having their children vaccinated.

In The Gambia, I met parents who saw things very differently. For them, infectious disease was not a bogeyman of the past but an ever-present threat. Malaria and gastroenteritis stalked their children every day, and they had no confidence that the under-resourced healthcare centres would be able to help. It was a rare parent in The Gambia who hadn't been to the funeral of a close relative's child. They knew what their own babies faced.

In the early 2000s, childhood vaccination had recently expanded dramatically across Africa, including The Gambia. Infant mortality rates were dropping so precipitously that their children had a much better chance of growing up than children born even a few years earlier.

Gambian parents did whatever was necessary to get their children vaccinated. Most mothers had to take their babies to a clinic in the back of a 'bush taxi': a battered old Peugeot estate car that bounced and creaked along roads riddled with potholes. When a bush taxi stopped to let someone in or out, the passengers often had to get out and push-start it. At the clinic, mothers were often told to come back next week because the vaccines had run out – and come back is what mothers did.

I went to The Gambia to run one study, but the nature of

research is that every question answered raises another dozen to be asked. I spent the next ten years digging into the immune system's interactions with infections and with vaccines, moving from The Gambia to Malawi to South Africa and back to Malawi before my research career was cut short by the machinations of my own immune system. With irony I wasn't inclined to appreciate, I developed a lymphoma: a cancer of my immune system's lymphocytes similar to that suffered by the son of the nurse who would give me the MMR years later. My failing health sent me back to Britain and into the merciful arms of the NHS.

That lymphoma toughed out more rounds of chemotherapy than I care to remember. The superb clinicians resorted to the nuclear option of a haematopoietic stem cell transplant, replacing all of my misbehaving lymphocytes with a donor's. My new immune system finally saw off the lymphoma, but my recovery came at a price. I lost all the immunity I'd accumulated from four decades of vaccines and infections. Worse, my new immune system was now in such a fragile state that, for the same reasons the nurse's son couldn't be vaccinated against yellow fever, it couldn't be trusted to handle the live attenuated vaccine strains in the MMR.

Meanwhile, measles was returning to Britain. It was a consequence of headlines like the one I'd found funny a decade earlier; enough parents had avoided the MMR that there were now enough unvaccinated children to allow measles to circulate. Measles is serious enough in an adult with a healthy immune system, and because it's a virus, antibiotics weren't going to help if I caught it. If a child with measles breathed on me, they could kill me.

That headline wasn't funny anymore.

Five years after the transplant, the doctors decided my immune system was ready to throw a few punches, which is why a man with two decades of medical research behind him was receiving a childhood vaccine.

The nurse's question made me realise that even people who work with vaccines every day don't always have a clear idea of how they work. That's hardly surprising; modern vaccines are the product of three centuries of trial and error and, for much of that time, trials were so poorly conceived that errors often went undetected.

At the time, I would also have said that even people who work with vaccines often forget how important infectious disease was for most of those three centuries. How much time do any of us spend wondering at the closed sewer that freed us from typhoid and cholera?

A year later, infectious disease reminded us of its importance. Thanks to COVID-19, I researched and wrote most of this book in lockdown, knowing that a donated immune system would never be as effective as the one I was born with, and that there was a strong chance I wouldn't survive if the COVID-19 virus found its way into my throat.

It gave me a strong sense of what drove the vaccine researchers of previous generations – or at least some of them. The research that brought today's vaccines was part of the last three centuries of history, and history is not always pretty. Many researchers were driven by humanitarian urges, but, like all aspects of science and technology, medical research has often been driven by the needs of army and empire. Some of the vaccines that are still in use were born of motives and methods that make for uncomfortable reading today.

By the time I entered medical research, the principle of informed consent was sacrosanct. Before I could accept a volunteer for a study, I needed to make sure they understood what they were volunteering for and that they knew they could unvolunteer at any time. If my studies involved children who were too young to give informed consent, their parents' consent was needed on their behalf. I was required to make very sure that any information I collected was kept strictly confidential, and every procedure needed to be approved by institutional ethics committees.

Research hasn't always worked like that. Until the 1970s, medical research often involved orderly lines of adults or children with no idea of what they were about to receive.

The world of today is built by choosing what we want to keep from the world of yesterday and discarding what we don't. If the sort of experiments that proved today's vaccines have no place in today's world, we can choose to keep the vaccine and make sure tomorrow's vaccines are proved with ethical experiments.

The first part of the book is a whistle-stop tour through the three centuries of discoveries – and more than a few blind alleys – that brought us to our current understanding of why we need vaccines, how they work and how we make sure they work.

The second part devotes one chapter to each of the vaccines routinely given in Britain. Not every country uses all of these vaccines, and some countries use vaccines that aren't used in Britain, but most of the vaccines used in any country will be covered by those chapters. The story of each vaccine begins with the story of the disease it protects against. However, at the time of writing, the story of many of those diseases is far from over.

The third part deals with the most common concerns about the safety of the vaccines, some of which do have some basis and some of which are as mythical as the monster under the bed.

The final section lists the references from which I have drawn my information. It's there as an invitation to check up on me. I don't ask you to believe what I say because I am a scientist. I ask you to consider what I say in the light of the knowledge from which I draw my conclusions.

When you do that, I am confident you will agree with me that vaccination is one of the great discoveries of human history.

I

How vaccines educate
the immune system

Chapter 1

The principles of vaccination: isolate, attenuate, inject

On one side is the human body. On the other are the microbes that might harm it. Between them stand the phagocytes, lymphocytes and antibodies of the immune system.

They don't stand alone. They have some help from the human mind.

Today's vaccines are a product of the human mind and of a very modern process, from the peer-reviewed papers that show a vaccine is safe and effective to the quality-control stamps that tell us a vaccine contains exactly what it should contain and nothing else. Yet the human mind has been giving the human immune system a helping hand since long before anyone thought of academic journals or pharmaceutical factories.

Human minds have been applying themselves to immunological processes since time immemorial, in the literal sense that the person who first found a way to work with the immune system has been forgotten. How they came up with their trick has been lost, along with their name. The earliest definitive evidence we have that their trick worked arose from a conversation between two men whose names, in the British colonial outpost that was Boston in 1706, encoded their relationship: Cotton Mather and Onesimus.

Mather was a puritan clergyman, owner of the largest library in England's American colonies, member of London's Royal Society and an authority on witch-finding who vocally supported the Salem trials.[1] The boundary between science and mysticism then lay in a very different place to where it lies now.

Onesimus was Mather's slave.

He was born somewhere in Africa, but beyond that, his origins are lost, along with his given name. He was only Onesimus for the few years between Mather receiving him as a gift from his congregation and selling him for disobedience.

It's unlikely that the man who taught Europeans how to fight one of their greatest scourges was ever thanked for it.

Europe wakes up to variolation

Mather asked Onesimus if he'd ever had smallpox, one of the most feared diseases of the eighteenth century. We now know that the smallpox virus infects the throat and is transmitted when someone breathes it out. It then spreads rapidly through the body, and anyone who survives its attack on their major organs is likely to be permanently scarred by the pustules it raises on the skin.[2]

In Mather's day, all that was known was that it was a fast-spreading harbinger of death and disfigurement, so when Onesimus answered, 'Yes and no,' Mather wanted to know what he meant.

Onesimus showed Mather a scar on his arm and told a curious tale. When he was a child, the pus from someone else's smallpox pustule was inserted under his skin. Onesimus endured a mild case of smallpox, hence his yes. It had been far less serious than naturally acquired smallpox, hence his no.

Mather knew that nobody caught smallpox more than once, but he didn't know there was a way to ensure that one time would be mild. Once his curiosity was piqued, he discovered that the technique Onesimus described was well known in Boston – but only among its African-born slaves. Their European owners had never heard of it, because before Mather, none had thought to ask.

Controlled exposure to a microbe that causes a disease is not vaccination, which uses an adulterated version of the microbe. The two approaches do, however, work in the same way: by triggering immune memory, the phenomenon by which the immune system can recognise a microbe it has encountered in the past and respond faster and more effectively the second time round.

In 1706, no one knew that microbes even caused disease, let alone how to adulterate them, but the technique Onesimus described was well known in much of Asia and Africa.[3] Mather couldn't know that there are written records from mid-1500s China,[4] when the practice was described as so commonplace that the unknown genius behind it may already have been forgotten. Europe had been somewhat slow on the uptake.

The learned men of Europe and its colonies called smallpox 'variola', so they called Onesimus's procedure 'variolation'.

Fifteen years after that conversation, smallpox arrived in Boston. In 1721, it tore through the town, reducing Bostonians to agonised wheezing for breath as the pustules encrusting their skin spread into their lungs. For possibly the only time in their lives, black Bostonians fared better than white. Many had been variolated and remained untouched.

Mather might have sold Onesimus by then, but he hadn't forgotten him. He appealed to Boston's medical men to try the technique that had protected their slaves, but only found one willing to give it a try. Zabdiel Boylston, a member of Mather's congregation, variolated his six-year-old son, his slave and his slave's son. All three recovered without serious illness.

Boylston and Mather offered to variolate anyone who wanted to be variolated. Some were willing but others took a view summed up in a note attached to a grenade thrown through Mather's window, which, fortunately, failed to explode: 'Mather, you dog, damn you, I'll inoculate you with this.'[5]

Mather had not only introduced the forerunner of vaccination to the European world. He had also inspired the forerunner of the anti-vaccination movement.

Nevertheless, his results were hard to argue with. Boylston inoculated 280 people, and all but six survived the 1721 epidemic, giving a death rate of one in forty-seven. Among Boston's population as a whole, the death rate was one in thirteen.[6]

Variolation became so widely used across North America that five decades later, George Washington had his entire continental army variolated, putting an end to the smallpox outbreaks that nearly stifled the American revolution at birth.[7] The first president of the United States of America probably had no idea that he owed his country's independence to the advice of a slave.

Lady Mary Wortley Montagu

Mather and Boylston were the first to use variolation in the European world, but only just. While they were fighting Boston's 1721 smallpox outbreak, Lady Mary Wortley Montagu introduced variolation to London.

Being the daughter of a duke, Lady Mary could get away with the occasional breach of protocol – and a century and a half before women were admitted to British medical schools, revolutionising medical practice was certainly a breach of protocol. In her youth, she was a celebrated beauty who caused a minor scandal when she broke her engagement to an Irish viscount called Clotworthy Skeffington by eloping with Lord Wortley Montagu. Her marriage endured but her beauty did not. A few years into her marriage, a bout of smallpox left her face eyebrowless and pitted with scars.[8]

The following year, her husband was appointed ambassador to the Ottoman Empire, and in Constantinople, she learned about variolation. She was so impressed with the practice that when her husband was away, she had their son variolated and presented his scar to her husband as a fait accompli. The boy recovered quickly, and when the family returned to London, she brought her knowledge of immunisation with her. In 1721, while smallpox was ravaging Boston, it also made an appearance in London, so Lady Mary enlisted the court surgeon to variolate her daughter.

Her title and connections protected her from the sort of vitriol that Mather received. Hans Sloane, president of the Royal Society, was an early convert to variolation and his patronage, combined with Montagu's aristocratic connections, did far more to make variolation respectable than the solid evidence provided by Mather. Variolation was taken up across Britain and subsequently Europe. It saved a lot of lives, albeit at the cost of a few. Deliberately infecting someone with smallpox could never be a completely safe process.

Respectability proved to be a mixed blessing. As European physicians adopted variolation, they also adapted it to fit their concept of how medicine should be practised.

Where Montagu had described a simple scratch to the arm with a pus-dipped needle, physicians prepared their patients with a course of bloodletting, laxatives and emetics. Physicians and surgeons charged by the procedure, and the more they complicated variolation, the more lucrative it became.

The preparations weakened their patients, leaving them

vulnerable to a more severe infection than they needed to endure. One man left with a particularly unpleasant memory of variolation was a Gloucestershire surgeon called Edward Jenner.[9] It may have been what inspired Jenner to come up with something better: vaccination.

The man from Gloucestershire

Jenner became a surgeon the hard way. He couldn't afford university fees, so he learned his trade through apprenticeship, starting when he was thirteen years old. When his mentors ran out of things to teach him, he learned by experiment.

At thirty-five years old, his experiments with unmanned hydrogen balloons were probably the first experiments in aeronautics conducted in Britain. At thirty-nine, his first manuscript to the Royal Society resolved a question that had bamboozled naturalists for centuries: where the cuckoo lays its eggs. At forty-five, he proved that a man had been poisoned by feeding his stomach contents to two dogs, which subsequently died. His foray into forensics failed to impress a jury, however, and the man's wife was acquitted of murdering him.[10]

At forty-eight he conducted the experiment that made him famous. In 1797, he enlisted a dairymaid called Sarah Nelmes, who had a cowpox pustule on her hand. Cowpox was a disease of cattle that occasionally infected dairy workers, but although cowpox pustules looked identical to smallpox pustules, they were no more than a minor irritation and did not spread across the body. Jenner took a scraping from Nelmes's pustule and used it to inoculate an eight-year-old boy called James Phipps. James later complained of a headache and a mild fever but quickly recovered. Jenner then variolated him, and recorded symptoms so mild that he would have expected them in someone who had already had smallpox. Cowpox had rendered James immune to smallpox with no need for weeks of bleeding and purging.

Jenner wrote a report of his experiment, but the Royal Society declined to publish it. Rejection is a common fate of manuscripts reporting revolutionary results, but the Royal Society's reason was solid: one small boy wasn't much of an experiment. Instead of repeating his procedure on more children, Jenner self-published his report as a pamphlet.

It attracted enough attention that other surgeons tried it. There was never a clinical trial of Jenner's technique but surgeons and physicians all over Britain, and subsequently Europe, concluded that it worked.[11]

Jenner's experiment replaced variolation with vaccination as we now understand it: he had triggered James's immune memory to smallpox without exposing him to the smallpox virus.

The word 'vaccination' was coined by Richard Dunning, Jenner's friend and fellow surgeon. He derived it from *vacca*, the Latin word for 'cow', so vaccination literally means, 'from the cow'.

From the cow to the world

Vaccination proved as effective as variolation and far safer. Physicians and surgeons around the world embraced it as a phenomenon that protected people from smallpox, but none could have explained how it worked, any more than Onesimus or Mather could have explained what underpinned variolation.

It was only decades after Jenner had vaccinated James Phipps that anyone delved into the possibility that vaccination might be more than a phenomenon, and looked for the principles behind it with the hope that understanding them might open the door to protecting against more than smallpox.

The discovery of those principles hinged on an 1879 experiment on chicken broth in the Paris laboratory of the man who, more than anyone else, turned vaccination into a practical approach to tackling multiple diseases.

Louis Pasteur started his career as a chemist and agricultural scientist on a mission to improve the quality of French wine. When he delved into the process by which grapes ferment, he realised he was looking not at a chemical process but a biological one. Fermentation did not simply *happen* to grape juice, but was *done* to it by yeast, a type of microbe. If a living microbe lay behind fermentation, Pasteur reasoned, then flash-heating it to kill the yeast could stop the fermentation at the moment when the wine was perfect.[12] 'Pasteurisation', as flash-heating became known, is now more widely associated with sterilising milk, but generations of oenophiles owe a debt to Pasteur's first major success.

His work on wine showed a process that would characterise Pasteur's career: he would investigate what lay behind a problem and use it to work out a practical solution. For Jenner, phenomenon had been the end of his process. For Pasteur, it was the beginning.

Pasteur reasoned that if fermentation was caused by microbes, perhaps putrefaction was as well. Having proved it, he went further. If microbes were what rotted dead flesh, perhaps microbes might also be behind the diseases that afflicted the living.

By then, Pasteur was in his late forties and had lost the use of one hand to a stroke.[13] With a Légion d'Honneur and a seat in the Académie des Sciences, he had reached the career stage where most scientists stepped back from the laboratory and dispensed their wisdom to the younger men who toiled in it. However, the distant sage was not a role that suited Pasteur. He preferred to stand next to his toiling assistants – or sometimes over them – while dispensing wisdom in the form of direct orders.

In 1873, he was elected to the Académie de Médecine, whose members thought they might benefit from the insights of a man versed in scientific thought. They got more than they bargained for. Once Pasteur had conceived his microbiological theory of disease, he wouldn't let it go – and he'd never learned the art of diplomatic disagreement.

His fellow academicians might have appreciated a tanner's son improving the quality of their wine, but that didn't mean they were going to listen to him telling them they were doing medicine all wrong. On one occasion, grey-bearded men had to physically intervene to prevent a punch-up that led to Pasteur being challenged to a duel.[14] Not everyone elected to the Académie gloried in drama, however, and cooler heads got everybody calmed down before any pistols were fired.

Between debates, Pasteur was gathering evidence. He'd returned to agricultural science and was working on a disease called chicken cholera, so-called because, like human cholera, it causes diarrhoea, although the microbe behind it would later prove to be unrelated.

There are two versions of the story of how the seminal experiment came about, and frustratingly, we don't know which is true.[15] One has Pasteur's assistants keeping the chicken cholera microbe alive in chicken broth. They periodically took a sample of the microbe to inoculate a fresh bottle of broth – a process called 'passaging' – before it got through all the nutrients in the first bottle. When Pasteur was away, his assistants paused the passaging, leaving the microbe in the same nutrient broth for much longer than usual. When he returned, the microbe could no longer make chickens fall ill, but it could protect them against fresh chicken cholera microbes.

The other version credits one of Pasteur's assistants, Émile Roux, with discovering the protective version of chicken cholera bacteria by passing pure oxygen through the cultures.

However it came about, the 1879 experiment showed that a microbe could be adapted to confer immunity without causing infection. In short, it could be turned into a vaccine.

Pasteur broadened the definition of the word 'vaccine' beyond smallpox by applying a similar approach to anthrax. Charles Chamberland, Pasteur's most adept assistant when it came to developing laboratory equipment, found that anthrax microbes treated with carbolic acid at exactly the right temperature protected livestock from infection with fresh anthrax.[16]

In 1881, Roux and Chamberland tested their anthrax vaccine on a herd of sheep and cattle in the village of Pouilly-le-Fort, a short train journey from Paris. By this time, the Académie debates had attracted widespread attention and quite a crowd gathered to watch. There were livestock breeders who wanted a successful experiment to end their problems with anthrax, detractors who wanted a failed experiment to make Pasteur shut up about microbes, and journalists who didn't care either way if they got a story out of it.

The Pouilly-le-Fort trial was a spectacular success. When anthrax killed all the unvaccinated animals and none of the vaccinated ones, vaccination in the modern sense had arrived. Pasteur and his assistants had shown that vaccination was not a one-off phenomenon, but followed principles that they had successfully applied to two different diseases, and could apply to many more.

It's thanks to Pasteur that we still call it vaccination, even though few modern vaccines have anything to do with cows. A few months after the Pouilly-le-Fort trial, Pasteur, with a recent promotion to his Légion d'Honneur that he insisted on sharing with Chamberland and Roux, presented his results at the International Congress of Medicine.

In his summing up, he said, 'I have given to the term vaccination an extension which science, I hope, will adopt as an homage to the merits and the immense services rendered by one of the greatest men England has ever produced, your own Jenner.'[17]

With this speech, he ensured that the word 'vaccination' would stick.

Isolate, attenuate, inject

Pasteur's experiments with chicken cholera and anthrax led him to codify his approach into the three-step Pasteur doctrine of vaccine development: isolate, attenuate, inject.

First, isolate the microbe causing the disease. Work out what it is and how to culture it.

Second, attenuate the microbe by finding a way to turn the disease-causing 'wild-type' into a vaccine strain that triggers the same immune memory without causing the disease.

Third, inject it into the chicken, cow or human that you're trying to protect, and, if you've got the isolation and attenuation right, you can stop worrying about that chicken, cow or human getting the disease in question.

The principle is simple. The practice is anything but. Nevertheless, vaccines are still developed using the broad outline of the Pasteur doctrine, albeit using techniques that Pasteur could only have dreamed of.

After his success with anthrax, Pasteur was keen to try his doctrine on a human disease, which presented a new problem. Until he injected his attenuated strain into someone, he couldn't be sure it really was attenuated. It was one thing to risk a chicken or a cow keeling over because the strain wasn't attenuated enough. It was quite another to risk a human being.

The dilemma led him to target rabies. Someone bitten by a rabid dog was already facing a painful death within a few weeks. If Pasteur could inject someone with an attenuated rabies strain soon enough after they were bitten, he might be able to save someone who was otherwise beyond hope. If something went wrong, it wouldn't make their situation any worse.

Pasteur couldn't know that he'd picked a particularly awkward disease to start with. Rabies is not caused by a bacterium, like chicken cholera and anthrax, but a fundamentally different type of microbe that would later be called a virus. At the time, it wasn't called anything, because nobody suspected the existence of viruses. It says a lot for Pasteur's confidence in his microbial theory that despite the microbe being too small to be seen through his microscopes, he was so sure it was there that he persisted in applying his isolate, attenuate, inject doctrine.

Pasteur and his assistants spent four years culturing rabies in rabbit spinal cords and experimenting on dogs and rabbits. By 1885, they had something they were confident enough to try on a human.

That human was nine-year-old Joseph Meister, whose parents had heard there was one man in the world who might save their son after he was bitten by a rabid dog. It was an anxious few weeks for everyone concerned, but when Joseph showed no sign of developing rabies from either the bite or the vaccine, Pasteur was confident enough to try it on a second patient.

That patient was a boy who became a hero. Fifteen-year-old shepherd Jean-Baptiste Jupille was bitten while defending younger boys from a rabid dog. He was rushed to Paris for Pasteur's groundbreaking treatment, and not only survived but was sent home with a thousand francs from the Institute de France to reward his courage.

Jupille's five minutes of fame helped to publicise the success of the vaccine, and before long, Pasteur was receiving patients from as far afield as the USA and Russia. His success was a key driver behind the establishment of the Institut Pasteur, so named despite Pasteur's objections. It was funded by charitable donations, ranging from a few francs from thousands of ordinary French people to bundles of cash from great names in finance, like Rothschild and Rockefeller, and emperors, like Dom Pedro II of Brazil, Tsar Alexander III of Russia and Sultan Abdul Hamid II of the Ottoman Empire.[18]

The Institut was decorated with statues of its major donors alongside a statue of Jean-Baptiste Jupille's epic battle with the rabid dog. When Jupille, like Joseph Meister, accepted a job as a concierge at the Institut, he gave the Institut the rare distinction of having a statue of a serving doorman.

Developing the Pasteur doctrine

Pasteur's idea of attenuation involved a series of injections, starting with a highly attenuated version of the microbe and ending with something close to the wild-type. The idea was to habituate the patient to progressively more virulent versions of the microbe until they could handle the real thing.

Many of today's vaccines are produced by attenuation, but, with the benefit of a century and a half of hindsight, Pasteur's way of doing it now looks over-complicated and unsafe.

Over-complicated because it depended on immune memory triggered by the first injections to cope with the more virulent strains used in later injections. If the immune system could handle those virulent strains, it could already handle the wild-type and there was no need for multiple vaccine strains. Unsafe because if it couldn't, those later injections were as dangerous as injecting with the wild-type.

Attenuation is still used, but these days an attenuated vaccine is a single highly attenuated strain of the microbe.

Ironically, Pasteur's attenuated rabies vaccine almost certainly wasn't working in the way he thought it was. He assumed that the more times he passed it between rabbit spinal cords, the more attenuated the microbe became, which gave him his selection of strains of different virulence. We now know that while viruses do become attenuated in culture, the process is nowhere near as predictable as Pasteur concluded. It's far more likely that the process was producing a lot of inactive virus, and that's what triggered the immunity that saved Meister and Jupille.

Modern vaccinology is built on the Pasteur doctrine but it does not use it in the way that Pasteur did. The building began with two of the more colourful characters of early vaccinology: Waldemar Haffkine and Almroth Wright.

In 1884, Haffkine earned his zoology doctorate from the University of Odessa not a moment too soon. Being a Ukrainian Jew, his youth had been punctuated by regular pogroms of rape and vandalism. Haffkine combined his studies with helping to organise his community's self-defence association which, by the time he graduated, made him a marked man.[19] He needed to leave the Russian Empire in a hurry, and his fascination with the emerging science of microbiology led him to the Institut Pasteur.

He quickly established himself and, using Pasteur's doctrine, developed an attenuated vaccine strain of the cholera microbe. It involved two injections, with the second being less attenuated than the first,[20] but even after he tested it on himself and several of his friends, the French authorities balked at the idea of injecting cholera microbes into healthy people.[21]

One of those friends saw the authorities' refusal as an opportunity. Ernest Hankin, an officer of the Indian Medical Service, promptly recruited Haffkine. In 1893, Haffkine arrived in Calcutta,* where he initiated the first large-scale roll-out of a vaccine since smallpox nearly a century earlier.

Haffkine met Wright when he returned to Europe in 1895, recovering from a bout of malaria. Wright was a dishevelled giant of a man with a voice one acquaintance described as the 'narrowest squeak possible'[22] and a solid track record in the study of blood.[23]

In 1892, Wright was appointed head of the British Army's

---

* Now Kolkata.

medical school at Netley, Hampshire. It was a controversial appointment for a man with no military background, especially as he had been promoted over the head of David Bruce, an army officer of nearly ten years. Bruce had proved his scientific chops in describing what he called Malta fever, which would later be renamed brucellosis in his honour. However, Bruce's drinking and womanising – and what was mysteriously described as 'an unfortunate incident with a railway porter'[24] – saw him passed over for promotion.

By 1895, Wright was trying to apply the Pasteur doctrine to typhoid, one of the many diseases that ran rampant through tightly packed army camps. He was persuaded by the microbiological theory of disease but didn't know how to apply it.

He invited Haffkine to advise him and their conversations must have been productive, because both men went on to invent vaccines by simply killing the isolated microbe, enabling them to develop vaccines much faster than they could have done using attenuation. Wright acknowledged Haffkine's input in the first sentence of the paper describing his typhoid vaccine,[25] and threw himself into a two-decade-long barney with the War Office until they started vaccinating soldiers upon recruitment.[26]

Haffkine's target was bubonic plague, which was spreading across central Asia and arrived in India at about the same time as Haffkine returned in 1896.[27] Instead of the attenuation he'd used against cholera, he did what Wright was doing with typhus: he simply killed the bubonic plague microbe.

Wright and Haffkine didn't so much 'isolate, attenuate, inject' as 'isolate, inactivate, inject'. Their development of Pasteur's doctrine enormously widened its possible application. It was a lot easier to kill a microbe than to maintain multiple strains at different levels of attenuation. Moreover, it avoided the danger of a microbe turning out to be less attenuated than it should have been and causing the disease it was supposed to prevent.

Simply killing the microbe didn't work with every disease, as Wright found out when he tried it with brucellosis. His disgruntled deputy had already done the isolating, so Wright inactivated it and injected it into himself. He tested it by injecting the wild-type microbe and nearly died of the subsequent infection.[28]

Bruce had his revenge.

More importantly, Wright had shown that there was no single approach to the middle part of the Pasteur doctrine. Killed vaccines might have worked against typhoid and bubonic plague, but that didn't prove they would work against anything else. Each microbe would require a bespoke approach.

Immunology

The most remarkable aspect of what men like Pasteur, Haffkine and Wright achieved is how little they knew while they were achieving it. They had only glimpsed the enormous diversity encompassed by the word 'microbe', and while they recognised that exposure to a microbe could confer immunity to it, they had only a vague idea of how immunity works.

The first step in unravelling immune memory was made by Paul Ehrlich, who worked for Pasteur's arch-rival Robert Koch.

Pasteur had loathed all things Teutonic since a Prussian artillery shell decapitated a stuffed crocodile in the Muséum National d'Histoire Naturelle.[29] For Pasteur, bombarding a museum was a direct assault on science and culture, but worse was to come. The 1870 Franco-Prussian War ended in humiliating defeat for France and, just to rub it in, the proclamation of the new nation of Germany in the Palace of Versailles. Koch had been an army surgeon in that war and was less than enamoured of France,[30] leading to a bitter rivalry between the two fathers of the microbial theory of disease.

Ehrlich discovered that if he injected mice with minuscule concentrations of plant toxins, their blood acquired the ability to neutralise those toxins.[31] He concluded the toxins were triggering the mice to produce a substance he called *antikorps*, literally translated into English as 'antibody'. It followed that if an animal could produce *antikorps* against a plant toxin, then an animal – or a human – could produce antibody against a disease-causing microbe.

Meanwhile, in Paris, Élie Metchnikoff, Pasteur's protégé and Haffkine's mentor, had discovered a type of cell called a phago-cyte that engulfed and killed microbes.[32] Their directors' rivalry dictated that both Ehrlich and Metchnikoff insist that they had found the basis of immunity while the other was mistaken. Almroth Wright showed that they were both right;[33] a phagocyte might be able to kill microbes, but it was a lot better at it when the microbe had been treated with antibodies. Wright had discovered a process we now call opsonisation, in which antibody molecules coating the microbe also bind it to the phagocyte.

He'd also shown that the immune system is made up of many different elements that interact with each other while attacking invading microbes in different ways. It would later emerge that Metchnikoff's phagocytes encompassed several different types of white blood cell. The other major type is the lymphocyte, which is central to immune memory.

Some types of lymphocytes produce the antibodies that Ehrlich first identified. Others, called killer T-cells, identify cells of the body containing invading microbes and destroy them. Still others regulate the immune response, preventing it from attacking certain types of microbe.

The immune system has been learning about microbes for as long as there have been immune systems and microbes, and it's got pretty good at it. At the same time, microbes have been learning about the immune system, and those that cause disease have got painfully good at slipping past it. That's where the human mind is needed to assist the human immune system. It can develop vaccines that use the mechanism it uses to remember microbes it has seen in the past to warn it of the ones it needs to be ready for in the future.

This leads us to the question of what exactly we're talking about when we talk about microbes.

Chapter 2

The adversaries: bacteria and viruses

'Microbe' is a catch-all term for anything alive that's too small to be seen with the naked eye. In the late nineteenth century, the idea that microbes could make people ill is what drove the three founding fathers of the microbiological theory of disease: Louis Pasteur, his hated rival, Robert Koch, and an English surgeon called Joseph Lister.

All three first got interested in microbes at a time when that interest placed them squarely against the prevailing medical opinion, hence Pasteur's frequent spats in the Académie de Médecine. All three contributed evidence that microbes did indeed cause disease, and all three spent a considerable amount of effort trying to persuade their peers to pay attention to that evidence.

A major turning point was the 1881 Seventh International Medical Congress in London, where Pasteur presented his anthrax vaccine trial to the great and the good of European medicine and expanded the word 'vaccination' to mean more than a scraping of cowpox.

Among his frock-coated audience were Koch and Lister.

Pasteur even found a few kind words for Koch's new method for microbial culture, in which he solidified liquid nutrient broth into a jelly using a substance called agar. It allowed him to watch bacterial colonies form on the surface, which Pasteur called '*un grand progrès*',[1]* one of the nicest things he ever said about Koch or any other German after the Siege of Paris.

Lister, who corresponded regularly with both Koch and Pasteur, was more interested in applying the microbiological theory in his operating theatre than in studying microbes. Spraying everything in sight with carbolic acid[2] lacked the elegance of Pasteur and Koch's experiments, but when surgery carried a fifty-fifty chance of fatal infection, Lister's near elimination of the problem[3] made the microbiological theory difficult to argue with.

If their peers took their time in coming round to the microbial theory, it wasn't because microbes themselves were a new idea. In the 1670s, an inquisitive Dutchman named Antonie van Leeuwenhoek discovered microbes when he put a drop of pondwater under a microscope.[4] For two centuries, natural philosophers regarded the cornucopia of squirming, wriggling, shimmering 'animalcules' as mere curiosities. The journey towards recognising them as agents of human disease only began when Pasteur recognised that a microbe was behind fermentation.

Meet the microbes

Follow in van Leeuwenhoek's footsteps and place a drop of pondwater under a microscope, and you'll glimpse how much is going on where we can't see it. Tiny animals munch on chains of algal cells, but you'll need to turn up the magnification to see

---

* A great step forward.

the squirming dots of bacteria. What you won't see with a microscope are viruses, which are too small to be seen with even the most powerful microscope.

To give an idea of how small a virus is, we'd have to scale it up 100,000 times for it to be the size of a full stop on this page. At that scale, a bacterial cell would be about the size of a marble and a cell of the human body would be as big as a grapefruit.

Today, we grow up with the axiom that tiny 'germs' cause disease, but for Pasteur's peers, microbes were tiny shapes that danced through drops of pondwater. The idea that such minuscule 'animalcules', as they were called, might threaten a human being was absurd.

Science had yet to understand that each of us is a walking bag of nutrients, gathered from fields, farms and fisheries and eaten into one body for the delectation of any microbe that can exploit it. That's why we need an immune system: to protect us from those hungry microbes.

The immune system staves off the vast majority before we even notice them, but it can't change the fact that each of us is a bonanza to any microbe that sneaks past it. Some microbes have become extremely adept at sneaking, and those are the ones that make us ill.

A microbe that causes disease is called a pathogen, and there are many different classes of microbe that qualify for the term. To cover all of them, this book would break the average coffee table, which is why I've restricted it to the vaccines on the British schedule. As all of those vaccines are against bacteria and viruses, we'll put fungi, protozoans and a horror of different worms to one side, and focus on those bacteria and viruses.

Bacterial friends and foes

Let's start with the bacteria, the marbles to the human cell's grapefruit. They're everywhere. Pour some of Koch's nutritious agar into a Petri dish, touch a swab to anything that hasn't just been disinfected, touch the agar with it and watch a colony of bacteria spread from where you touched it.

Bacteria cover the planet, from the deepest oceans to the highest mountains. Weigh all the bacteria on earth and they'd outweigh the animals, human beings included, thirty-five times over.[5] Wherever there is a source of nutrients for a bacterium to metabolise into more bacteria, there will be a bacterium metabolising it.

We're very good at living in a world dominated by bacteria. If we weren't, we wouldn't be living at all. We're so good at cohabitation that our bodies are coated, inside and out, with a bacterial community that we're still a long way from fully understanding. Most of the bacterial cells we're carrying are in our bowels, but they're also on our skin and in our mouths, throats and throughout our digestive systems. There are so many that men typically have as many bacterial as human cells, while women, who have proportionally larger bowels, have twice as many bacterial as human cells.[6]

That doesn't mean that if we look in a mirror, we're seeing a bundle of bacteria looking back at us. Because bacterial cells are so much smaller than human cells, bacteria only make up around three grams of every kilo of our body weight. What we can see of ourselves is all human.

In the century after Pasteur, Koch and Lister argued their microbiological theory into being the dominant paradigm of medicine, relations between human and bacterium were seen as inherently antagonistic. We might not be able to avoid being swarmed with bacteria, the reasoning went, and we might even need some bacteria to digest our food, but we were never more than one misstep away from some mischievous bacterium slipping past our defences and making us ill.

That began to change in 1989, when David Strachan, an epidemiologist at the London School of Hygiene and Tropical Medicine, noticed that more British children were developing hay fever and eczema than they had in the 1950s.[7] Strachan suggested that children were living in such clean environments that their immune systems, products of the age-old battle against bacteria but deprived of enough bacteria to battle, were reacting to things they should be ignoring.

It happened less often in children who shared their home with other children, which, Strachan suggested, might be because children exchanged bacteria with the children they mixed with outside the home and then exchanged those bacteria with their siblings. More children meant more diversity among their bacteria, and perhaps a diverse bacterial community was a healthy bacterial community.

Strachan's 'hygiene hypothesis' reframed our interactions with bacteria as more of a balance than a battle. However, different studies that explored the hygiene hypothesis came up with different results. Some found clear associations between bacterial exposure and health but others did not.

The hygiene hypothesis is one of the few concepts in microbiology to be widely recognised by people who are not microbiologists. However, it does not tell the whole story.

In 2010, Graham Rook of University College London suggested that among the many species of bacteria that we might share our bodies with, some are 'old friends'[8] that have been with us since our ancestors were hunting antelope on the East African savannah, hundreds of thousands of years ago. Our old friends have been with us for so long, Rook suggested, that they've become 'as essential to health as our liver or kidneys'.[9] Conversely, a body that is not hosting its old friends is effectively missing a critical organ. The 'old friends' hypothesis suggests that bacterial diversity is important not for diversity's sake, but because the more bacteria we meet, the more likely we are to be reacquainted with those old friends.

The problem with the old friends hypothesis is that we don't understand enough about the bacteria we share our bodies with to know if it's true. If it is, we certainly don't know which bacteria are the old friends that are – hopefully – a part of me as I write this, and part of you as you read it, and which we can happily live with or without.

If we can live in harmony with our bacteria, it's thanks to the immune system maintaining a sometimes precarious balance. The difference between peaceful cohabitation and conflict is often a matter of where the bacteria are. For instance, a bacterium that we need to keep our bowels healthy might cause serious disease if it finds its way into the bloodstream.

As well as policing that balance, the immune system stands between us and a select list of bacteria with which there is no balance to be found. That's where vaccination comes in. It gives our immune system advance warning so that when those bacteria arrive, they find us suffused with antibodies that rip open their surfaces or bind them to phagocytes that engulf and destroy them before they can do any harm.

The viruses: unseen murdering ultra-microbes

Being one of the first to culture bacteria in the laboratory, Pasteur was also one of the first to encounter a perennial problem in bacterial culture: making sure the bacteria you put in your nutrient medium are the only ones in it. He needed a way to sterilise the medium, and when Pasteur needed a solution to a technical problem, he turned to Charles Chamberland.

Chamberland, the man who had worked out how to attenuate anthrax, invented a porcelain filter too fine for bacterial cells to pass through.[10] When he published his design, the 'Chamberland filter' became an essential piece of equipment for anyone exploring the new science of microbiology.

Among those nascent microbiologists was Martinus Beijerinck, a botanist at the Polytechnic School of Delft* in the Netherlands. Beijerinck recognised that if microbes caused human and livestock disease, they may also cause diseases of economically important plants. His particular interest was tobacco mosaic, a disease named for the mottled pattern it causes on the leaves of the tobacco plant.

Beijerinck started by looking for a bacterium. He didn't find it, but when he passed the sap of an infected plant through a Chamberland filter, the filtered sap caused tobacco mosaic in unblemished plants.

Beijerinck concluded that if sap could carry tobacco mosaic after he'd filtered out any bacteria, then something much smaller than a bacterium must be causing it.

He considered a toxin, but when he took a drop of sap from a plant with tobacco mosaic, that drop was all that he needed to infect an unblemished plant. However many times he passed tobacco mosaic from one plant to another, the effect remained undiluted, which showed he was not dealing with a toxin. Whatever was causing tobacco mosaic, Beijerinck concluded that it could replicate in the plant it infected. Every time he took a drop of sap from a plant he had infected, it had as much of the tobacco mosaic agent in it as the drop of sap he had used to infect the plant in the first place.

His 1898 paper describing what he called a *contagium vivum*

---

* Now Delft University of Technology.

*fluidum** is a classic example of how something invisible can be described by its effects.[11] He proposed some sort of living liquid, which, given what he was able to observe, was a reasonable supposition.

Scientists soon realised that *contagium vivum fluidum* was a phenomenon that occurred in animals, including humans, as well as plants. There was, as one author put it, 'an ultra-microbe, too immensely small for the strongest lens to uncover, revealing its existence only by the murdering of men with its unseen mysterious poison'.[12]

Beijerinck's dilution experiment showed that it was not a poison, but the unknown ultra-microbe nevertheless acquired the Latin word for poison: 'virus'.

We now know that a virus is a fragment of rogue genetic code. When that code gets into a living cell, it hijacks the processes of the cell to replicate itself. That's the fundamental difference between bacterial and viral infections: a bacterium uses the human body as a source of nutrients, while a virus repurposes the machinery of a cell that it slips into.

It's also why nobody had any chance of properly understanding a virus for more than fifty years after Beijerinck's seminal paper. Nobody knew how genes were coded. The fundamentals of virology only became visible after 1953, when James Watson and Francis Crick at Cambridge University were celebrated around the world for describing the structure of deoxyribonucleic acid, or DNA as it became universally known. Less celebrated was Rosalind Franklin, whose expertise in X-ray crystallography had made their breakthrough possible.

Watson, Crick and Franklin all saw describing DNA's structure as the beginning of a scientific adventure rather than the end of one. Describing the molecule that carries the genetic code

---

* Contagion of living fluid.

didn't explain how to read it, let alone how it controlled the machinery of every cell it lies at the centre of.

The three of them spent the next few years simultaneously cooperating and competing in their efforts to understand DNA. Franklin started with a clear advantage as the only one with a solid grasp of X-ray crystallography, the technique used to directly visualise DNA. When they were working on DNA's structure, she'd been hobbled by her position as a postdoctoral assistant at King's College, where the idea of a woman doing science was still so outlandish that she was barred from the men-only common room. While Watson and Crick's paper was rolling off the presses, Franklin moved up the Piccadilly Line to Birkbeck College, where, as the head of her own research group, she had a much freer hand.

Franklin developed a close friendship with Crick and his wife, even travelling through Spain with them after a symposium in Madrid. She would never be as friendly with the notoriously difficult Watson, who once wrote of her that 'the best place for a feminist is in someone else's lab',[13] but they kept in touch and Watson advocated on her behalf when she ran into funding difficulties.[14]

By the time Franklin was in her own lab rather than someone else's, scientists could at least see viruses directly. The 1940s saw the emergence of the electron microscope as an important tool in biology; this device gives a magnification a thousand times better than the best microscopes that Beijerinck had peered through.

Franklin knew she was dealing not with a living fluid but with a particle so tiny it could pass through the pores of a Chamberland filter. She also knew that it contained a genetic code. Over the next few years, she went a long way towards establishing how the genetic code forms those tiny particles.

For most living things, 'genetic code' is synonymous with DNA, the molecule that carries that code for all animals, plants, fungi and bacteria. However, viruses are so different from each other that they can't even agree on one molecule with which to encode their genes. Some use DNA, but others use ribonucleic acid, abbreviated to RNA. Viruses do share a similar life cycle: they enter a cell, replicate themselves, leave the cell and find another cell to replicate in. That other cell is usually right next to the cell the virus emerged from, but a virus won't be around for long unless it can find a way into someone other than the person it last replicated in. It needs a way to transmit from one person to another.

When a virus is between cells, or between people, it takes the form of those tiny structures that can only be seen with an electron microscope. Those structures became very familiar during the COVID-19 pandemic, when news anchors used their studded spheres as backdrops to their sombre reports. However, those pictures showed not the virus itself but a vehicle for it.

The studded sphere is a coat of protein molecules called the capsid, which protects the virus's DNA or RNA when it's outside a cell. Until those studs bind a target cell and insert the DNA or RNA into it, the virus is completely inert. How long a virus can last outside a cell depends on the virus. Most decay within hours, although some can last for days or even weeks. If it finds a cell to infect before it decays, the virus discards the capsid and its genetic material initiates the processes that make a virus viral.

One of the immune system's main weapons against viruses is the killer T-cell, which kills cells that viruses are replicating inside. When the rogue genetic code that is a virus hijacks a cell, the cell itself goes rogue. The virus turns it from a functional part of a human being into a factory for viral replication. Killing the cell is the quickest way of shutting down that replication.

Franklin started with plant viruses, but was quick to apply what she learned to human disease. She did not live to see her work come to fruition. She had barely started work on the poliovirus when she died of ovarian cancer at only thirty-seven years old.

Franklin's work went on without her. Aaron Klug, one of her postdoctoral researchers, completed the structure of the poliovirus, and his insights into how the genetic code is read won him the 1982 Nobel Prize.[15] He always acknowledged that his work was built on Franklin's, and had she lived, they would have shared it.

If the battle against microbial disease were a drama series, the unveiling of the ultra-microbes at the end of Franklin's short life would be the first season's finale. More than half a century later, we are still a long way from the final season, but thanks to scientists like Pasteur, Beijerinck and Franklin, we have the principles we need to understand the microbial pathogens that harm us.

If you're heading for a clinic where you or your child will be vaccinated, the past and the future of vaccinology may look like rather abstract concepts. You're more likely to be interested in how we know that vaccine will help you or your child to stay healthy. To answer that, we need to take a look at where vaccinology stands today.

Chapter 3

Vaccines today: what vaccines mean to us

In the 1930s, polio was to American microbiologists what Baby Face Nelson and John Dillinger were to the FBI, but while the FBI could produce mugshots of its designated public enemies, microbiologists had only a vague idea of what a virus was.

Uncertainty didn't stop John Kolmer of Philadelphia's Temple University. He claimed to have cultured the poliovirus in monkey spinal cords and attenuated it into a vaccine strain with a mercury compound and a castor bean extract called ricin. Quite how he got the idea that mercury and ricin would attenuate poliovirus remains a mystery, but Kolmer believed he was following the Pasteur doctrine of isolate, attenuate, inject.

He injected his supposed vaccine into forty-two monkeys, himself and twenty-five children – in that order – and when none showed any sign of harm, he decided it would put an end to polio and distributed it to doctors all over the USA and Canada.[1]

If Kolmer's approach seems reckless, it was far from the weirdest thing to fly the banner of medicine in Depression-era America. Men who believed themselves infertile were beating a path to the door of one John Brinkley, who treated them by surgically implanting goat testicles inside their scrotums.[2] Brinkley's treatment didn't cause a baby boom, but it made Brinkley very rich at the same time as Kolmer's vaccine enterprise ended in tears.

Of around 11,000 children who received Kolmer's concoction, ten developed polio within a week of being injected and five died.[3] The American Medical Association, who were trying to put clear water between medical practice and quacks like Brinkley, were not impressed by Kolmer's freewheeling approach. They took the view that Kolmer's vaccine was not as attenuated as he thought, and that far from protecting children from polio, it had caused it in those ten.

Kolmer stood by his vaccine and insisted the ten children must have been infected before they were vaccinated. He may have been right. There was a lot of polio about, but nobody knew how much, so it wasn't possible to say whether ten cases among 11,000 children was disturbingly high or encouragingly low.

Kolmer faced his critics at a 1935 meeting of the Southern Branch of the American Society of Public Health in St Louis. No punches were pulled. Kolmer was accused of being a murderer, and while he never accepted that his vaccine was responsible for the deaths, it was the end of both his vaccine and his reputation.[4]

This is why we don't do vaccine development like Kolmer anymore.

From Kolmer to COVID-19

Today, Kolmer's idea of vaccinology looks closer to Brinkley's testicular shenanigans than serious research, but before condemning him too harshly, we should remember that he had no framework to guide him. If he made up his procedures as he went along, so did everyone else doing medical research in the 1930s. If no one thought to stop him until after it had all – possibly – gone wrong, that was typical of the prevailing suck-it-and-see attitude.

Today's vaccine development follows a structured process to test first whether a vaccine is safe and then whether it is effective. Standardised procedures spare vaccinologists the need to reinvent them for every new vaccine, and produce a standard set of results for regulatory authorities to evaluate.

The best way to understand those procedures is to follow a recent vaccine from concept to clinic, and, at the time of writing, they don't come any more recent than the AZD1222 vaccine against COVID-19 developed by Sarah Gilbert's team at Oxford's Jenner Centre.

AZD1222 is one of several names it's been known by. It was originally called ChAdOx1 nCoV-19, and when the pharmaceutical giant AstraZeneca got involved, they branded it as Covishield and Vaxevria. To most of the world, it's the Oxford/ AZ vaccine.

Gilbert had set her team to work on a COVID-19 vaccine within weeks of the virus being identified,[5] but they weren't starting from scratch. For years before COVID-19 appeared, Gilbert had been working on the new technology of viral vector vaccines.

A viral vector is a virus that infects humans without doing any harm. Slot a gene from another microbe into the viral vector, and when it infects a cell, it produces a protein from that microbe along with its own. As far as the immune system is concerned, that protein is part of the invading virus, so it retains a memory of it. That's the vaccine.

Gilbert's vector was a virus called ChAdOx1, an acronym of the three words that sum up the virus's history: 'chimpanzee adenovirus Oxford'. It was derived from a type of virus called an adenovirus that had been isolated from a chimpanzee. In Oxford, Gilbert's team made a critical adjustment before they put it into a human being: they removed a gene so it can't replicate itself.[6]

It can infect a human cell, but then it's stuck in there until the immune system rallies its killer T-cells to root it out.

Once they'd rendered ChAdOx1 harmless, Gilbert's team could slot a gene from any microbe into it. They first tried a gene from the virus that causes Middle Eastern Respiratory Syndrome, or MERS, a virus carried by domestic camels that causes a particularly nasty disease when it infects humans. They chose the gene that codes for the spike protein, which attaches the virus's capsid to a cell so it can infect it. If a vaccine could trigger the immune system to produce antibodies to the spike protein, the logic went, they would block the attachment, and a virus that can't attach itself to a cell can't infect it.

Gilbert's MERS vaccine had looked promising,[7] but no one had stepped up to fund its further development. It fell into the 'biotech valley of death',[8] a financial chasm between the small-scale trials that suggest a vaccine might be useful and the much larger-scale trials needed to prove it. At the time of writing, the MERS vaccine languishes among countless vaccines and treatments littering the bottom of the valley, and it will remain there unless and until someone ponies up the cash needed to pull it out.

The COVID-19 virus is very closely related to the MERS virus. When it appeared in 2019, ChAdOx1 was still a solution looking for a problem, and it had shown at least the potential to solve a very similar problem. If slotting the MERS virus's spike protein into ChAdOx1 triggered immune memory to the MERS virus, there was every reason to expect the COVID-19 virus's spike protein to do the same.

From mice to men: preclinical studies

Like Kolmer, Gilbert tested the new vaccine on animals before letting it anywhere near human beings. Any experiment involving human beings is classed as 'clinical', and no ethics committee will allow a clinical trial of a vaccine until they can scrutinise 'preclinical' results from animal studies.

Kolmer didn't need to worry about ethics committees. Kolmer is part of the reason why today's vaccinologists do.

As with most vaccines, the first preclinical studies were on mice. As different as mice are to humans, they're similar enough that if a vaccine can't trigger a mouse's immune system, it probably won't trigger a human's. Gilbert would know her team's time and effort would be better spent elsewhere.

Gilbert's vaccine triggered both antibodies and killer T-cells that responded to the COVID-19 virus.[9] So far, so good. Now Gilbert needed to know if that immune response could protect against the COVID-19 virus.

For that, she needed an animal a lot more similar to a human than a mouse. Like Kolmer a century earlier, and most vaccine developers since, she opted for a monkey called the rhesus macaque. Macaques are not endangered and are susceptible to many human diseases, making them an oft-used intermediate between mice and humans.

The idea of experimenting on monkeys – or even on mice – makes a lot of people queasy. I happen to be one of them. Since I left zoology for medical research, I've avoided jobs that involve animal experiments. I am far from the only medical researcher more comfortable being forbidden from harming my subjects than being compelled to do so.

Lacking the stomach for animal experiments does not make me opposed to them. On the contrary, I recognise them as essential. Without them, we would be forced to choose between seeing medicine stuck where it is, with no new treatments ever being developed, or having every new medication tested on human beings without weeding out the dangerous ones through preclinical studies on animals. Given the stark choice between human suffering and animal suffering, I will choose animal suffering every time.

If the battle against human suffering requires animal suffering, that suffering can be minimised by not using more animals than are necessary. Where Kolmer used forty-two monkeys to conclude they looked fine – which was as scientific as Kolmer's description got – Gilbert only needed eighteen to show that the vaccine could trigger an immune response, that two doses could trigger a better immune response than one, and that this immune response protected the monkeys from COVID-19. By properly designing her experiments, Gilbert gleaned considerably more information with half the number of monkeys.

The results from the preclinical studies were as good as Gilbert could have hoped, but an oft-quoted truism of vaccinology is, 'mice lie and monkeys exaggerate'.[10] The only way to find out if the vaccine was as safe and effective in humans was to give it to human volunteers. It was time to move on to clinical trials.

The four phases of clinical trials

A vaccine must pass through four phases of clinical trial:[11]

Phase 1 trials involve giving the vaccine to a small number of healthy people to make sure it doesn't cause any nasty side effects that didn't show up in the preclinical studies.

Phase 2 trials involve larger numbers of people to test whether the vaccine triggers an immune response.

Phase 3 trials test whether the vaccine protects against the disease it is designed for, which involves a large number of people at risk of being infected.

Phase 4 is not a formal trial, but involves ongoing monitoring of the vaccine after it has been rolled out.

If preclinical trials are a vaccine's infancy, clinical trials are its adolescence – and, like most self-respecting adolescents, most vaccines don't follow conventions to the letter.

The first clinical trial of the Oxford/AZ vaccine combined phases 1 and 2. That's a common practice, because if you're going to inject people with the vaccine to test its safety, you may as well evaluate their immune response, and once you've done that, you've done the phase 2 trial.

The Oxford/AZ vaccine had a somewhat precocious adolescence because, unlike most vaccines, that first human trial did not involve dose-escalation. Usually, the first few volunteers get a very low dose, and if they suffer no serious ill effects, the next group get a slightly higher dose. If they're fine, the next group get a higher dose again, and so on.

One reason for doing this is that if you're exposing people to a vaccine for the first time, it's sensible to start with very little of it. Another is that higher doses usually trigger stronger immune responses, but only up to a point. Raising the dose beyond that point is likely to make the side effects worse without improving the immune response.

Dose-escalation finds the ideal dose with minimal risk, but Gilbert had already done a dose-escalation trial with her MERS vaccine. She decided that the ideal dose for ChAdOx1 carrying a MERS spike protein would be the same as the ideal dose for ChAdOx1 carrying a COVID-19 spike protein. Nevertheless, similar is not identical, so she still needed that phase 1 and 2 trial to see if the vaccine was as safe and effective in humans as it had been in rhesus macaques.

The double-blind placebo-controlled clinical trial

The gold standard for testing a vaccine, or indeed any medical intervention, is the double-blind placebo-controlled trial:

placebo-controlled because some volunteers are given a fake vaccine to compare to those given the test vaccine; double-blind because neither the volunteers nor the trial clinicians know which is which.

Every clinical trial designer must decide what to use as a placebo. Some trials use a syringe full of saline solution, but everyone knows that a vaccine gives you a sore arm. Saline solution doesn't. If word got around that some people were getting sore arms and some weren't, the volunteers would know whether they'd got the vaccine or the placebo, which would defeat the object of double-blinding.

Gilbert needed an active placebo; something that would make an arm as sore as the test vaccine. Vaccine ethics committees take a dim view of injecting volunteers with something purely to make them feel ill, even if it only causes mild inflammation. Gilbert's solution was a vaccine against the meningococcus bacterium that, as we'll see in the chapter on meningococcal disease, has been given to British fourteen-year-olds since 2015. Anyone injected with it would feel like they'd been vaccinated because they had, and their sore arm wouldn't be for nothing, because they'd gain immunity to meningococcal infection.

The meningococcal vaccine also provided a baseline for an acceptable level of side effects with which to compare the COVID-19 vaccine. However, a paradox of vaccine trials is that to evaluate side effects, investigators have to assume they don't know them when they see them.

Not side effects, but adverse events

Vaccines cause side effects. A sore arm for a few days, a slight headache, maybe a raised temperature. We accept them as a price worth paying for protection, but before a vaccine can be rolled out, we need to know that's as bad as it gets.

However, if a doctor or nurse working on a trial were to try to measure them, they'd probably get it wrong.

Put yourself in their position. Yesterday, someone had either the vaccine or an active placebo. You don't know which. Today, they're running a fever. You'd probably be comfortable calling that a side effect.

Someone else had the vaccine or placebo six weeks ago, and today, they're in A&E with a broken nose. It *could* be a side effect, but you'll probably blame it on the dozen pints of Guinness they sank before mouthing off at a passing rugby team.

Now consider someone who got the vaccine or placebo a week ago, and today, they're vomiting so badly they've been hospitalised with dehydration. Vaccines sometimes cause nausea and vomiting, but it would be an extreme case to hospitalise someone. A week is a long time for a side effect to take to kick in, but not an impossibly long time. How do you decide whether it's a side effect or if that person ate something that disagreed with them?

The answer is: you don't.

You record it as an 'adverse event', along with the fever that you thought was a side effect and the broken nose that almost certainly wasn't. An adverse event is any and every medical problem experienced by a volunteer. Later on, you can work out whether the vaccine caused more adverse events than the placebo, but to do that, you need to have recorded every single one of them.

The adverse events are constantly monitored by an oversight board. Its members are not blinded, so they can watch out for obvious red flags. If a vaccinee becomes seriously ill, the oversight board usually orders a pause in vaccinations while they investigate.

Their job is to err on the side of caution, so it's a rare trial that doesn't get paused now and again. If there's evidence that a vaccine caused a serious adverse event, it's usually the end of the trial and the end of the vaccine. However, vaccines are usually given to thousands of volunteers before they're rolled out. There's bound to be the occasional medical emergency that has nothing to do with the vaccine.

During the Oxford/AZ vaccine trials, journalists who had never covered a clinical trial before breathlessly reported every pause as if it might be curtains for the vaccine. In fact, those pauses were simply due diligence.

At the end of the trial, the investigators have a comprehensive list of who got sore arms, headaches, fevers and broken noses. The investigators can then use that list to see whether the more serious adverse events were more common among volunteers who got the vaccine than volunteers who got the placebo.

Even something as unlikely to be vaccine-related as a broken nose could be part of a pattern. One volunteer getting into a drunken punch-up is unfortunate; half a dozen would be a worrying pattern if everyone in the placebo group remained unpunched. There has never been a vaccine that makes someone obnoxious after a few drinks, but vaccine developers can't assume they've anticipated every possible side effect. As long as all adverse events are recorded, they don't have to; they'll be in the data even if no one was looking for them.

Nothing dramatic happened in the Oxford/AZ vaccine's first clinical trial.[12] It caused the usual sore arms and an occasional fever but nothing out of the ordinary.

The Oxford/AZ vaccine had passed phase 1 and phase 2 at the same time. It was time for phase 3.

It's safe, but does it work?

Just because a vaccine triggers an immune response, it doesn't necessarily follow that the immune response will protect against the pathogen. That's a lesson that HIV has repeatedly and painfully driven home, where one candidate vaccine after another has triggered beautiful immune responses only for a phase 3 trial to show they don't protect anyone.

Phase 3 trials need to be much larger than phase 2. The larger the better. The more people in the trial, the sooner the infection rate among the placebo recipients outstrips the infection rate in the vaccinees – or the sooner it's obvious that it isn't going to – and the sooner the trial returns an answer. The Oxford/AZ vaccine passed phase 2 with 1,077 volunteers. A phase 3 trial would need tens of thousands. It was going to be expensive.

Gilbert's vaccine had arrived at the biotech valley of death.

Unlike her MERS vaccine, it didn't fall into it. With most high-income countries in lockdown, governments were willing to build a solid-gold bridge across the valley of death if that was what it took. The phase 3 trial was funded by various sources, including British government agencies, charitable foundations and AstraZeneca.

In the event, four phase 3 trials were run in parallel. None was large enough to show a clear discrepancy between the vaccine and placebo groups, but between them, a clear answer emerged.

The first was a simple expansion of the phase 1 and 2 trial already underway in Britain. The transition happened in the spring of 2020, as we were emerging, blinking dazedly, into a short summer of respite. We badly needed the breather between lockdowns, but Britain was no longer the ideal testing ground for the vaccine because, at the time, there wasn't much COVID-19 around for it to protect volunteers against.

Instead of waiting for the next surge, parallel trials were funded in Brazil, South Africa and the USA, where a lot more COVID-19 was circulating.

In the rush to phase 3, a few details fell through the gaps. Instead of an active placebo, the South African investigators opted for saline solution, while the Brazilian investigators ended up using the meningococcal vaccine for the first dose and saline for the second.

Another problem was that while most trials of two-dose vaccines aim for rigid consistency in the scheduling of the doses, the interval varied between two and three months. Then, after the trials had been running for several months, the British trial team uncovered a manufacturing glitch that had led to 3,500 people getting a half-dose of the vaccine.[13]

None of these problems added to the risk – a half-dose was safer than a double-dose – but they risked making the results harder to interpret. The oversight board could have excluded the results from anyone whose dose regime had not followed the intended protocol, but instead, they opted to roll with it and treated the problems as unintentional trials of the dose regime.

In a phase 3 trial, the oversight board periodically reviews the data to see whether there have been enough infections to evaluate a vaccine's efficacy: how effective the protection it gives is, if, indeed, it gives any protection at all. By November 2020, they had an answer. Not *the* answer. The trial is still ongoing as I write this. But *an* answer.

The headline result was that for every three people who were infected after being given the placebo, only two were infected after being given the vaccine.[14] That was good news. It showed the vaccine was protecting people, even if the protection wasn't as strong as Gilbert – and by then, most of the world – might have wanted.

Much better news was that only around half the infected vaccinees noticed they'd been infected. Their immune systems had fought off the virus before they became ill, and they only knew they'd been infected because they'd had their throats swabbed every week. The vaccine wasn't putting up an impenetrable wall of protection, but it was keeping people well who would otherwise have been ill.

It was an interim rather than a final analysis, but it was enough to apply for an emergency licence. Different national regulators took different views of the application. The British Medicines and Healthcare products Regulatory Agency (MHRA) and the European Medicines Agency (EMA), recently separated by Britain's departure from the EU, were quick to grant the emergency licence. In the USA, the regulators took a different view and withheld it.

It's unusual for different regulators to take different views of the same data, but it's unusual for regulators to be presented with an interim analysis in the middle of a pandemic. If the American regulators took a more cautious view, it may have been because the USA had secured supplies of other COVID-19 vaccines that had been developed at the same time.

The emergency licence allowed the Oxford/AZ vaccine to be rolled out in Britain and across the EU, but even if the phase 3 trials had been completed by then, it wouldn't have been the end of the testing.

The Oxford/AZ vaccine was still in its phase 3 adolescence, but amid the COVID-19 pandemic, the world needed it to grow up fast. It was time to enter phase 4.

Where vaccine roll-outs go right and wrong

However well a phase 3 trial is designed, tens of thousands of volunteers are never going to capture the complexity encompassed by the potentially billions of people who receive a vaccine after it is rolled out. Some of those people will have rare medical conditions. Some will accept the first dose and not turn up for the second. Some will be pregnant, barring them from volunteering for a clinical trial in the first place.

Somewhere among those billions, there may lurk a few people

who, through some combination of genetics, underlying conditions and sheer bad luck, will have a particularly nasty reaction to the vaccine. The Oxford/AZ vaccine's interim analysis showed no such reaction had happened among the 12,000 people who had received it by then, but that only proved that nasty reactions were rarer than one in 12,000. It didn't prove they could never happen.

Rare adverse events are what keep vaccinologists awake at night. Maurice Hilleman, Merck's legendary head of vaccine development, who was involved in developing around half the vaccines on the childhood schedule, once said that he could only relax when a vaccine had gone into 3 million people without a serious incident.[15]

This is where phase 4 comes in.

National regulators depend on reports of adverse events suffered immediately after receiving a vaccine, made either by the person who suffers from them or by their doctor. In Britain, reporting is through the Yellow Card scheme,[16] originally set up in 1964, although the eponymous yellow cards have since been replaced with a website tinted to stay on brand. It allows anyone or their doctor to report a side effect from a vaccine or any other medication directly to the MHRA.

Most high-income countries have a similar scheme, and by March 2021, the EMA had received thirty reports of blood-clotting disorders from the 5 million Europeans who had received the Oxford/AZ vaccine.[17] The EMA didn't say the vaccine had *caused* the blood clots. Blood clots happen for many different reasons, and among 5 million unvaccinated people, thirty would not have been an unusually large number. The report was simply raising a possible concern, although the Danish Health Agency was less sanguine than the EMA; they had already suspended the Oxford/AZ vaccine.

The rare adverse event is the bane of any vaccine regulator. A side effect as rare as thirty in 5 million, or one in 167,000, wouldn't have shown up among 12,000 people. However, thirty reports didn't necessarily mean thirty blood clots. For all the EMA knew, those thirty could be the tip of an iceberg of cases that no one had thought to report.

On the other hand, just because something happened soon after a vaccination doesn't mean the vaccine caused it. One paediatrician told me how easy it is to mistake coincidence for cause through the story of a child he treated for epilepsy.[18] The child's mother had taken him for a vaccination, but arrived to find the clinic was running late. Rather than sit in the waiting room, his mother pushed his buggy to a nearby café. In that café, the child had his first epileptic seizure.

If the clinic had been running on time, he'd have had that seizure immediately after being vaccinated. His mother would have been convinced that the vaccine caused the seizure and quite possibly that it caused his lifelong epilepsy. His GP, not knowing if it was a coincidence of timing or part of a pattern, would have made a Yellow Card report, and would have been right to do so. The first sign of a worrying pattern is a series of events that, taken individually, look like coincidences.

This was the conundrum that Kolmer and his critics tried to resolve with a shouting match in St Louis. The EMA opted for a more constructive approach: they called in the epidemiologists.

Epidemiology is the study of disease within a population. It covers everything from the genetics of addiction to how pathogens spread to whether the Oxford/AZ vaccine really caused blood clots.

The epidemiologists tasked with the latter problem looked at the data from across the whole of Denmark and Norway to see if the Oxford/AZ vaccine increased the chances of ending up in hospital with a blood clot.

They found that it did.

For every 100,000 vaccinations, they found between five and seventeen people developed blood clots who would not have done without the vaccination.[19] Later studies, which could look at many more vaccinations, have confirmed that the Scandinavian study was in the right ballpark.[20]

However, the news from Scandinavia wasn't all bad. Around half the people who suffered the blood clots recovered, and receiving the Oxford/AZ vaccine still cut someone's overall risk of death by two thirds. The risk from COVID-19 was far higher than the risk from the vaccine.

As so often happens with health-related scares, the risk was widely reported without context. We deal with risks every day and between five and seventeen cases per 100,000 people is only meaningful if we compare it with those everyday risks. The most compelling comparison was provided not by an epidemiologist but by a medical student, one Rebecca Lonergan, whose letter to the *British Medical Journal*[21] pointed out that the risk of blood clots associated with the contraceptive pill is around seventy to 120 per 100,000: around a hundred times the Scandinavian estimate. Her comparison was widely referred to in technical discussions but widely ignored by the media.

Nevertheless, finding that a vaccine was causing blood clots was disturbing news. Feeling off-colour for a day or two after vaccination is one thing. Risking a blood clot is something else, even if it's only a very small risk.

At the time of writing, the Oxford/AZ vaccine is still in phase 4, and regulatory authorities around the world are still working out how to get the maximum effectiveness out of it for the lowest risk.

The Oxford/AZ vaccine has become a celebrity among vaccines. It's been in the public eye since its adolescence spent in phase 1 and 2 trials, it grew up through phase 3, and now it's been rolled out, it's had more headlines devoted to it than any other vaccine. As with many a child star who has matured into a diva, some of those headlines have been less than flattering. It's still very much in phase 4, so it remains to be seen whether it will age well.

II

The UK childhood vaccine schedule

Chapter 4

Diphtheria

It was a peaceful August weekend when the strangling angel called on Charles Sherrington's nephew.

Sherrington was at his London home when he received his brother-in-law's telegram. 'George has diphtheria. Can you come?'

In 1894, most men would read that as an invitation to a child's deathbed.

Sherrington was not most men. He had studied the microbial theory of disease under Robert Koch in Berlin, and, at the time, he was trying to reproduce a treatment for diphtheria pioneered in Koch's institute. He had cultured the diphtheria bacterium, filtered out the bacterial cells and injected the liquid he was left with into a horse called Tommy. If the papers he was working from were to be believed, Tommy's blood would gain the ability to cure a child with diphtheria.

The papers were thin on specifics, and Sherrington had to make a lot of it up as he went along. He'd planned to inject the long-suffering Tommy a few more times, but George couldn't wait.

Seizing a syringe and a lantern, Sherrington took two litres of Tommy's blood and left it to clot. He removed the serum – the liquid fraction of blood – and boarded that morning's first train to Lewes, a small town in Sussex best known for burning politicians in effigy on Guy Fawkes Night.

Dr Fawsett, who had been attending George, picked up Sherrington from Lewes Station. Sherrington's talk of horse serum must have sounded like witchcraft, but Fawsett took it philosophically.

'You can do what you like with the boy,' he said, without meeting Sherrington's eye. 'He will not be alive at teatime.'[1]

They arrived to find the servants 'scared and silent'. George was struggling to breathe and so insensible that he didn't recognise his uncle.

Sherrington gave no more detail on George's condition, but as no one doubted the diagnosis of diphtheria, he was probably suffering from its signature feature: a grey mass forming over the back of his throat. The texture of this mass, which is now called the pseudomembrane, is what gives diphtheria, the Greek word for leather, its name.

George's pseudomembrane was probably accompanied by the characteristic 'bull neck' swelling, caused by inflammation of the lymphoid glands in his neck. No wonder he was breathing with difficulty. The swelling and the pseudomembrane were slowly closing his windpipe. That's why diphtheria was called the strangling angel.

Tommy's serum had a dramatic effect on George. By teatime, he was not only still alive but breathing more easily. Two days later, he had recovered sufficiently that Sherrington felt able to return to London. No sooner had he arrived than he was ushered into a dinner party given by Joseph Lister, by then one of the greatest of the great men of British medicine, who insisted Sherrington regale his guests with the first successful treatment of diphtheria in Britain.

Sherrington would soon move on from diphtheria to research the nervous system, earning a Nobel Prize and a knighthood.

George would grow up to be a strapping young man of six feet and win the dubious honour of a commission in the First World War.

Tommy the horse was memorialised by having one of his hooves preserved and mounted at the Institute that would later bear Lister's name.

The discovery of the diphtheria toxin

The technique that Sherrington and Tommy used to cure George was based on a discovery by Émile Roux, Louis Pasteur's assistant-turned-evangelist.

In 1888, Roux found that when he infected animals with diphtheria bacteria, they caused disease that seemed more severe than the number of bacterial cells warranted. He hypothesised that the disease might be caused not by the bacteria themselves, but by some toxin they were producing. He filtered the bacterial cells out of the liquid in which he'd cultured them, and sure enough, the medium alone caused diphtheria.

Roux had discovered the diphtheria toxin that caused the pseudomembrane that nearly polished off George a few years later. It was the first proven example of a microbial toxin causing a disease, and the first of many advances driven by the strangling angel.

Roux was not the only one interested in diphtheria. In 1890, while Roux was winding up the first phase of his diphtheria research, Robert Koch was opening the Prussian Institute of Infectious Diseases in Berlin.

One of his Institute's first breakthroughs was Paul Ehrlich's discovery of the antibody, or rather of its effects. It would be decades before Ehrlich's *antikorps* would be identified as a soluble protein that latches on to other proteins, but his colleague, Emil

Behring, found a way to use it without having more than a vague idea of what it was. When Behring found that animals produced *antikorps* to Roux's diphtheria toxin,[2] he set out to transfer it from an animal to a diphtheria-stricken child, where, he hoped, it would neutralise the toxin and save the child.

Koch, who was more interested in cholera and tuberculosis, gave Behring a spare sheep and left him to it. Legend has it that Behring saved his first child with sheep antibodies on Christmas Day 1891, when 'a child desperately sick with diphtheria cried and kicked a little as the needle of the first syringe full of antitoxin slid under its tender skin'.[3] The tale of the Christmas Day miracle may be fanciful; there's evidence that Behring had started his treatments earlier in December,[4] and two of the eleven children he treated died nonetheless.[5] However, diphtheria had a fatality rate of around 65 per cent, so nine survivors out of eleven showed that he'd lowered the fatality rate to 18 per cent. Behring was on to something.

Behring moved on from sheep to horses, which could yield a lot more serum,[6] pioneering the approach that Sherrington was trying to reproduce when he was summoned to Lewes. However, neither Behring nor Sherrington was working at the scale needed to treat diphtheria-infected children *en masse*.

Proving antitoxin with randomisation

Behring wasn't the easiest man to get on with. He was abrasive towards his colleagues and was perennially convinced that he wasn't getting enough credit for his work. One biographer believes he would today be diagnosed with bipolar disorder.[7] Whatever the reason, he belonged to that species of modern researcher that colleagues classify as a 'difficult bugger'.

One man he did not quarrel with was Roux, who, despite being Pasteur's disciple in all matters scientific, had never shared his mentor's Germanophobia. Defying their directors' antipathy, Roux and Behring corresponded regularly and generously acknowledged each other in their publications. They got on so well that Roux stood as godfather to one of Behring's children.

By 1894, Roux was working with Joseph Grancher, a paediatrician at Paris's Hôpital des Enfants Malades* and one of the first practising doctors to embrace Pasteur's microbiological theory of disease. Grancher was making a start by introducing hygiene standards that were still lacking in most hospitals. If the microbial theory suggested horse serum might cure a hitherto untreatable disease, Grancher was willing to give it a try.

Horse serum halved the death rate among Grancher's diphtheria patients, which made a strong argument for treating patients with the serum of immunised animals, or serotherapy as it became known. Serotherapy was based on the same principle as vaccination: when Roux or Behring injected diphtheria toxin into a horse, they were effectively vaccinating the horse against it. The horse's immune system responded by producing antibodies that bound the toxin, and the binding worked just as well if the antibodies were transferred to a child as if they were left in the horse.

They had yet to learn that what applied to the single molecule of a toxin applied equally to the many molecules that compose a microbe; indeed, the medical world was still digesting the idea that disease was caused by microbes. For many doctors, concoctions of horse serum seemed downright bizarre, and the gaps in Roux and Grancher's knowledge left them ill-equipped to defend serotherapy against its detractors. Their experiments with antitoxin had, after all, been done at the same time as Grancher's hygiene crusade. If more diphtheria patients were recovering, how could they be sure it was antitoxin that made the difference and not the better hygiene?

---

* Now the Hôpital Necker-Enfants Malades.

Nor was antitoxin without its risks. I can attest to that from painful experience, having received antibody therapy twelve times myself. Eleven times, I sat quietly reading a book, but on one occasion, the words blurred on the page and a rocketing temperature left me shivering and vomiting. That was with a modern preparation of purified antibody dripped into me over several hours, watched over by nurses ready to shoot me full of antihistamines and antiemetics that had me back to my book in less than an hour.

Roux's method was to inject crude horse serum straight into the vein of a very ill child, with no way to treat any possible reaction. No wonder some doctors wanted to be sure it was worth the risk.

One man whose misgivings outweighed his enthusiasm was a Professor Sørensen at Copenhagen's Blegdamshospitalet. One of his junior physicians, Johannes Fibiger, suggested they test antitoxin by only treating children admitted with diphtheria on alternate days. They'd see whether the treatment made a difference soon enough.

In an era where Roux and Grancher's approach of simply trying a new treatment to see what happened was the norm, Fibiger's idea was groundbreaking. He was suggesting what's now called randomisation: allocating patients to receive or not to receive a treatment so its effect can be compared between two similar groups of individuals.

Fibiger's results were unequivocal: the strangling angel killed one of every eight untreated children, but only one in thirty of the treated children.[8]

Sørensen's reservations had been answered but also validated. Untreated children at the Blegdamshospitalet[9] proved more likely to survive diphtheria than the children Roux and Grancher treated with antitoxin at the Hôpital des Enfants Malades,[10] proving that it took more than an improved recovery rate to show a treatment was successful. As antitoxin became more widely used, such discrepancies between hospitals, or between different years in the same hospital, were often reported and seldom explained.

Whatever the reasons, Fibiger's trial showed that antitoxin was the treatment the world needed against diphtheria – and also why the world needed randomised trials. The world would learn the former lesson quicker than the latter.

Behring's ideas had been proved but, being Behring, he felt unappreciated and left Koch's institute in 1895. He finally received the recognition he craved in 1901, when he received the inaugural Nobel Prize for Physiology or Medicine and was elevated to the Prussian nobility,[11] to become Emil von Behring. When he died in 1917, even the British *Lancet* published a glowing obituary without mentioning that he was on the other side of a war that was getting bloodier by the day – although it pointedly avoided mention of his ennoblement.[12]

Gaston Ramon's refolded *anatoxine*

By the dawn of the twentieth century, horses around the world were being co-opted into battle against diphtheria. Death rates plummeted among children who made it to hospital but only up to a point. Antitoxin didn't save every child and many didn't make it to a hospital in the first place.

Children needed to be protected against diphtheria *before* they were infected.

Logic dictated that if injecting a horse with diphtheria toxin triggered *antikorps*, then injecting a child with the toxin should do the same. The catch was that no one was keen to inject children with a deadly toxin in order to find out how small that small amount needed to be.

As it was medical doctors who first injected diphtheria toxin into horses, it adds a pleasing symmetry that a man trained as a vet worked out how to detoxify diphtheria toxin and make it safe to inject into children. In 1923, Gaston Ramon of the Institut Pasteur found a combination of heat and formaldehyde treatments that turned toxin into what he called an *anatoxine* – later translated into English as 'toxoid' – that didn't harm the animals he tried it on but did trigger antibodies against the unmodified toxin.

Ramon had found a way to turn diphtheria toxin into a diphtheria vaccine.

In the 1920s, biochemistry depended more on trying different things to see what happened than applying underlying principles. Ramon could show that what happened was the diphtheria toxin had lost its toxicity, but it would be decades before biochemistry matured enough to explain how.

The diphtheria toxin belongs to the class of molecules called proteins, and like any protein, it's made of a chain of amino acids. The twenty amino acids are to a protein what the twenty-six letters of the English alphabet are to this book. As every word is defined by which letters appear in which order, a protein is defined by which amino acids are arranged in which order.

Yet there's more to written language than letter order. Meaning also depends on the structure of the sentences and paragraphs that contain the words. Similarly, there is more to a protein than the order of its amino acids. The amino acid chain is folded into a structure that's as important to the protein's function as the amino acid order.

Ramon's formaldehyde treatment leaves the chain of amino acids untouched but rearranges the folding, which changes the protein enough that it can no longer carry out its function. If the protein in question is diphtheria toxin, then the function it loses is its toxicity.

The effect of Ramon's treatment on diphtheria toxin is similar to the effect of randomly moving the spaces and paragraph breaks on this page. The letters would be in the same order, but they would no longer make sense.

However, antibodies don't care how a protein is folded. They respond to amino acids in a certain order, like a search function that looks for letters and ignores spaces and paragraph breaks. Just as such a search function would see no difference between 'diphtheria toxin', 'dip htheriatoxin', 'diph ther iato xin' and 'diphthe riatoxin', an antibody latches on to an amino acid sequence whether it's folded into a lethal toxin or a harmless toxoid.

Ramon was introducing a new approach to making vaccines. Pasteur's original doctrine had been based around attenuating the pathogen, Wright and Haffkine had shown that sometimes it was enough to inactivate it, and now Ramon showed that sometimes, the whole pathogen wasn't needed. An immune response to a single molecule was enough to protect against diphtheria.

Ramon paved the way for much simpler vaccines but he never received the sort of recognition that Behring did. He was nominated for the Nobel Prize 155 times but never won it, making him the most oft-refused nominee in history.[13]

Backward Britain

When Ramon made his breakthrough, French children were routinely vaccinated against smallpox and only smallpox. His diphtheria vaccine began the expansion of vaccination from a one-off procedure to the schedule of vaccines against a plethora of diseases that it is today.

It wasn't only in France. Diphtheria toxoid was rolled out in many European countries, but Britain was not among them. Britain might have been the birthplace of vaccination, but it was also the birthplace of the anti-vaccination movement which, in the first half of the twentieth century, was at the height of its influence.

It had started as a backlash to the government's often cack-handed attempts to make smallpox vaccination mandatory at a time when smallpox vaccines were neither reliable nor particularly safe. It was only at the end of the nineteenth century that anyone worked out how to purify and preserve the cowpox virus. Before that, what was actually in a vaccine preparation was something of a lottery – and, as if that wasn't bad enough, it occurred to few pre-Pasteurian doctors to sterilise their lancets between patients.[14]

By the 1920s, smallpox vaccine production had improved dramatically and sterility had become a watchword of the medical profession.[15] Protestors were no longer throwing things at vaccinators or burning Edward Jenner in effigy,[16] but anti-vaccine sentiment had not gone away, and some of vaccination's most strident opponents spoke from inside the medical establishment. Some were motivated by genuine concern for their patients, but many feared that a national vaccination programme would be the thin end of a wedge that would place their profession under government control.[17]

During a 1935 visit to Britain, one Canadian doctor received a cool reception when he told his British colleagues how vaccination had all but eliminated diphtheria from Canada: 'A few openly scoffed; others were politely amazed or quietly incredulous; some mutely dismissed me as some sort of apostate who had broken faith with the Old Country.'[18]

Diphtheria remained so rife that Ramon spoke despairingly of *Angleterre refractaire*, which might be generously translated as 'refractory Britain' – or less generously as 'backward Britain'.[19]

It all changed in 1940. As the fall of France brought the Second World War to the British doorstep, the government took control of healthcare almost overnight, and with that control came a nationwide diphtheria vaccination programme. It took some time to implement, but by the end of 1942, a third of English children and half of all Scottish under fifteen years old had received the toxoid.[20] Uptake rose through the wartime and post-war years, and the plot on page 72 shows that by the time systematic nation-wide reporting began in 1966, three quarters of children had been vaccinated by their second birthday. It also shows that the number of cases dropped precipitously well before that, as the vaccine reached more and more children through the 1940s.

Records of diphtheria deaths are less systematic, but we do know that before 1940, between 2,500 and 5,500 British children died of diphtheria every year.[21,22] By the late 1950s, deaths were in the single figures and have stayed there.[23]

Backward Britain was a thing of the past – at least in the sense that Ramon had meant it.

How *Corynebacterium* becomes diphtheria

Given how little was known about diphtheria itself when they were developed, it's extraordinary that antitoxin and the toxoid vaccine have proved so enduringly successful.

Behring, Roux and Ramon could recognise the diphtheria bacterium under a microscope because it looked like a club or a truncheon. They couldn't know that *Corynebacterium diphtheriae*, as it's now called, often lives up the noses of people who don't develop diphtheria. You or I may well have some *Corynebacteria* up our noses right now, behaving themselves as peaceably as all the other species up there.

The trick of turning *Corynebacterium* from a peaceful house guest into a strangling angel is pulled off by a phage: a virus that infects a bacterium. The phage carries the gene for the toxin, which it slots into *Corynebacterium*'s genome.[24] *Corynebacteria* are peaceful enough if left to their own devices, but when they're infected with the phage, they start producing a toxin 300 times more potent than cobra venom.[25] It only takes a tiny amount to reduce a child to the pitiful state from which Tommy helped Charles Sherrington rescue his nephew.

How long does immunity last?

Potent as the toxin is, children are not helpless against it. In one of the few studies on unvaccinated children, a 1923 study of children in New York showed that more than half of five-year-olds had some immunity to the diphtheria toxin,[26] which was a lot more than had been ill with diphtheria. The phage-infected *Corynebacteria* up their noses must have been secreting the toxin in quantities too small to do any damage but large enough to trigger an immune response.

Unfortunately, the protection didn't last. Once the children passed five years old, every year saw more of them become susceptible to diphtheria as their immunity waned. It begs the question of whether the immune response to the toxoid vaccine lasts longer than the response to the toxin itself.

The answer is probably not.[27,28,29]

The problem of immunity being short-lived is why the NHS schedule delivers five diphtheria vaccinations by the age of fourteen.

The first three are given early, at eight, twelve and sixteen weeks, as part of the '6-in-1' vaccine that combines diphtheria with tetanus, whooping cough, hepatitis B, polio and *Haemophilus influenzae* type b in one injection. Diphtheria immunity is boosted at three years and four months in preparation for going to school, and again at fourteen years with the adult dose, which is a tenth of the childhood dose to avoid triggering too much inflammation by injecting it into someone already immune.[30]

As the plot on page 72 shows, British vaccine coverage has stayed above 90 per cent since the 1990s. Diphtheria has become such a rare disease that most people have only a vague idea of what it is. However, there is no room for complacency, because while the antibodies triggered by the vaccine neutralise the toxin, they do not stop us from carrying the *Corynebacterium* that secretes it.[31]

It ties the strangling angel's hands, but it cannot banish it. We saw how quickly it can break free when the collapse of the Soviet Union disrupted the diphtheria vaccination campaign.

The worst diphtheria epidemic since the Second World War saw 150,000 cases and 4,000 deaths across the former Soviet countries.[32] The most disturbing aspect of that epidemic was that despite the economic crisis of the 'hungry nineties', to use the Russian term, the effect on the vaccination programme was never that bad. Even at the worst of the disruption, two thirds of children were still receiving all three doses.[33]

The epidemic was ended by restoring the vaccination programme. The diphtheria vaccine is now so widely available that since 2010, more than 85 per cent of the world's children have received at least one dose.[34] As more children have received the vaccine, fewer have caught diphtheria, with cases dropping from 90,000 in 1980 to below 10,000 per year since 2005.[35]

We know how to protect ourselves against diphtheria, but we can't ever drop our guard. The ex-Soviet epidemic shows us that it can return whenever a vaccination programme falters, and indeed, recent years have seen its return in the wake of the Yemeni Civil War[36] and among Burmese Rohingya people forced into refugee camps in Bangladesh.[37]

We'll always have to share the world with *Corynebacterium*, and all it takes is the combination of a bacteriophage and a missed vaccination for diphtheria to be back among us.

Children vaccinated by their second birthday

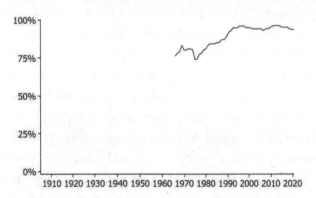

Diphtheria cases

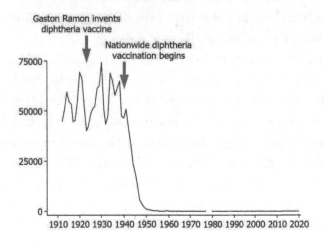

The top panel shows the number of children vaccinated by their second birthday. The bottom panel shows the number of people diagnosed with diphtheria.

Both plots show data from the beginning of systematic records until 2020. Data on vaccine coverage are from England and Wales until 1978 and from England only after 1978.[38,39] Data on cases are all from England and Wales.[40]

Chapter 5

Tetanus

Head westward from the Scottish coast into the North Atlantic, past the Isle of Skye and the Outer Hebrides, keep going for another 65km and, if you've read your compass right, you'll see the cliffs of St Kilda rise ahead of you. It's a tiny archipelago, not quite 9km² at low tide, and for centuries, it's been home to one of the most remote communities in the British Isles.

In 1886, the island's sole schoolteacher, George Murray, wrote about a particular affliction of the babies of that community. 'This one was 13 days except one and a half hours ... the first signs of its being dangerously ill was at the end of a week, when it ceased to suck the breast, but still sucked the bottle. The following day, the jaws fell ... when all hope of its recovery were given up ... It was pitiful to see the poor little things in the pangs of death.'[1]

The baby was probably unnamed. The 'jaws falling' happened so often that St Kildan parents resisted emotional attachment until their newborns survived their first couple of weeks.

In the 1880s, there was nothing unusual about children dying young, but St Kildan babies were dying at a rate that horrified a mainland Scot like Murray. 'One man, not yet 50 years old,

I should say, pointed to the place to me where he buried nine children ... Sad to think of the like. Bad treatment at birth must have been the cause of so many dying.'[2]

Murray's vague 'bad treatment' was one of several explanations put forward, along with the inevitable 'consanguinity' in such a small community and a divine plan to prevent overpopulation.[3] None suggested a solution until 1892, when St Kilda's clergyman, Angus Fiddes, sought advice from the Glasgow Obstetrical and Gynaecological Society. He was advised that when a baby's umbilical cord was cut, the stump should be covered with gauze soaked in iodine. On St Kilda, the usual practice was to cover it with fulmar oil, so-called because it comes from a seabird called the fulmar that projectile vomits its stomach contents at anyone who ventures too close to its nest. Far from being deterred by the stink of semi-digested fish, the St Kildans believed it had medicinal properties.

Replacing fulmar oil with iodine dramatically improved the survival of St Kildan babies, suggesting that the falling jaws were caused by a microbial infection. We now recognise the lethal falling jaws as neonatal tetanus.

The Glasgow surgeons who Fiddes consulted probably didn't recognise it from his description. The tetanus bacterium had only just been discovered and it was seen as a disease of livestock that occasionally infected humans. However, they didn't need to identify the microbe to recognise that fulmar oil was a less than ideal disinfectant.

Of herbivores and soldiers

Part of the reason why the falling jaws remained mysterious for so long is that, unusually among bacterial diseases, tetanus is not contagious. Without the tell-tale cluster of cases that pop up when an infection passes from one person to another, an early follower of Pasteur's microbiological theory wouldn't have looked for a microbiological cause.

The bacterium in question is *Clostridium tetani*. It lives mostly in the intestines of herbivores, including farm animals like cattle, sheep and horses. Most of the time, it's an inoffensive member of the complex microbial community that helps the animal digest its food. Like any intestine-dwelling microbe, *C. tetani* is occasionally expelled in the animal's faeces.

For most of the 'anaerobic' bacteria living in the oxygen-free environment of an animal's intestine, being dumped into the open air is fatal. The tetanus bacterium doesn't like oxygen any more than the next anaerobe, but it has a particular trick to survive. It forms a structure called a spore and shuts down its metabolism.

Becoming a spore enables *C. tetani* to do nothing, which is more difficult than it might sound. From microbe to man, living things need complex molecules that don't react well to fluctuating temperatures and the constant bombardment of radiation from the sun. Their vulnerability makes life a constant process of repair and renewal that, if it ever stops, cannot be restarted because too many of those complex molecules will have deteriorated. That's why viruses don't last long when they're outside a cell.

Maintaining the molecules fundamental to life without life to maintain them is a trick that only a few bacteria have pulled off. Unfortunately for us, *C. tetani* is one of them. Its spores preserve their molecular machinery so well that they're among the most resilient of all biological structures. They can survive being frozen, boiled, treated with household disinfectants, or, more relevant to survival in the wild, spores can lie dormant in soil for years until they're swallowed by a grazing animal. As soon as they're back in their happy place in the animal's intestine, they germinate and pick up where they left off.[4]

If that was all *C. tetani* did, it would never have filled St Kilda's graveyard with babies. Its dark side is revealed when it finds its way into an open wound. Once it's in there, it has a nasty habit of secreting a toxin that makes diphtheria toxin look feeble. Tetanus toxin is 500 times more potent than diphtheria toxin, making it 150,000 times more potent than cobra venom.[5]

The sliver of good news is that once the spore germinates, C. tetani loses its resilience. If Fiddes's iodine-soaked gauze protected the babies he applied it to, it was because the iodine penetrated deep enough to kill the germinated bacteria.

Quite why C. tetani is an inoffensive guest in an animal's intestine but secretes a lethal toxin if it gets into a cut on that same animal's leg remains a mystery. Laboratory experiments have shown that it switches the toxin production on or off according to what nutrients it's getting,[6] but that doesn't explain what, if anything, C. tetani gains by poisoning its host.

Tetanus toxin attacks the nervous system, driving the muscles into spasms that were vividly depicted by a nineteenth-century surgeon called Charles Bell. In 1809, Bell attended wounded soldiers evacuated to Portsmouth after the Battle of Corunna in Spain.[7] The time it took to get them to Portsmouth fell within the three-day to three-week window between a wound being infected with tetanus spores and the toxin taking hold.

Bell, a gifted artist, captured the effects of tetanus in the painting titled Opisthotonus, which was what the spasms of tetanus were then called. The man depicted on page 84 is a soldier undergoing spasms so violent they have probably fractured some of his vertebrae, which, if he'd had any hope of surviving, would have left him permanently disabled. He had no such hope; Opisthotonus is a portrait of a man dying in agony.

His facial rictus is behind Murray's description of jaws falling and another common name for tetanus poisoning: lockjaw.

By the time of the Reverend Fiddes's trip to Glasgow, the connection between opisthotonus and C. tetani was known, but no one had realised that its spores could find their way into an unhygienically cut umbilical cord as well as into bullet or bayonet wounds. The advice to use iodine was based on sterilisation being a generally good idea rather than being specifically targeted at C. *tetani*.

It was only in 2004 that microbiologist Ian Poxton confirmed that St Kilda's falling jaws were caused by neonatal tetanus, more than seventy years after the last St Kildans resettled in Argyll. Poxton found their abandoned houses riddled with C. *tetani* spores, deposited there by the cattle the St Kildans shared their homes with and probably the peat they brought in to burn on their open fires.[8] No wonder neonatal tetanus was rife. Babies were being born besieged by spores.

Shibasaburo Kitasato's antitoxin

In 1868, the Meiji Restoration ended Japan's centuries of self-imposed isolation and made the world of sixteen-year-old Shibasaburo Kitasato a lot bigger. He seized its opportunities with both hands, joining one of the new University of Tokyo's first intakes of medical students and then travelling to Berlin to study with Robert Koch.

Berlin must have been a confusing and exhilarating place for the boy from a Kyushu village, which was provincial even by the standards of a country closed to the world. If he was disorientated by working in a research group that was revolutionising medicine in one of the world's great metropolises, he didn't take long to catch up. He proved himself equal to any of Koch's team when he found a way to culture C. *tetani*, which was no simple task given its objections to oxygen.

Having isolated the bacterium, he purified the toxin and, working with Emil Behring, who was doing much the same thing with diphtheria, Kitasato developed an antitoxin. He and Behring co-published their respective successes in 1890, showing the world how to cure diphtheria and tetanus within the same few pages.[9]

Although they started working in parallel, it was Behring who turned Kitasato's tetanus antitoxin into a treatment. Two years after their joint paper, Kitasato returned to Tokyo, where he spent the rest of his life building medical research and education in Japan. In 1914, he founded the Kitasato Institute,* which remains one of Japan's leading medical research institutions.[10]

While Roux and Grancher led the rush to get diphtheria antitoxin into hospitals, Kitasato's tetanus antitoxin was seen primarily as a veterinary treatment. It was widely used to treat injured livestock, especially horses, which were as vital to the functioning of late-nineteenth-century Europe as motor vehicles are in the early twenty-first century, but was only rarely used to treat tetanus in humans.

At the time, nobody realised how many people were dying of tetanus. Neonatal tetanus still wasn't recognised and, decades later, epidemiologists found that until a government mandates reporting of tetanus deaths, they are invariably underestimated.[11] Because it's not infectious, authorities don't watch out for outbreaks to clamp down on, so even a large number of cases spread across a large area rarely attracts attention unless someone is looking for them.

The most malicious weapon

The year that Kitasato founded his research institute was also the year that the world gave itself a reason to sit up and pay attention to tetanus and, by extension, to Kitasato's antitoxin.

---

* Now Kitasato University.

The First World War was a monumental human tragedy driven by a revolution in military technology, but it was also a triumph of medical technology. For most of the major powers involved, it was the first war in which more soldiers were killed by enemy action than disease.[12]

Part of the reason is that new weapons, like artillery, machine guns and poison gas, stacked up the bodies that could be tallied to enemy action. However, it was also the first war that saw both sides deploy a professional medical corps. Keeping men from dying of disease before the enemy had a chance to kill them was now a priority for military planners, as was keeping them from dying of infection when they were wounded – and no wound infection was more feared than tetanus. One German nurse called it 'the smallest, most cruel and most malicious weapon of this war',[13] which, from someone who must have seen the effects of mustard gas, is quite an accolade.

The British Army fought its first battles of the war in the pastures of northern France, where grazing livestock had so thoroughly seeded the soil with tetanus spores that many farmers injected their horses with antitoxin at the beginning of every summer. Artillery blasted that spore-laden pastureland into dust and drove it deep into the bodies of soldiers on both sides. When they had fought each other to a standstill, the opposing armies dug deep into spore-laden mud that got into every wound, and also into the open sores of 'trench foot', the inevitable consequence of being permanently cold and wet in ill-fitting boots.[14]

Behind the front lines, doctors in field hospitals were finding that by the time a man developed the first spasms of tetanus, it was often too late for antitoxin to do any good.[15] They quickly learned not to wait for the spasms, but to treat every wounded man with antitoxin.

The effect of pre-emptive treatment was spectacular. The

British Army's records showed that in October 1914, one in every thirty wounded men was developing tetanus. By November, getting antitoxin in first dropped the figure to one in 590, and it stayed low for the rest of the war.[16]

Amid the mud and misery of the Western Front, antitoxin proved itself as potent against that most malicious weapon as it was against diphtheria. However, as with diphtheria, treatment was never going to be as good as prevention.

Another war, another defence against tetanus

When Gaston Ramon found a way to turn the lethal diphtheria toxin into a harmless toxoid, he immediately realised the same approach could be used with the tetanus toxin.[17] It was his colleague, Pierre Descombey, who published the technique, but as with antitoxin, the vaccine was initially used more in animals than in people. Ramon and Descombey all but eliminated tetanus from the French cavalry's horses,[18] but when the European nations were once again calling their young men into uniform, the idea of mass human vaccination came to the fore.

Major John Boyd had been in the Royal Army Medical Corps since the beginning of the First World War, so he must have seen what tetanus could do. In 1938, with the British Army facing the prospect of being sent back to France, Boyd pushed for British soldiers to be given Ramon and Descombey's vaccine. Thanks largely to Boyd, British troops went to the Second World War immune to tetanus toxin.[19]

Neither Ramon, Descombey nor Boyd carried out any sort of comparison between vaccinated and unvaccinated people. It seemed to work on horses and, with war looming, Boyd persuaded the army that it was better to be safe than sorry. He took it as a given that the vaccine worked, and he also provided the best evidence we have that he was right, although he provided it inadvertently.

The 1944–5 advance from Normandy into western Germany saw hundreds of thousands of British servicemen injured, many in the same tetanus-riddled pastures where their fathers had fought the First World War. Among those hundreds of thousands, only six developed tetanus, which, by the morbid logic of military medicine, was a resounding success.

The near elimination of tetanus from the British Army contrasted with the German Army's experience. German soldiers were not vaccinated against it, and while Boyd was never able to find out how many wounded Germans died of tetanus, there was no question that there were a lot. One hospital reported over 100 cases. The fabled Nazi efficiency was often less than it was cracked up to be, but in this case, its failure provides us with the closest to a clinical trial that the tetanus toxoid vaccine has ever been subjected to.[20]

Tetanus today

At the end of the Second World War, tetanus was still seen as an affliction of soldiers and horses, but in the post-war era of nationalised healthcare systems, its wider importance began to get noticed. Neonatal tetanus was finally recognised, and wherever cases were looked for, they were found. Nor was it only babies who were affected. Neonatal tetanus often goes hand in hand with maternal tetanus, in which the mother is infected while giving birth.[21]

A modern hospital has a battery of treatments that it can throw at a case of tetanus. Antitoxin neutralises the tetanus toxin, antibiotics kill the bacteria, muscle relaxants control the spasms and intensive care units can take over a patient's breathing if either the tetanus toxin or the muscle relaxants stop the patient from doing it for themselves. However, all of those treatments only offer a fifty-fifty chance of survival.[22]

For survivors, recovery can be a slow process. Seizures, tremors and cognitive impairment can last for months or years.

Tetanus is one of the few infections for which it is not too late to vaccinate after the initial infection, which is why people are often vaccinated after an injury that may have been contaminated. Because the bacterium may take as long as three weeks before it secretes the toxin, vaccination can give the immune system time to beat it to the punch.

The best way to beat tetanus is still to vaccinate before getting infected, and since the 1950s, more and more countries have been adding it to their routine vaccination schedules – although Britain, where much of the medical establishment remained unenthusiastic about vaccination, didn't add tetanus to the childhood vaccine schedule until 1961.[23]

Since then, the tetanus vaccine proved to be equally effective when combined with other vaccines, allowing several to be combined in the same syringe and cutting the number of injections needed to deliver them. It is now so commonly combined with diphtheria and pertussis (whooping cough) vaccines that it's almost synonymous with abbreviations like DTP, DPT or occasionally TdaP (to specify the use of the acellular pertussis vaccine that is the subject of the next chapter).

The current NHS schedule gives DTP five times during childhood. The first three are given as part of the '6-in-1' at eight, twelve and sixteen weeks, combining DTP with the hepatitis B, polio and *Haemophilus influenzae* type b vaccines in a single injection. The DTP and polio are boosted in the pre-school '4-in-1' vaccine given at three years and four months, and DTP is given again at fourteen years.

The combination leaves children thoroughly protected, although the protection is not lifelong. It typically lasts for thirty years after the last vaccination,[24] so there is an argument for booster vaccinations for anyone likely to be exposed to spores.

Most of the world's health services, including the NHS, offer another booster to pregnant women.[25] That's partly to protect her, but also because antibodies are among the many gifts that a mother gives her unborn child. They cross the placenta into the foetus's bloodstream, where they remain for several months after the child is born, protecting the child until he can be vaccinated to produce his own antibodies.

Uptake of the tetanus vaccine in Britain has remained above 94 per cent since 1992,[26] which has made tetanus a very rare disease. At the time of writing, the last year with more than ten cases was 2004.[27] Among those cases, fewer than one in ten had received the full vaccination schedule.[28]

Britain's success is not exceptional. Around the world, the number of children who receive three doses of the tetanus-containing DTP vaccine rose from 20 per cent in 1980 to 84 per cent in 2010, where it remains stable.[29] The global vaccine roll-out has led to an equivalent fall in tetanus deaths, from an estimated 340,000 in 1990 to 57,000 in 2015.

Tetanus is now a rare disease all over the world, but because the bacterium remains ubiquitous, it can never be eradicated. Wherever animals graze, there may be tetanus spores that can get into a cut. Nor do they stay confined to the countryside. Not even the most committed city-dweller can avoid contact with them. If tetanus is now a vanishingly rare disease, it's because the tetanus toxoid vaccine gives us a shield that we won't ever be able to drop.

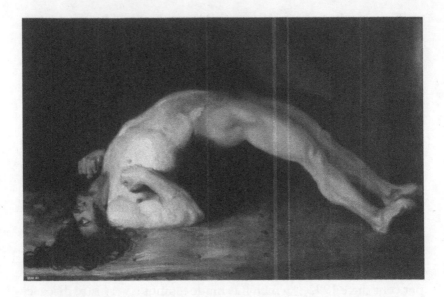

Opisthotonus by Charles Bell, depicting a man dying of tetanus poisoning. Reproduced with the kind permission of the Royal College of Surgeons of Edinburgh.

Chapter 6

Whooping cough

Paul Bordet was only a few months old when he caught whooping cough. In 1906, any Belgian parent would have recognised the explosive coughing that went on and on until Paul, exhausted and possibly turning blue, could finally suck in a breath with the 'whoop' that gives the disease its English name.

In early-twentieth-century Europe, childhood was a trial by endurance. One baby in four didn't live to see their first birthday,[1] and of all the infectious diseases, whooping cough was believed to be the biggest killer.[2] It killed one in every fifty children who caught it,[3] and it was a very lucky child who didn't catch it. Every parent would know someone whose child had died of the paroxysms convulsing Paul's tiny body.

All Paul's parents could do for him was offer a few prayers, but his father was thinking about what he could do for the children of the future.

Jules Bordet had been fascinated by science since he was a boy. His family lived in terror of the fumes and fires emanating from his improvised laboratory in their attic, but at sixteen years old, he turned away from chemistry to study medicine at the

Université Libre de Bruxelles.* He graduated in six years instead of the usual seven and while he was at it, he published his first paper on a bacterium called *Vibrio metchnikovii*.[4] In those early days of medical microbiology, one could do groundbreaking research before even graduating.

He impressed enough people that the Belgian government sent him to Paris to study under Élie Metchnikoff, discoverer of the phagocyte and the man whom the bacterium in Bordet's study was named for, at the Institut Pasteur.

He spent the next seven years learning the researcher's craft and, in a rare break from his laboratory, marrying a woman called Marthe.[5] Work and family occasionally coincided, such as when the Bordets' daughter caught whooping cough. Bordet put some of the sputum she coughed up under a microscope and became the first to set eyes on the bacterium that would one day bear his name. We now call it *Bordetella pertussis* but at the time, all Bordet could do was stare impotently at the microbe tormenting his daughter.

She recovered, and in 1901, Bordet and his family returned to Brussels, where he founded what he called the Institut Pasteur du Brabant, choosing a name that reflected his mentors in Paris.

When little Paul caught whooping cough, Bordet determined to get more than a glimpse of the bacterium – but to study it, he needed to find a way to culture it. Working with his colleague and brother-in-law Octave Gengou, he mixed potato extract and rabbit blood with agar so it formed a jelly-like substance in a glass culture plate. When Paul coughed droplets on to the agar, the bacterial cells found the mix of nutrients they needed and started dividing.

Bordet and Gengou, with a little help from Paul, had completed the first step of Pasteur's 'isolate, attenuate, inject' doctrine.

---

* Brussels.

The discovery would win Bordet the 1919 Nobel Prize in Physiology or Medicine, but, more importantly to a man devoted to his family – even if he occasionally used them as sources of samples – Paul made a full recovery.[6]

Paul Bordet's whoops

We now know that Paul must have inhaled some bacteria-laden droplets that an infected person had exhaled, and that he must have breathed them at least two weeks before he started whooping. The bacteria attached themselves to the inside of his throat and spent the first week dividing, dividing and dividing again, spreading down his respiratory tract toward his lungs.[7]

After a week, he would have developed a mild fever and perhaps a cough, but it would have looked no worse than an ordinary cold. It would take another week to turn into what we now call the paroxysmal stage of the disease, or pertussis: the fits of coughing and gasping for breath that give whooping cough its name.

The paroxysmal stage can go on for weeks. It must have been torture for Paul's parents, who knew that every day until he recovered, he could become that one in fifty who it killed.

Most whooping cough deaths are from inflammation raising the blood pressure in the lungs and rendering a child unable to breathe. Pulmonary hypertension, to give the condition its medical name, is often fatal, even in children who are treated in a modern intensive care unit.

Surviving whooping cough is one thing. Full recovery is another. The paroxysms can stop a child from breathing for long enough to starve his brain of oxygen, causing permanent brain damage.[8]

We still lack a solid understanding of the eponymous cough. In words co-authored by four of the world's leading experts on whooping cough, 'we still don't know why infection makes people cough!'[9]

In the dry prose of scientific journals, that exclamation mark is a scream of frustration. The bacterium secretes a witch's brew of toxins that probably have something to do with the cough, but we don't know exactly how.

Even more perplexing is that Paul would have had more bacteria in his respiratory tract when it looked like an ordinary cold than when he started the potentially fatal whooping cough. By then, his immune system was already clearing out the bacteria. After six weeks, there wouldn't have been a whooping cough bacterium left in his body, but he was probably still whooping and coughing.[10] In Japan, China and Korea, it's called the 100-day cough,[11] but it often lasts much longer than that.

Because the cough persists long after the infection, antibiotics are of only limited help. They kill the bacteria, but by the time a child's illness is clearly whooping cough rather than a cold, his immune system already has that task in hand. Antibiotics can head off brain damage and death, but they don't end the whooping cough.

While Paul's immune system was purging the whooping cough bacteria, it was forming an immune memory of it. Long after he recovered, his lymphocytes would go on secreting antibodies into the mucus lining his windpipe. If only lymphocytes would keep secreting those antibodies, whooping cough wouldn't be so dangerous to babies.

Unfortunately, they don't.

Immunity to *Bordetella* wanes over time, which occasionally allows it back in. How occasionally is yet another unknown, because a lot of those reinfections don't cause symptoms.[12] The bacterium hangs around in someone's throat for a few days until their immune memory kicks back in, leaving the infected person oblivious to the bacteria they exhale wherever they go. That's probably how Paul was infected in the first place: from an adult who didn't know they were infected.

This 'silent transmission' makes whooping cough a particularly difficult disease to get rid of, and it's also why it infects babies when they're so young. Most childhood diseases are passed around children old enough to play together and infect each other, by which time they're a lot more robust than a baby. The early-to-mid childhood years, from around five years to puberty, are the best time to catch an infectious disease, because that's when we're best equipped to handle them.[13]

Babies tend to have less contact with other children and more with adults, who are immune from most childhood diseases. However, those adults give the whooping cough bacterium a direct route into the throat of a baby who has yet to reach the robust years of childhood.

Worse, whooping cough is one of the most infectious of the infectious diseases. It's about ten times more infectious than influenza,[14] a level only matched by measles and chickenpox.

Whooping cough is a difficult disease to tackle, but that hasn't stopped a lot of people from trying.

The killed-bacteria vaccine

In the early twentieth century, potatoes and rabbit blood were easy enough to get hold of, so Bordet-Gengou agar, as their culture medium was called, allowed researchers around the world to isolate the bacterium and try to turn it into something they could inject.

Gaston Ramon's approach of detoxifying toxins, which had proved so effective against diphtheria and tetanus, wasn't going to work. Ramon had started with two bacterial diseases that could be stymied by an immune response to a single toxin molecule, but in that respect, diphtheria and tetanus are exceptions. Whooping cough, like most bacterial infections, requires a more multifaceted immune response to contain it. Early-twentieth-century vaccinologists had no way to work out what those facets were, so most followed Waldemar Haffkine and Almroth Wright's approach of simply killing the bacteria, injecting it and hoping for the best.

Sometimes their killed-bacteria vaccines worked, and sometimes they didn't. Their fundamental problem was that a culture plate is a much friendlier environment for a bacterium than a human being. Culture medium gives bacteria all the nutrients they can metabolise, and they don't need to duck and dive around an immune system to get at them.

When a microbiologist takes some of the bacteria to inoculate a fresh culture plate, the sample is inevitably dominated by the bacteria that divide fastest in the bonanza of free nutrients, which are also the ones that have adapted furthest from the disease-causing wild-type. That's how microbes in culture become attenuated, but after enough passages, bacteria can adapt so far from the wild-type that an immune memory triggered against the cultured bacteria won't recognise the wild-type and won't protect against it.

The problems don't end with the culture. In the early twentieth century, vaccinologists usually killed their bacteria with chemicals like formaldehyde, but then they needed to separate the dead bacteria from the killing chemicals. The purification process often removed a lot of the killed bacteria along with those chemicals.

By the time they had something ready for the 'inject' stage, they didn't know what they were injecting or how much of it.

The Furniture City takes on whooping cough

Killed-bacteria whooping cough vaccines produced a few successes and a lot of failures, and nobody knew what made the difference between them. Nobody, that is, until Pearl Kendrick entered the fray.

Kendrick's ultimate success was based on two things: her meticulous attention to detail and her enlistment of an entire city into her battle against whooping cough.

That city was Grand Rapids, Michigan, nicknamed the 'Furniture City' for the furniture factories that drew people from across America and beyond to work in them. When Kendrick arrived in 1932, half the population was foreign-born, mostly Dutch or Polish,[15] but the Depression had turned Grand Rapids from a boomtown into an impoverished, disease-ridden city of slums.

Kendrick arrived as associate director of a new laboratory of the Michigan Department of Health. It was a promotion after her recent doctorate, but screening water and milk for bacterial contamination hardly taxed her skills.

She asked for permission to work on whooping cough and her director replied with a one-sentence memo: 'If you are having any fun working on whooping cough, go ahead.'[16]

He could give his permission, but when state bureaus were struggling to keep the lights on, he couldn't give her any funding. Kendrick had to look to the city itself for resources – and Grand Rapids stepped up.

The city commission and local businesses chipped in to pay for laboratory supplies, while doctors, nurses and laboratory staff volunteered their time after their day's work. Kendrick's right-hand woman was Grace Eldering, who later wrote, 'When the workday was over, we started on the research because it was fun.

We'd come home, feed the dogs, get some dinner and get back to what was interesting.'[17]

It may have been fun, but Kendrick and Eldering's drive came from seeing so many children who were very sick and very poor.

'We learned about the disease and the Depression at the same time. Our watchword became "round to the back and up the stairs",' Eldering wrote. 'We collected specimens by the light of kerosene lamps, from whooping, vomiting, strangling children. We saw what the disease can do.'[18]

Thanks to their army of volunteers, Kendrick and Eldering obtained a steady supply of whooping cough bacteria. They found they could kill bacteria with a new chemical called Merthiolate at concentrations harmless to humans, avoiding the purification problem that had tripped up earlier attempts to make a vaccine. When their killed bacteria could consistently trigger an immune response in rabbits, they had a vaccine worth trying in children.

A child who developed whooping cough quickly gave it to any brothers and sisters. Kendrick reasoned that if they vaccinated some of the exposed siblings but not others, they would find out whether the vaccine worked.

Their problem was that whooping cough always beat them to the punch. By the time they heard of a whooping child with healthy siblings and found time to visit, the siblings were already whooping.[19]

If they could have paid dedicated staff, they might have been quicker off the mark, which, ironically, would have been disastrous. They didn't know that an infected child appeared healthy for at least a week before showing any symptoms. Their original plan would have led to the vaccine being given in that week, when it was already too late to do any good, and they would have concluded that it didn't work. Instead, they adapted their approach to their resources, matching every vaccinee with a control of the same age and sex who lived in the same district.[20]

In the 1930s, there was no playbook for testing a vaccine. Kendrick and Eldering had to work out everything from scratch. Their solution was similar to some modern epidemiological techniques, and if it wasn't quite how today's vaccine trials are done, it was a lot better than much of what passed for clinical trials in the 1930s.

Progress was slow, not least because they had to put the whole operation on hold whenever they ran out of money. Nevertheless, Kendrick's volunteer army persisted, and by 1937, they had around 4,000 recruits – and a result.[21] Vaccinated children were one-seventh as likely as unvaccinated children to develop whooping cough, and when they did, it was rarely a severe bout.[22]

Now they had to convince the American Public Health Association. Kendrick was a member, but not the only member to be testing a whooping cough vaccine. The other was James Doull, whose killed-bacteria vaccine hadn't worked,[23] and he was sceptical of Kendrick's claim to have succeeded where he had failed.

Doull was a medical doctor, an epidemiologist and a professor at Case Western Reserve University. He was firmly inside the American medical establishment, while Kendrick, a woman who ran a state lab in a backwater city and fiddled with vaccines in her spare time, emphatically was not. Doull could have stifled Kendrick's results, but instead he and Kendrick agreed to refer the dispute to the Association's chairman, Wade Hampton Frost at Johns Hopkins University.[24]

Frost wasn't eager to get involved. Reviewing Kendrick's results would mean travelling to Grand Rapids, which was a long journey from Baltimore for a man whose health was being eaten away by tuberculosis. Moreover, Frost thought it was a fool's errand. He firmly believed that only an epidemiologist could design a trial, and John Kolmer's polio vaccine debacle* was

---

* See Chapter 4.

recent enough to be fresh in his mind. When a bacteriologist in a city he'd barely heard of said she'd cracked the problem that had defeated Doull, it can't have sounded promising.

Neither Doull nor Frost appear to have realised that Kendrick being a bacteriologist instead of an epidemiologist was the key to her success. While Doull had paid little attention to how his bacteria were cultured, Kendrick had improved on the Bordet-Gengou agar, made sure her bacteria were cultured and killed in exactly the same way, and, critically, she had tested every batch on rabbits. Any batch that didn't trigger antibodies in the rabbits went in the bin.

Quality control isn't glamorous and only makes headlines when it goes spectacularly wrong, but it was central to Kendrick's success in developing a consistently successful vaccine.

Two trips to Grand Rapids dissolved Frost's scepticism. He became an enthusiastic supporter of Kendrick's, even arranging for a statistician to help her prepare her data for publication. Between Frost's concerns and carrying out the statistical analysis, the paper wasn't published until 1939,[25] two years after the end of the trial.

Frost didn't live to see it. He succumbed to his tuberculosis the year before.

The Michigan Method

The Kendrick-Eldering trial, as posterity has remembered Grand Rapids's war on whooping cough, introduced the 'Michigan Method' to the world. Its strength lay in its simplicity; any microbiology laboratory that could get hold of whooping cough bacterium could apply the Michigan Method to turn it into a vaccine. Around the world, government laboratories and pharmaceutical companies alike used it to produce what became called the whole-cell whooping cough vaccine.

In Britain, the Medical Research Council (MRC) had started testing whooping cough vaccines in 1942 with resources that Kendrick could only have dreamed of, but what they discovered with those resources was that their vaccines were among the many that didn't work. When they tried again in 1946, they asked Kendrick to send them some of her vaccine and compared it with four other candidates.

The MRC may not have been very good at making whooping cough vaccines, but they were writing that much-needed playbook for clinical trials. It was MRC scientists who invented the double-blind placebo-controlled clinical trial in 1943, when they used it to reach the conclusion that a fungal extract called patulin was utterly useless as a treatment for the common cold.[26]

Patulin was a disappointment, but the trial design was far more rigorous than anything anyone else had come up with. The MRC's second round of whooping cough vaccine trials were the first to apply it to testing a vaccine, making it far more rigorous than either Kendrick's or Doull's trials had been. The results were unequivocal; Kendrick's vaccine worked, and it worked better than any of the other candidates.[27]

The British medical establishment still harboured an enduring distrust of vaccination, and as the late 1940s brought antibiotics and a National Health Service to deliver them, the death rate from whooping cough started to fall, even though, as the plot on page 102 shows, the number of children getting whooping cough didn't. Anything from 65,000 to 175,000 British children caught it every year,[28] and it was still a disease that lingered for months.[29]

The MRC kept running trials until 1956, long after they'd convinced the rest of the world that whole-cell vaccines made by Kendrick's Michigan Method worked. By then, most high-income countries had already rolled them out in childhood vaccine programmes.

Britain finally added whooping cough to the childhood vaccine schedule in 1957, combined with diphtheria and tetanus in the DTP, or DTwP as it is now called to reflect the use of the whole-cell vaccine.[30] When systematic records of vaccine coverage began in 1968, over 75 per cent of children were being vaccinated and whooping cough was in retreat. Cases had been below 20,000 since 1965 and deaths were down to double figures.

By the mid-1970s, few new parents had ever known the dread of hearing their child's coughing paroxysm. As fear of whooping cough faded into folk memory, parents started to look askance at the whole-cell vaccine itself.

The cerebral cry

The whole-cell vaccine is a mash of the thousands of proteins, carbohydrates and everything else that makes up the whooping cough bacterium. That's a lot of different things for the immune system to react to, and it's why vaccines made of whole killed bacteria tend to trigger more inflammation than other vaccine types.

Most killed-bacteria vaccines have been intended for soldiers, whose commanding officers preferred them knocked off their feet for a couple of days rather than decimated by typhoid or meningitis. They have rarely been given to babies unless there was an epidemic already underway, when unpleasant reactions were the lesser of two evils.

The whole-cell whooping cough vaccine is the only killed-bacteria vaccine to have found its way into routine childhood vaccination. It raised few objections when parents were familiar with the ravages of whooping cough, but as whooping cough was slowly forgotten, some started wondering if the side effects were worth it.

In a few cases, those side effects were worse than a swollen arm and a couple of days of fever. There were rare cases of the fevers causing convulsions or a grating, high-pitched crying sound that tore at the nerves of babies' parents. It was only around one vaccination in a thousand that caused a 'cerebral cry',[31] and there were no lasting effects once the babies recovered – at least to the babies themselves. The parents were never likely to forget it.

In 1973, a British paediatric neurologist called John Wilson announced that the whole-cell whooping cough vaccine could cause permanent brain damage. He was later proved wrong but, in a saga covered in detail in Chapter 20, he dissuaded many parents from having their children vaccinated.

With a disease as infectious as whooping cough, what happened next was entirely predictable. The outbreak of 1977 swept through unvaccinated children, myself among them. Tens of thousands of children were left struggling for breath, which scared parents back to their GPs to get their children vaccinated. There was another major outbreak in 1982 and several smaller ones through the rest of the 1980s, but enough parents returned to vaccine clinics to get whooping cough back under control.[32]

It wasn't only in Britain. The same pattern of vaccine scare, vaccine refusal and whooping cough outbreak played out in several other countries, including Japan, where it provoked a more constructive response. It inspired a vaccine that caused less unpleasant side effects.

Acellular vaccines

In December 1974, a one-year-old Japanese girl died within two hours of receiving the DTwP vaccine. A month later, a seven-year-old girl died suddenly within a day of receiving her DTwP.[33]

There was no reason to suppose that the vaccine had caused either death, and critically, no evidence that children were more likely to die suddenly after a DTwP vaccination than at any other time. However, caveats do not sell newspapers. The headlines shouted that two healthy children had dropped dead from a vaccine against diseases that no longer mattered.

Japan's Ministry of Health initially responded to the public outcry by suspending vaccination, and later by delaying it until children were two years old. They reasoned that by then, children are past the age when they're likely to develop unexpected medical problems that might be blamed on a vaccine and put even more parents off vaccinations.

The Japanese approach got parents back to vaccine clinics, but it allowed whooping cough the run of the under-twos, the age group most likely to die of it. In 1974, the year before the suspension, Japan had seen only 206 whooping cough cases, none of which had been fatal. In 1979, there were over 13,000 cases and over 200 deaths.[34]

The idea of a better vaccine wasn't a new one. Yuji Sato of the Japanese National Institutes of Health had been working towards it since 1960, in collaboration with Margaret Pittman at the American National Institutes of Health (NIH). Pittman was a fixture at the NIH, and indeed of American medical research, for much of the twentieth century. She joined the NIH in 1936[35] and was still there in the 1990s when, at more than ninety years old, her eagerness to get to work got her pulled over for speeding.[36]

Pittman and Sato started by working on the witch's brew of toxins that *Bordetella* produces. They reasoned that if they could identify enough toxins, they could come up with a cocktail that would stop an infection from taking hold. If the immune system only had to deal with a few proteins instead of the whole bacterium, perhaps it would trigger less inflammation and avoid the fevers that caused the convulsions and the cerebral cry.

Sato did most of the detailed work needed to see which molecules triggered which effects in mice. He identified two different toxins and found that once he turned them into harmless toxoids, they worked as an effective vaccine without causing the side effects of the whole-cell vaccine.[37]

Japan's Ministry of Health used Sato's acellular vaccine to replace the whole-cell vaccine from 1981, although, still worried about the vaccine being blamed for early childhood illnesses, Japanese children still had to wait until they were two years old before being vaccinated. Whooping cough slowly subsided through the 1980s,[38] but it was only after 1995, when the Ministry readjusted the schedule to start vaccinating three-month-olds,[39] that Japan beat whooping cough back to the levels it had been before the 1974 scare.

However, Sato's two-toxin vaccine only went so far. It soon emerged that some strains didn't produce the toxins in Sato's vaccine,[40] and the race was on to add more components. We now know that a vaccine needs at least three different toxins to be effective,[41] and some have as many as five.

Whooping cough in Britain

By the 1990s, few of the new generation of British parents had heard of the scare of the 1970s, which is why, as the plot on page 102 shows, around 90 per cent of children were being vaccinated[42] even though the NHS was still using the whole-cell vaccine with all of its side effects.[43]

British infants were given DTwP at eight, twelve and sixteen weeks, but in 2001, acellular pertussis was introduced into Britain as a pre-school booster given to three-year-olds. The acellular vaccine only completely replaced the whole-cell vaccine in 2004, but not because of the side effects. The Joint Committee on Vaccination and Immunisation (JCVI), whose advice to the Ministry of Health is key to shaping vaccine policy, wanted to combine the DTP with an inactivated polio vaccine. The only off-the-shelf combination available happened to use the acellular rather than the whole-cell whooping cough vaccine.[44]

The spirited debates of the 1970s and 1980s were yesterday's news, and the media gave the change so little coverage that few parents were even aware of it.

Another problem emerged some years after the change. Immunity triggered by the whole-cell vaccine didn't last as long as immunity to natural infection, and immunity to the acellular vaccine proved to have an even shorter duration.[45]

That doesn't mean that the acellular vaccine is pointless. On the contrary, vaccinating babies protects them when they are at their most vulnerable. If their immunity wanes and they get whooping cough as adults, it will be milder than if they hadn't been vaccinated.[46]

The problem is that as those babies become children, they can carry the whooping cough bacterium and infect their younger siblings before their eight-week vaccination.[47] In 2012, an outbreak put hundreds of children in hospital and killed fourteen.[48] A hundred years before, in Bordet's time, that would have been a quiet week for whooping cough, but it's not what we expect in the twenty-first century.

A new strategy was needed, and it was needed fast. Vaccinating at an earlier age wasn't an option, because babies don't reliably respond to the whooping cough vaccine until they reach six weeks.[49] The solution was to give the vaccine before the child was born.

Vaccinating a pregnant woman raises the level of antibodies in her bloodstream, boosting her own immunity to the whooping cough bacterium and ensuring that enough find their way across the placenta to the foetus that the baby is protected until his eight-week vaccination.

This strategy got whooping cough back under control, but

the fact remains that the acellular vaccine is not as effective as the whole-cell vaccine. A few new vaccines have been developed, but at the time of writing, none have made it out of the biotech valley of death. Whooping cough is no longer a priority for the governments and pharmaceutical firms that can afford to develop them.

For now, we need to do the best we can with what we have – and the 1977 and 2012 outbreaks warn us of what to expect if we don't do it diligently.

The top plot on page 102 shows the percentage of children vaccinated against whooping cough by their second birthday. The middle plot shows the number of reported whooping cough cases. The bottom plot shows the number of deaths attributed to whooping cough.

All three plots show data from the beginning of systematic records until 2020. Data on vaccine coverage are from England and Wales until 1978 and from England only after 1978.[50,51] Data on cases and deaths are from England and Wales.[52]

Children vaccinated by their second birthday

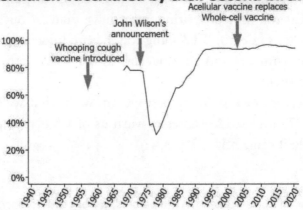

Whooping cough cases

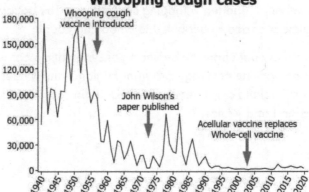

Whooping cough deaths

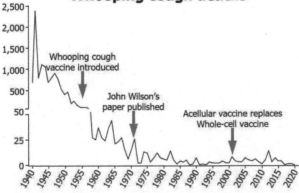

Chapter 7

Haemophilus influenzae type b (Hib)

Helena is a very lucky woman.[1]

At eighteen months old, she developed what both her mother and her GP thought was a cold. This was 2000. The days when a sniffle could herald some deadly disease lay in the past.

Didn't they?

The following day, it no longer looked like a cold. Her father later described Helena as 'floppy and grey-looking'. At the Royal London Hospital, the nurses' expressions tipped off her parents that something was seriously wrong. Paediatric nurses know meningitis when they see it.

Helena was rushed to intensive care because of a bacterium called *Haemophilus influenzae* type b, usually abbreviated to Hib. At that point, her chances of survival were pretty good. A modern hospital like the Royal London saves nineteen out of every twenty children with Hib meningitis.[2] However, there's more to recovery than survival. One in ten survivors is left with a major disability like deafness or cognitive impairment. For children under five years old, like Helena, the risk is closer to one in five.[3]

Not that her parents were calculating the odds. The words her father used were 'total despair'.

Helena's luck held with a lot of help from the intensive care team. She made a full recovery, but her illness evidently triggered some soul-searching in her parents, who hadn't had her vaccinated against Hib. They hadn't even known a vaccine was available, which is why they shared Helena's story with the *Daily Telegraph* to raise awareness of how dangerous Hib is.

The art of being wrong

There's an oft-repeated maxim, usually attributed to physicist Wolfgang Pauli, that very little of science is right and most of it is wrong, but the worst sin a scientist can commit is to be 'not even wrong'. Conclusions drawn from today's evidence are often disproved by tomorrow's, but when there's no roadmap to the truth, not every detour is a blind alley.

The Pauli dictum acknowledges that sometimes, being wrong is an achievement halfway to being right.

Soon after Richard Pfeiffer qualified as a doctor in 1879, a typhoid outbreak gave him a crash course in medical microbiology. He based a thesis on his experiences, which caught the attention of Robert Koch, who recruited him to study cholera at Berlin University.[4] Two years later, Pfeiffer became more interested in a plague of coughing and sneezing that often led to fatal pneumonia. The 'Russian flu' had arrived in Europe.

Pandemic influenza is covered in detail in Chapter 17, but in 1889, doctors had no idea what caused it, even if they had no difficulty in recognising it.

Pfeiffer was among the first to approach influenza with what we'd now recognise as scientific method. Mixed with the green phlegm coughed up by influenza sufferers, he found a bacterium he recognised. A few years earlier, Koch had identified the same bacterium from a case of conjunctivitis.

Pfeiffer's next move was to look for it in the lungs of people who had died of influenza. Sure enough, he found it. In 1893, with the pandemic subsiding, Pfeiffer published his grand conclusion: he'd found the microbe that causes influenza.[5]

He hadn't.

It wasn't until forty years later that influenza was finally proved to be a virus. By then, Pfeiffer's mistake had borne fruit, even if the fruit was of a different variety than he originally believed it to be. Isolating 'Pfeiffer's bacillus', as *Haemophilus influenzae* was originally called, was no easy task, and Pfeiffer had needed to carry out the first systematic study of how to culture a bacterium in a laboratory.[6] In drawing the wrong conclusion, he showed many medical microbiologists how to get to the right one.

He also prompted other scientists to research a bacterium that would prove important in disease, even if it wasn't the disease that Pfeiffer thought it was.

The first breakthrough was made by the young Margaret Pittman, then at New York's Rockefeller Institute, who noticed that Pfeiffer's bacillus was more diverse than Pfeiffer had realised. When she followed Pfeiffer's culture techniques, she found that the colonies it formed might look either rough or smooth under a microscope. The difference, she found, was that the bacteria forming the smooth colonies were coated in a polysaccharide capsule.

The polysaccharides are a broad class of molecules made up of long chains of saccharides that most of us know best as components of sugar; white sugar is made up of two saccharides joined together, one called glucose and one called fructose. A long chain of glucose molecules stuck together makes the polysaccharide called starch.

There's more to polysaccharides than food groups. Pittman's colleagues at the Rockefeller, Alphonse Dochez and Oswald

Avery, had recently found that some bacteria build capsules of polysaccharides around themselves. They were working on the pneumococcus, and we'll come back to them in Chapter 8, but their findings pointed Pittman towards the first of her many seminal discoveries.

She found Pfeiffer's bacillus could have six different capsule types, which she labelled 'a' to 'f', with all the type 'b' capsules isolated from post mortems of people who had died of meningitis.

Pfeiffer had mistakenly thought he'd made a fundamental discovery about influenza. When Pittman found that all her type 'b's came from meningitis patients, she *did* make a discovery that was far more fundamental than she could have realised at a time when *Haemophilus* was regarded as a possible cause of influenza.

When influenza was found to be caused by a virus in 1933, *Haemophilus* ceased to be a priority and Pittman left the Rockefeller to start her six decades at the NIH. Her 1931 paper is still quoted as the seminal work on categorising polysaccharide-encapsulated bacteria, and underpinned later research on the pneumococcal and meningococcal bacteria as well as Hib.

By then, Richard Pfeiffer had semi-retired from a career so illustrious that he'd been honoured by having a genus of bacteria named after him – although, appropriately for a man who had associated his bacterium with the wrong disease, a clerical error gave the name *Pfeifferella* to a bacterium Pfeiffer never worked on.[7,8]

The drama of the throat

We now know that Hib is one of the commonest causes of serious meningitis in young children.[9] The doctors who treated Helena would have been unsurprised to find it was what brought her to them.

Its lethal nature is born of the microbial soap opera that plays out in every child's throat. That throat is an appealing place for a bacterium. It's lined with nutritious carbohydrate-rich mucus supplemented by passing food whenever the child eats. The catch is that there's only so much space in there, and a child's immune system does not roll out the welcome mat.

When *Haemophilus* joins the scramble for space in a throat, it must contend with all the other bacteria drawn to the same place for the same reasons. One of its rivals is *Streptococcus pneumoniae*, the pneumococcus, which tries to kill it with hydrogen peroxide.[10] *Haemophilus* can't win a straight fight with the pneumococcus, but it can direct the attention of a child's immune cells.[11] The cells in question are the phagocytes, which seek out and engulf bacterial interlopers.

That's where those polysaccharide capsules come in handy. They make Hib a lot less conspicuous to the phagocytes than pneumococcus is.

It's as if a brawl between two gangs of football hooligans ends with the weaker running away when the police turn up, leaving their stronger but slower adversaries to get arrested.

The human body may be the home of a thriving bacterial community, but harmonious it is not.

Haemophilus only manages to enjoy the bounty of the child's throat for so long. After a few months, her immune system rumbles it and secretes antibodies into the throat mucus. When that happens, it's all over for *Haemophilus*. The nutritious mucus becomes toxic and clears *Haemophilus* from the child's throat.

If it hasn't found a way into another child's throat by then, *Haemophilus* has reached the end of its line. Not that the child cares one way or the other. She remains healthily and happily oblivious to the drama playing out in her throat – as long as it stays in her throat.

Haemophilus becomes dangerous if it slips out of her throat and into her bloodstream. Most *Haemophilus* types don't last long in the blood because they run afoul of complement, a cluster of proteins that latch on to their polysaccharide capsules and punch holes in them.

Unless it's the Hib-defining capsule that Pittman called type b.

Type b polysaccharide doesn't give complement anything to latch on to, enabling Hib to circulate around the body unmolested. Unfortunately, it often finds its way out of the bloodstream into the meninges, which is where children like Helena least want it.

The meninges are the membranes that enclose the brain and spinal cord and, like many encapsulated bacteria, Hib has a particular affinity for them. Once in the meninges, the immune system's attempts to root it out inflame the meninges and cause them to swell. In the confined space of the skull or the spine, that swelling puts pressure on the brain or the spinal cord.[12]

Hib disease usually affects children, because, without vaccination, Hib itself is very common. It passes through most children's throats before their sixth birthday,[13] and whether it causes disease or not, their immune systems will make sure it doesn't come back.

Polysaccharide vaccines prove their worth

That most children spend a few months bouncing around with Hib in their throats tells us two things.

First, it tells us that Hib meningitis is an abnormality, albeit a particularly nasty abnormality. Hib persists by riding respiratory droplets to another child's throat. Any Hib that gets into the bloodstream or the meninges has no way back out. Meningitis happens when the immune system loses control of bacterial squabbling rather than being inherent to Hib's behaviour.

Secondly, it tells us that a child's immune system can clear Hib out of her throat. Her antibodies act as an intermediary, with one end attaching to Hib's capsule and the other forming an attachment point for complement proteins that otherwise skate past it. We need both complement and Hib-specific antibodies to get rid of Hib,[14] but we're born with complement and even very young children are capable of producing antibodies.

When Hib was identified as a major threat to children, it looked like a relatively simple matter to trigger those antibodies by purifying and injecting the polysaccharide.

The first test of a Hib polysaccharide vaccine was part of a trial of a vaccine against a different bacterium altogether. In 1973, Finland was in the throes of an outbreak of childhood meningitis caused by a different encapsulated bacteria called the meningococcus.* Based at Finland's Central Public Health Laboratory, Helena Mäkelä and her protégé, Heikki Peltola, responded with a clinical trial of a vaccine made from the meningococcus polysaccharide.

They first took an interest in the Hib polysaccharide because they needed an active placebo; something that would replicate the side effects of the meningococcus vaccine without protecting against meningococcus.

A group at the Harvard Medical School had recently developed a Hib polysaccharide vaccine[15] and shown it to safely induce an antibody response.[16] They were still looking for the funding to test it in a large trial, but Mäkelä and Peltola weren't concerned about protection. They simply needed another polysaccharide that they knew was safe.

Their trial proved that the meningococcus vaccine was what Finland needed to counter the meningococcus outbreak,[17] but when it was complete, Mäkelä and Peltola wondered if they might

---

* See Chapter 9.

have also collected useful data on the Hib polysaccharide. They went back to their data and found that the Hib polysaccharide triggered an antibody response so effective that in the two years following vaccination, it slashed the number of children developing Hib disease by a factor of eight.[18]

However, they also found that the polysaccharide vaccine didn't trigger an antibody response in children under eighteen months old.[19] It was a serious limitation, because children under a year old are at the greatest risk.[20]

The problem would prove common to all polysaccharide vaccines: from the moment a child is born, she's perfectly capable of deploying her lymphocytes against proteins, but she won't be very good at deploying them against polysaccharides until she's two years old.

The first two years are when a child encounters most of the bacteria that will be with her for the rest of her life. There's something to be said for not starting a fight with every newcomer, especially if some of them are likely to be the microbial 'old friends'. However, the price of that forbearance is that she can't respond to polysaccharide vaccines.

Something better was needed.

Conjugate vaccines: a gift from the NIH to the world

One of John Robbins's colleagues said he 'never met a polysaccharide he didn't like'.[21] For a man who spent his career showing immune systems how to destroy the polysaccharide capsules of bacteria, 'like' may not have been the operative word, but he was certainly fascinated by them. His focus was legendary – and it wasn't confined to polysaccharides.

Rachel Schneerson, his colleague at the US National

Institutes of Health, once recounted a visit to the State Department when the patterns on a Persian carpet caught his attention. Completely forgetting where he was and why, Robbins followed the patterns down a corridor and into a room lined with gilt and mirrors. With his attention firmly on the carpet, the significance of the mirrors didn't occur to him until a security guard demanded to know what he was doing in the ladies' bathroom.[22]

The Polish-born and Israeli-educated Schneerson was a kindred spirit when it came to polysaccharides, if not Persian carpets. When they started working together in 1969, top of their to-do list was to get a Hib vaccine to work in babies too young to respond to the pure polysaccharide.

If a baby's immune system recognised proteins but not polysaccharides, they reasoned, perhaps it would recognise a polysaccharide combined with a protein. They bound Hib polysaccharide to the diphtheria toxoid protein,[*] and when they tested it in mice, their protein-conjugate molecule triggered antibodies to both its protein and polysaccharide components.[23]

Schneerson and Robbins published their conjugate vaccine without patenting it.

'We had a notion – a wrong notion, maybe – that public money went into making it, so it should be free to the public,' Schneerson said years later, when conjugate vaccines were being used around the world. 'Why wrong? Because immediately someone else did a little modification and applied for a patent.'[24]

She was referring to the alacrity with which several pharmaceutical firms picked up their protein-conjugate technology and ran with it, producing several different Hib vaccines using different carrier molecules. Whatever Schneerson's reservations

---

[*] See Chapter 4.

about commercialisation, conjugate vaccines have proved a spectacularly successful addition to the public health toolbox.

The British trial of the tetanus toxoid carrier

In 1991, the USA became the first country to roll out a Hib conjugate vaccine[25] – but only just. By then, the British medical establishment was dominated by a new generation who had shed their predecessors' suspicion of vaccination. The NHS wanted to include Hib vaccination on the childhood schedule but needed to choose which conjugate vaccine to use.

Their problem was a recent finding that replacing diphtheria toxoid as the carrier protein with tetanus toxoid triggered more antibodies.[26] It looked like the better option, but with antibodies, quality is more important than quantity. Unless the antibodies target the pathogen in the right place, they won't do any damage to it. The tetanus-Hib conjugate *looked* like the better vaccine, but until it proved its mettle in a phase 3 efficacy trial, there was no way to know if it worked at all.

A JCVI sub-committee was tasked with making the choice.[27] Their dilemma was that once they'd chosen a vaccine and rolled it out, it would be unethical to switch it for a placebo to test a vaccine that national policy would mandate as an essential protection against meningitis.[28]

Robert Booy and Richard Moxon of Oxford University came up with the solution: a pilot roll-out in a few regions before the national roll-out. If the vaccine was indeed effective, they would see a lower rate of Hib disease in those regions than in neighbouring regions where the vaccine had not been used. If not, they would need to rethink the choice of the tetanus toxoid-Hib conjugate.

The choice of vaccinated and unvaccinated regions was

not as random as Booy and Moxon might have liked. Some local health authorities were using computer systems so anti-quated that they couldn't add a new vaccine to the records issued to parents,[29] so they could only be the unvaccinated control regions.

In the spring and summer of 1991, the pilot roll-out began in local authorities running northward from West Berkshire through Oxfordshire and Northampton to Kettering. They were compared to neighbouring regions with aged computers, running from East Berkshire through Wycombe and Aylesbury up to Milton Keynes.

The results were convincing. There was only one Hib case in a vaccinated child, and the roll-out regions saw less than a third as many cases as the unvaccinated regions.[30] The paper reporting the study contains a graph showing Hib cases in the early vaccine districts falling off a cliff between 1991 and 1992. The control districts started vaccinating when the nationwide roll-out began in July 1992, presumably having used the time to upgrade their computers, and the same plot shows a similar plummet in cases between 1992 and 1993.

The plot on page 117 shows the same pattern across the whole country. Unfortunately, cases were only recorded systematically for a couple of years before the 1992 roll-out, but the pattern seen in Britain is not unusual. Wherever the conjugate vaccine has been introduced, far fewer children end up in hospital with Hib disease.

While the polysaccharide vaccine protected against menin-gitis by triggering antibodies in the bloodstream, the conjugate extends the immune response to the throat. It not only protects a child from falling ill, but also makes her unable to infect anyone else,[31] something that the polysaccharide vaccine was never able to do.

By 1996, one British paediatrician was able to write, 'many

junior doctors today have not had occasion to treat a child for [Hib] disease'.[32]

It didn't last. The plot on page 000 shows cases starting to rise again in 1999,[33] and in 2000, Helena became one of the victims of Hib's return. There were nowhere near as many cases as there had been before the roll-out, but there were enough to show that something had changed.

The difference lay not in the Hib vaccine itself, but in what had been given alongside it. Initially, Hib had been combined with DTwP containing whole-cell whooping cough vaccine. In 1999, a shortage of the whole-cell vaccine had led to its being temporarily replaced with the acellular vaccine. It turned out that the difference mattered. The Hib vaccine triggered a much stronger immune response when combined with the whole-cell vaccine than with the acellular.[34]

The explanation has never been nailed down, although there's good reason to suspect the same cause as the unpleasant side effects of the whole-cell vaccine. Those side effects are caused by the immune response kicking in a little too enthusiastically, but that same enthusiasm might enhance the immune response to any vaccines given along with it. The acellular vaccine avoided the side effects but at the cost of the 'adjuvant' effect on the Hib vaccine.

Meanwhile, France had also run out of whole-cell vaccine but didn't see Hib come back.[35] The difference lay in the scheduling of the doses. Like most countries, Britain was using three doses given at two, three and four months of age to ensure that a baby is producing her own antibodies by the time she loses protection from maternal antibodies.[36]

So far, so sensible.

The difference was that French children received a fourth dose between their first and second birthdays. The three-dose schedule proved effective in leaving a child with immune memory, but memory alone isn't enough to protect from Hib. A memory response can take a day or two to kick in, but once Hib is in the bloodstream, it invades the meninges within hours. To be protected, a child needs her lymphocytes to be continuously secreting antibodies into her bloodstream. The fourth dose was needed to ensure that continuous secretion.[37]

Britain introduced the fourth dose in 2003, and the resurgence quickly subsided. Hib became a rare disease once again, and remained so even after the whole-cell whooping cough vaccine was completely replaced with the acellular vaccine in 2004.

Hib on the retreat

Twenty-five years after Helena Mäkelä and Heikki Peltola proved the Hib polysaccharide vaccine, Peltola reviewed Hib disease around the world and came to an equivocal conclusion: conjugate vaccines were extremely effective against Hib, but they weren't being used where they were most needed. Hib had always killed more children in countries that could not afford conjugate vaccines than in high-income countries where most children were now protected.[38]

One exception was The Gambia. In return for its hosting a trial showing the Hib conjugate was effective in a low-income setting,[39] the manufacturer Pasteur Mérieux had supplied the country with vaccines that all but eliminated Hib.[40]

The Gambia is exactly the sort of country that badly needed Hib conjugate but lacked the public funds to pay for it. The complex manufacturing processes behind conjugate vaccines do not come cheap.

In 2000, the year that Peltola reported the global vaccine disparity, the Global Alliance for Vaccines and Immunization

(GAVI) was incorporated to funnel money from international donors into vaccination programmes in low-income countries. Hib vaccine was one of GAVI's early priorities, and the WHO recommended that all children should receive three doses of it.[41] It took time to build momentum, but half the countries classed as low-income had introduced the vaccine by 2008 and nearly all by 2010.[42]

Wherever the vaccine has been rolled out, Hib meningitis cases have dropped as precipitously as they did in Northampton and Kettering. In 2000, only 13 per cent of the world's children were receiving three doses of Hib conjugate vaccine. By 2010, it was 40 per cent.[43] At the same time, estimated deaths from Hib nearly halved, from 363,000 in 2000 to 199,000 in 2008. With global vaccine coverage reaching 72 per cent in 2019, there's every reason to expect the next estimate will find it much lower.

However, Hib is so infectious that near-universal global vaccination will be needed to eliminate it. We won't see that any time soon, but that's no reason for any child to face the same odds that faced Helena when she was rushed to the Royal London Hospital.

Hib has the distinction of being the bacterium that introduced conjugate vaccines to the world, which matters because Hib is not the only bacterium that hides behind a polysaccharide capsule. Pneumococcus and meningococcus both use the same trick, and Robbins and Schneerson gave us the tool we need to deal with them.

Hib vaccine coverage

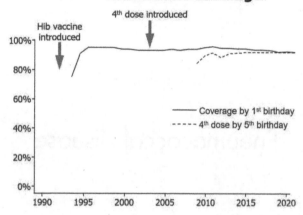

Laboratory confirmed Hib cases

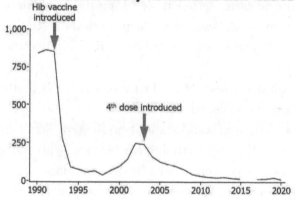

The top plot shows the percentage of children vaccinated against Hib by their first birthday from the 1992 roll-out to 2020. The bottom plot shows the number of laboratory confirmed cases of Hib from the beginning of systematic records in 1993 until 2020.

Vaccine coverage data is from England.[44,45] Laboratory reports are from England and Wales for 2014[46] and 2015,[47] but from England only in all other years.[48,49,50]

Chapter 8

Pneumococcal disease

Jacques Hervieux was sick of watching mothers die. Again and again, women came into Paris's Hôpital Lariboisière to give birth, only to waste away with a mysterious fever. In an 1879 presentation to the Académie de Médecine, his frustration boiled to the surface.

'I have a terrible fear which I cannot shake ... that I will die before this vibrio is found,' he said.

One man listening could stand it no longer. 'What causes the epidemic is ... the physician and his helpers, who transport the microbe from a sick woman to a healthy woman.'

Louis Pasteur's interruption was probably met with a groan. The venerable academicians were heartily sick of Pasteur pontificating about how their poor hygiene killed their patients based on nothing but his upstart theories of microbiological disease.

Pasteur strode to the blackboard and sketched a chain of bacterial cells that he'd isolated from many victims of childbed fever. 'This is what it looks like.'[1]

It was the first public description of the bacterium that would become known as the pneumococcus, a name it would acquire in 1886 when Albert Fränkel at the University of Berlin identified it as a frequent cause of pneumonia, from the Greek *pneumon* for lung and *coccus* for 'berry', in reference to the bacterium's spherical structure.[2] Most scientists still call it the pneumococcus, although its full name is now *Streptococcus pneumoniae*.

Hervieux hadn't expected his gloomy prediction of dying in ignorance to be disproved so quickly, but faced with Pasteur's sketch, he proved himself more open-minded than many of his colleagues. He accepted Pasteur's argument and introduced improvements to hygiene that saved more lives than anyone ever counted.

At the time, improving hygiene was all Hervieux could do about the pneumococcus. The first attempt at a vaccine came two decades later, and is one of the more ignoble chapters in the story of vaccination. Its object was not to prevent disease for its own sake but to facilitate the mistreatment of migrant workers.

Almroth Wright and South African gold

In 1886, the same year that Fränkel named the pneumococcus, another discovery was made that would become inextricably linked with the development of pneumococcus vaccines: the world's largest gold deposit was discovered under the Witwatersrand scarp, known as the 'Rand' to the generations of men it has made or destroyed.

When its gold was discovered, it was in the Transvaal Republic, a country built by Afrikaner farmers' faith in what one historian described as 'God and the Martini-Henry',[3] the rifle they had used to take the land from the Zulu, and to discourage the British Empire from taking it from them.

Discouraging as a well-aimed Martini-Henry could be, it would take more than bullets to put British mining magnates off the Rand's gold. They certainly weren't put off by the tens of thousands of deaths in the Anglo-Boer War that saw the British Empire gulp down the Transvaal.

The one thing they balked at was offering decent pay and working conditions to their miners. People who lived close to the mines quickly learned not to work in them, so the magnates recruited labour from Portuguese East Africa.* They were neither the first nor the last to recognise that the further a labourer is from home, the harder it is for him to object to being mistreated.

Gold miners were so plagued by disease that as many as one in ten never returned home. Chief among their diseases were pneumococcal infections of the lungs, meninges and the membrane surrounding the heart: today's terminology, pneumonia, meningitis and pericarditis.[4]

When the Union of South Africa attained limited self-government in 1910, that government started to pay attention to what was going on under the Rand.

The magnates argued that 'tropical natives', meaning recruits from north of the Union's border, were inherently more susceptible to disease because they were 'a different class of boy to the East Coast boys south of latitude 22'.[5] This was eugenics – then very much in vogue – deployed in service of the bottom line: according to the magnates, migrant labourers fell ill because they were predisposed to fall ill and not because they were poorly fed, quartered in crowded hostels without sanitation, and, at the end of a long working day of breathing silica dust, were soaking wet and denied so much as a change of clothes.[6]

The Minister of Native Affairs didn't buy it. He pushed for something to be done until the chairman of the Transvaal Chamber of Mines promised to vaccinate all miners against pneumococcus. There was one obstacle to keeping his promise: no such vaccine existed.

---

* Now Mozambique.

The magnates needed someone who could invent a vaccine in a hurry, so they turned to the inventor of the typhoid vaccine, Sir Almroth Wright.

By 1911, Wright had left the Army Medical College to head St Mary's Hospital's pathology department. Being as committed a controversialist as ever, he was better known publicly for polemics against women's suffrage that had led to clashes with the playwright George Bernard Shaw and the *enfant terrible* of Edwardian politics, Winston Churchill.[7]

Wright approached pneumococcus in the same way he'd approached typhoid: by isolating the bacterium, killing it and injecting it. He tested his killed-bacteria vaccine by randomising miners into vaccinated and unvaccinated groups, which, at a time when new medications were rarely tested at all, was an unusually rigorous approach.

His ethics remained distinctly Edwardian. Wright described how 'the natives were lined up' and alternate men were vaccinated. He didn't record adverse events, but killed-bacteria vaccines usually cause swellings and fevers. It's safe to assume that Wright's experimental vaccine made the miners' lives even more miserable for a few days.

Nevertheless, his vaccine did have some success. Vaccinated miners were less likely to develop pneumonia, at least in the first few months after starting work. Because pneumonia was most common among new miners, Wright thought it 'more probable that the progressively increasing resistance in both the inoculated and uninoculated groups is achieved by processes of self-immunisation consequent upon minor infections which affect practically the whole mass of the population'.[8]

Wright's self-immunisation hypothesis would prove to be remarkably astute given how little was known at the time.

He left South Africa in 1912, pausing in Cape Town to give a lecture in which he delivered the far less astute conclusion that 'one can hardly suggest a disease which is not bacteriological' and returned to London to resume his clashes with anyone who cared to clash with him.

Wright came down on the right side of history in some matters and the wrong side in others, but whichever side he chose, he was never less than decisive about it. No wonder his colleagues nicknamed him Sir Almost Right or, if they were feeling less charitable, Sir Always Wrong.[9]

A multitude of serotypes

Wright handed over his vaccine work to his assistant, the British-born footballer-turned-doctor Spencer Lister (no relation to his more famous contemporary, Joseph Lister). Lister soon made a key discovery: the blood from a pneumonia patient was usually lethal to pneumococcus isolated from that patient, but only occasionally to the pneumococcus from other patients.[10] The human immune system was seeing differences between pneumococci that appeared identical under Lister's microscope.

At the same time, Alphonse Dochez at New York's Rockefeller Institute was finding the same thing. When he inoculated mice with killed pneumococcus isolated from a human patient, the inoculated mouse would be protected against that same pneumococcus, but only sometimes against a pneumococcus isolated from a different patient.

Dochez noticed something that Lister missed. There was a distinct pattern to whether inoculating with one pneumococcus could protect against another. The immune systems of his mice were recognising four distinct types of pneumococcus. A mouse inoculated with a pneumococcus was protected against all pneumococci of that type but not from any of the others.[11]

To the immune system, the pneumococcus is not one bacterium but many.

Dochez had invented the concept of the serotype: a way of classifying microbes based on the antibodies produced against them. The previous chapter described how his colleague, Margaret Pittman, applied his technique to type *Haemophilus influenzae*. Dochez had opened a window into how diverse the bacteria bundled together and called pneumococcus actually are.

To Lister, the discovery of serotypes explained the shortcomings of his killed-bacteria vaccine. If the vaccine didn't work, it must be because the serotype in the vaccine was different to the serotype it failed to protect against. What he couldn't know was how many different serotypes he was up against. Nearly a century later, ninety-seven pneumococcus serotypes[12] have been discovered, and we're still not sure that's all of them.

Lister persevered, but he fell into conflict with one Alexander Orenstein, who came up with a radical solution to the Rand's pneumococcus problem: treat the miners like human beings.

Orenstein faced an uphill struggle, but after the government banned recruitment of 'tropical natives' in 1913, the magnates had no choice but to implement his suggested improvements to living and working conditions. Lister never did come up with a vaccine that worked consistently, and Orenstein's grudgingly implemented reforms saved a lot more miners' lives.

It would be unfair to define Lister's legacy purely in terms of his failures with the pneumococcal vaccine. He was a pioneer of medical research in South Africa and played major roles in establishing the South African Institute of Medical Research and the University of the Witwatersrand, both of which are among the world's leading research institutes today.

Oswald Avery's brooding forehead

Much of what we now know about the pneumococcus is thanks to Oswald Avery. When he started work at the Rockefeller, Avery shared an apartment with Dochez, and between working together in the laboratory during the day and long conversations late into the night, Avery and Dochez applied their shared knowledge of chemistry to take the pneumococcus to pieces.[13]

They found that like *Haemophilus influenzae*, the bacterial cell was encased in a polysaccharide capsule[14] that hides its proteins from the immune system. We now recognise pneumococcus as one of several encapsulated bacteria that follow essentially the same life cycle as *Haemophilus*, bouncing from one person's throat to another and hanging on until the immune system notices them.

Avery found the polysaccharide capsule was the target of the antibodies Dochez had been working with,[15] meaning that serotypes are in fact different types of capsule. Soon after, Dochez moved on to Johns Hopkins Medical School, leaving Avery to continue beavering away at pneumococcus without one of the few close friends he'd ever had.

Avery was a congenial colleague whose eloquence earned him the nickname of 'the Professor', or simply 'Fess', long before he ascended to the formal title. However, those closest to him knew a more complex and perhaps more troubled man. One colleague described 'a brooding forehead that appeared too heavy for the frail body, a gaze focused inwardly as if unconcerned with the surrounding world, a melancholy figure whistling gently to himself the lonely tune of the shepherd song in *Tristan and Isolde*'. For all his bonhomie, Avery would cheerfully turn down any social invitation due to what the same colleague ascribed to 'an acute need for privacy, even if it had to be bought at the cost of loneliness'.[16]

At work, Avery found that not only were there many different types of pneumococcus capsule but some forms had no capsule at all. If that seemed weird, it was about to get a lot weirder.

In 1928, Frederick Griffith at the British Ministry of Health found that only encapsulated pneumococci caused disease in mice.[17] So far, so logical. If the capsule helps a bacterium hide from the immune system, it followed that the immune system could clobber an unencapsulated bacterium before it did any damage.

Then Griffith found that the different types were not as distinct from each other as he'd thought. Sometimes, pneumococci lost their capsules while he was culturing them. That made a certain amount of sense; they didn't have to contend with an immune system while they were being pampered on a laboratory culture plate. All the capsule was doing was soaking up nutrients that could be used for dividing into more bacterial cells.

When Griffith ripped those pneumococci out of their comfortable laboratory life and injected them into mice, they quickly adapted to an irate immune system by producing their capsules again. There was no inherent difference between encapsulated and unencapsulated types. Griffith's pneumococcus was producing its capsule – or not – depending on its circumstances.

Then Griffith took pneumococci that had stopped producing capsules in culture and mixed them with killed encapsulated pneumococci. The living pneumococci started growing capsules again – but not the ones they had grown before they got used to laboratory life. Instead, their new capsules were of the type of the killed pneumococci. They had adopted a characteristic of the killed pneumococci that they had never possessed themselves.

Griffith tried the same experiment in live mice, injecting them with live pneumococci that had lost their capsules and killed pneumococci with capsules of another type. Once again, the live pneumococci adopted capsules of the killed type.

Reading Griffith's paper, one can almost see him sitting at his typewriter with his head in his hands, periodically hammering out a few paragraphs of a possible explanation before adding a few more about why the explanation doesn't add up. At one point, he suggests the existence of an 'S substance' carrying the capsule blueprints from one bacterium to another. It was a fleeting glimpse of a truth that would make others famous, but Griffith didn't linger on it.

Avery became obsessed with it. Undeterred by his official retirement or an autoimmune condition called Graves's disease,[18] he spent fifteen years breaking pneumococci into their constituent chemicals in search of what he called the 'transforming chemical'. It led him to perhaps the most fundamental discovery in biology.

He wrote: 'The evidence presented supports the belief that a nucleic acid of the desoxyribose type is the fundamental unit of the transforming principle of Pneumococcus.'[19]

Almost hidden in Avery's modest prose is the discovery of the substance carrying the information that makes the pneumococcus a pneumococcus – and that also, we now know, makes everything from a bacterium to a blade of grass to a blue whale what it is. Avery's 'nucleic acid of the desoxyribose type' is what we call DNA.

Today, DNA is indelibly associated with the fractious team of James Watson, Francis Crick, Rosalind Franklin and Maurice Wilkins, who established its structure. It takes nothing from their groundbreaking work to say that without Avery, they wouldn't have known what to work on.

Pneumococcal fratricide in a child's throat

Dochez and Avery discovered bacterial capsules, serotypes and DNA, three discoveries that are fundamental to what we know about bacteria, infectious disease and life in general, but they only began to unravel the complexities of the pneumococcus.

We now know that the pneumococcus behaves in a very similar way to *Haemophilus* in that its comfort zone is a child's throat, it passes from one child to another through respiratory droplets, and its capsule buys it time before the immune system wakes up to what's going on.

The immune system isn't its only problem. It needs to fight for the coveted real estate of the throat lining, and it is armed for this fight with hydrogen peroxide,[20] a chemical we use in disinfectants for the same reason: it kills bacteria. Except, that is, for pneumococci, which can secrete it with impunity because they themselves are resistant to it.

Different pneumococcal strains are as ready to fight each other as any other species. They've even developed chemicals called pneumocins to kill each other.[21] They don't stop at killing; when two types fight to the death, the winning side sometimes scoops up DNA fragments from the losers and incorporates them into his own. That's the trick that left Griffith perplexed and pointed Avery towards DNA.

It's also a trick that makes the pneumococcus a very slippery customer. The victor of a pneumococcal dust-up can end up with a capsule different to either of the types that started the fight.

As long as the bacteria are fighting each other, they don't do the child any harm. The problem comes when they find their way out of his throat to somewhere they're not supposed to be.

My mother always used to tell me that if I didn't wear a coat, I'd catch my death of pneumonia. I went through my childhood thinking that pneumonia was a particularly nasty sort of cold that lurked in wait for insufficiently wrapped children, and although my mother was no medical microbiologist, she wasn't far wrong. A common cause of pneumonia is a cold virus damaging the lungs and letting in the pneumococcus.[22]

Pneumonia is bad news, but it's not the worst thing the pneumococcus can do. Like *Haemophilus*, it occasionally finds its way into the bloodstream, where it can cause potentially fatal sepsis. That's bad, but not as bad as if it gets into the pericardium lining the heart or the meninges lining the brain and spinal cord.

The most likely victim of a pneumococcus is a young child, simply because the longer a child lives, the more types pass through his throat and leave him immune to a repeat visit. At two or three years old, children are constantly carrying one strain or another,[23] usually without suffering any ill effects. As they build a repertoire of antibodies to the most common strains, they become less likely to carry them, but the repertoire is never complete. Even as adults, one in ten of us is carrying a pneumococcus at any given time.[24]

That explains Almroth Wright's self-immunisation hypothesis. Mineworkers arriving from Portuguese East Africa would have encountered types they had never encountered before, and they were encountering them under the worst possible circumstances. Their lungs were damaged by silica dust and they were weakened by the appalling conditions. No wonder a lot of them developed some form of pneumococcal disease.

If they survived the first few months, they would have built up a repertoire of antibodies to those new types and were unlikely to be troubled by them.

Sir Almroth had, true to form, been almost right.

In less arduous conditions, the pneumococcus is rarely a danger to adults below the age of sixty-five, but in later years, we start to lose our hard-won immunity to it. People whose immune systems have kept pneumococcus out of their throats for decades start carrying it again, and if they're unlucky, the pneumococcus finds its way into their lungs. Pneumococcal pneumonia in the elderly was once so common that one Victorian textbook described it as 'the natural end of the old man',[25] and it remains a major concern in elderly care.

The first polysaccharide vaccines

When Dochez and Avery discovered that antibodies bind pneumococcus's polysaccharide capsule, they paved the way for capsule polysaccharides to be used as vaccines. The first pure polysaccharide vaccines were produced on much the same ad hoc lines as Lister's killed-bacteria vaccines. Doctors and scientists facing an outbreak would isolate a pneumococcus from one of its victims, culture it and use it as a source of polysaccharide to purify and inject. Those early vaccines were rarely compared to an unvaccinated control group,[26] leaving it unclear whether they did any good.

The US Army approached the problem more systematically. Military recruits often had the same problems with pneumococcus as migrant gold miners, and for much the same reason. Young men drawn from different parts of the country brought different types with them and shared them in the close confines of a barrack room, exposing many to new types.

In 1945, army scientists found that a four-type vaccine protected against two thirds of the pneumococcal disease circulating in an Army Air Force technical school.[27] It didn't completely solve their pneumococcus problem but it showed they were on to something.

By 1946, vaccines against six different pneumococcus types were rolled out for children and adults in the USA. It looked like the dawn of pneumococcal vaccination had arrived, but then what appeared to be an even brighter dawn outshone it: antibiotics. Almost overnight, pneumococcal infections were transformed from a potentially lethal disease into something that could be treated in a few days.

The new vaccines were withdrawn. It would prove a costly mistake.

Robert Austrian's dangerous lady

There is a hypothetical medicine called the magic bullet. It cures the disease it's aimed at within hours of being administered, it works every time and it has no side effects. It is a medicine with only one drawback: it doesn't exist.

For a short time in the 1950s, it looked like antibiotics might be the fabled magic bullet, but it's an unwise doctor who believes in fables, and no one ever accused Robert Austrian of lacking wisdom. He's often described as the nemesis of the pneumococcus, having once said, 'I've had a wonderful affair with the pneumococcus which I tend to anthropomorphize as a dangerous lady with whom I hope my relationship will continue.'[28]

Many medical researchers will recognise the sentiment. When you devote your career to studying a pathogen with the ultimate intention of exterminating it, you develop a somewhat ambiguous relationship with it.

When Austrian joined Philadelphia's University of Pennsylvania in 1962, he was painfully aware of the limitations of antibiotics against pneumococcal disease in general and pneumococcal meningitis in young children in particular. Even today, nearly a third of pneumococcal meningitis cases are fatal despite everything that modern medicine can throw at them.[29]

Austrian dragged pneumococcal polysaccharide vaccines off the shelf where they were languishing, dusted them off and spent much of his career persuading the world to use them. The 1960s and 1970s have even been called 'the Austrian era'[30] of pneumococcal vaccination in recognition of his dogged determination.

Austrian's problem was twofold. He needed to know which

pneumococcal types to put into a vaccine, and he needed someone to pay for a large enough trial to show whether they worked.

The first part of the problem was solved when the National Institute for Allergy and Infectious Diseases (NIAID) got on board. In 1967, NIAID started cataloguing which types were sending people to hospital.[31] Austrian and his team made a vaccine from the polysaccharides of those types, and he persuaded the pharmaceutical firm Eli Lilly to solve his second problem by opening their very deep pockets.

To test his vaccine, Austrian followed in Wright's footsteps. He took pneumococcal vaccines back to the Rand.

In the sixty years between Wright's arrival and Austrian's, South Africa had changed beyond recognition, introducing Apartheid in 1948 and cutting its last ties with Britain in 1961 to become a fully independent republic.

One thing hadn't changed: the Rand's gold miners were still plagued by pneumococcal disease. One man in five caught pneumonia in their first year working the mines.[32]

Working conditions were better than in Wright's time, but by the early 1970s, the mines again depended on migrant labour that was mostly recruited from Portuguese East Africa and Malawi, the only southern African countries to retain diplomatic relations with South Africa.

Austrian's polysaccharide vaccine trials produced some encouraging results, but before he had enough data to definitively show whether they worked, his permission to work in the gold mines was revoked. The new generation of magnates had never been enthusiastic about hosting clinical trials, even if they might dramatically improve the health of their workforce, and now they decided they weren't worth the potential distraction.

At the same time, Austrian lost Eli Lilly's backing.[33] Even if he could have found somewhere else to test his vaccines, he didn't have the funding.

Austrian did what any Philadelphia-based scientist with an orphaned vaccine would do: he took it to Maurice Hilleman.

Hilleman was the head of vaccine development at Merck and a legend in the field of vaccinology. While most medical researchers would regard developing a vaccine as the crowning achievement of their career, Hilleman is credited with about forty.[34] For Austrian, it was almost as important that Hilleman's department was only a few miles from his laboratory.

Hilleman persuaded Merck to back Austrian's vaccine and managed to get the magnates to rethink their objections to having it tested on the Rand. By 1977,[35] Merck had a fourteen-type version of Austrian's vaccine ready to go.

In 1983, it was superseded by PPV23, the polysaccharide vaccine used around the world today.[36] The PPV stands for pneumococcal polysaccharide vaccine, and the twenty-three refers to the twenty-three types it contains.

Austrian had resurrected the polysaccharide vaccine – and, it turned out, not a moment too soon.

Vaccines against antibiotic resistance

In 1967, while Austrian was trying to drum up support for the idea that antibiotics alone could not tackle the pneumococcus, a penicillin-resistant pneumococcus turned up in Papua New Guinea.[37] It was the first of many.

Pneumococcus's antibiotic resistance arises from rare mutations, and before antibiotics became widely used, they stayed rare. Unless a pneumococcus encounters an antibiotic, maintaining resistance to it only takes resources away from fighting off competitors and dividing to make more bacteria.

That changed when antibiotics became the treatment of choice against bacterial diseases. Throwing antibiotics into the battle for space in a throat is rather like the backstory to a post-apocalyptic film; whoever is left alive gets to claim the living space. When the living space is someone's throat, whoever is left alive is whoever is resistant to antibiotics. It doesn't matter whether it was the pneumococcus or something else that was making the child ill in the first place. For an antibiotic-resistant pneumococcus, what matters is that antibiotics clear out the competition.

Once there's one antibiotic-resistant pneumococcus in circulation, there will soon be many. If a susceptible strain wipes out a resistant strain and helps itself to its DNA, that DNA may make the susceptible strain resistant before it ever encounters an antibiotic.[38]

The best way to avoid the spread of antibiotic resistance is to minimise antibiotic use, which is easier said than done. No doctor is going to withhold antibiotics from a patient because of the less immediate threat of antibiotic resistance. Nor should she. The whole point of stemming the spread of resistance is so that antibiotics work when someone needs them. Withholding them from someone who needs them would defeat the object of stemming resistance.

Polysaccharide vaccines offered a solution: someone immune to pneumococcus won't get infected and need antibiotics. However, it was only a partial solution, because the most vulnerable age for pneumococcal disease is between six months and one year, which is too young to respond to a pure polysaccharide vaccine.

John Robbins and Rachel Schneerson's work on Hib pointed the way forward: conjugating capsule polysaccharides to carrier proteins. During the 1990s, several different pharmaceutical firms tested pneumococcal conjugate vaccines,[39] but given the complex interactions of pneumococci with other bacteria, the human body and each other, simply throwing a vaccine into the mix was never going to lead to straightforward results.

Pneumococcal vaccination in Britain

The British experience epitomises the struggles of even a well-resourced healthcare system to contain childhood pneumococcal disease.

Britain was a relatively late adopter of the polysaccharide vaccine. In 2003, it was rolled out for everyone over sixty-five and quickly dropped the number of pneumococcal cases. It was soon apparent that while it was effective in protecting people in their late sixties, its effects diminished with age. In people over eighty, it didn't do much at all.[40]

Children had to depend on antibiotics until a seven-type conjugate vaccine was introduced in 2006. Serious pneumococcal disease in children under two dropped from over 1,500 cases every year[41] to under 500 by 2008.[42] In 2010, the seven-type vaccine was replaced with the current thirteen-type vaccine, Pfizer's Prevenar-13,[43] which dropped the annual number of cases to below 300.[44]

So far, so predictable.

Then strange things started happening. The first oddity was when pneumococcal cases in older people dropped in a way they had stubbornly refused to do when the older people themselves were vaccinated.[45] The likely reason is that the pneumococci were surviving by bouncing between the throats of children who weren't yet immune to them, only occasionally breaking out to infect older people. Vaccinating children denied pneumococci anywhere to circulate and protected their grandparents.

Another complication was that by taking some strains out of circulation, vaccination clears the way for others. 'Strain replacement'[46] is not altogether a bad thing. The types chosen for the vaccine are the ones that are most likely to make us ill, so the strains that replace them are more likely to behave themselves when they're in our throats. Vaccinating children dramatically dropped the overall number of pneumococcal disease cases, but among the few cases that did end up in hospital, the types not covered by the vaccine became a little less rare.[47]

Unfortunately, not every complication was as benign.

In the USA, the roll-out of the seven-type conjugate was closely followed by the appearance of an entirely new type. Type 19A combined three different traits that made it an ugly customer: it was adept at crossing the throat lining into the bloodstream, its capsule was not recognised by the immune memory triggered by the available vaccines, and it was often resistant to at least some types of antibiotic.[48]

The immediate problem of type 19A was solved by including it in the thirteen-type vaccine, but its unexpected appearance warns us that the pneumococcus is a moving target. Because of pneumococcus's trick of exchanging DNA, we have to assume that new types arise fairly often. Pneumococcal vaccines contain no DNA, so they cannot create a new type, but if one arises naturally, vaccination can make children immune to some of its competitors and give it space to thrive.

Type 19A was the first new pneumococcal strain to take advantage of the vaccination programme but it won't be the last.

Finding the right dose

We might ask why we can't include all ninety-seven types in a vaccine. If every throat is protected by antibodies against every type, then no type can cause disease.

The problem is that the immune system needs a certain amount of polysaccharide from each type to trigger a response, but there's only so many different polysaccharides it can cope with at once. Even the minimum amount of too many types will overwhelm it so it won't respond to all of them.[49] That's why today's polysaccharide vaccines are limited to the twenty-three most dangerous types.

There's an even bigger problem with conjugate vaccines, which trigger a response not only to the polysaccharide but also to the protein it's conjugated to. When there's a high level of antibodies to the protein, the immune system takes it out of circulation without reacting to the polysaccharide.

The original dose regime for conjugate vaccines was for three doses given in the first six months of a child's life, which was very effective at protecting children through their vulnerable first year. A booster shot was then given between the first and second birthday, which extended the protection through childhood.

The problem is that it's also four doses of the same carrier protein. In Prevenar-13, and many other formulations used around the world, the carrier is a non-toxic derivative of the diphtheria toxin,[50] which is recognised by the antibodies triggered by the diphtheria toxoid vaccine.

We now know that three doses in six months was overdoing it. The first indication of that came by accident, due to a shortage of vaccines in the USA. Children who missed doses proved no more vulnerable to pneumococcal disease than those who got all doses on schedule.[51] The finding was explored more systematically in a trial led by Marilla Lucero at the Research Institute for Tropical Medicine in the Philippines, who found that one dose was as good as three.[52]

Lucero's trial only followed children until they were nine months old, which covered much of the most vulnerable period, but it left the question of whether those children stayed protected as they got older. The issue was picked up by David Goldblatt at London's Institute for Child Health, who led a series of trials showing that one dose in the first six months is as protective as three, as long as it's boosted when the child is one year old.[53]

By showing that the number of doses could be cut, Lucero and

Goldblatt may have opened the door to adding more types to the conjugate vaccine. That matters because if pneumococcus is a moving target, vaccines will need to move with it.

Wright tested his first pneumococcal vaccine in 1911, the year the *Titanic* was launched. I write this at a time when robots are exploring the surface of Mars, but we are still far from having seen the last word in pneumococcal vaccines.

Global vaccination against a global disease

Most of the detailed research on the pneumococcus has been from high-income countries, but it kills a lot more children where there are no hospitals capable of treating meningitis.[54] Moreover, conjugate vaccines used in The Gambia[55] and South Africa[56] have proved less effective than they are in the USA and Europe.

One reason is that the types chosen for the vaccine are based on which types cause most pneumococcal disease in the USA, which are very similar to the types that cause most disease in Europe but miss some of the types most important in Africa and South Asia.[57] Another problem is simply that conjugate vaccines are too expensive for many low-income countries.

Despite those difficulties, the last decade has seen pneumococcal vaccines being used more and more widely, saving the lives of around a quarter of a million children between 2000 and 2015.[58] By 2019, the WHO estimated that nearly half the world's one-year-olds had received at least one dose of a pneumococcal conjugate vaccine.[59] There's still a lot of catching up to do, but pneumococcal conjugates are finding their way to more and more of the children who need them.

One place where pneumococcal pneumonia remains rife is in the gold mines of the Rand, where many workers still live without running water or flush toilets.[60] Such living conditions combine with widespread HIV and silica dust to make South African mines a hotbed of tuberculosis, which has largely overshadowed the common but more treatable pneumococcal pneumonia.[61] Nevertheless, the problem that drew Almroth Wright to South Africa more than a hundred years ago has never been solved, and in describing the conditions of the men who feed the world's hunger for gold, one 2013 report said they create a 'perfect storm' for an unmitigated public health disaster.[62]

Chapter 9

Meningococcal disease

Clair Michna was having the time of her life. She was loving school, preparing for her GCSEs and planning to study law at university. She couldn't know that she was having her last experience of good health.

When a headache put her in bed, she thought it was a cold. The following day, when her mother opened her bedroom door, Clair complained that light was painful. It worried her mother enough to call a doctor for a home visit. By the time he arrived, Clair was seeing double, and when he lifted her head, she screamed in pain. The doctor recognised the symptoms of meningitis and sent her straight to hospital.[1]

Her meningitis was caused by the group B meningococcus bacterium, which, once it gets into the meninges, can divide so fast that it doubles the number of bacterial cells in less than an hour. Clair's lymphocytes and phagocytes were charging after it, inflaming her meninges to the extent that she was barely conscious by the time the ambulance got her to the hospital.

She was diagnosed with not only meningitis but also septicaemia, meaning that her immune system was battling the bacteria throughout her bloodstream and inflaming the lining of the blood vessels.[2]

Her memory of the next few days is dominated by screaming pain whenever someone opened the door to her hospital room. Even through two pairs of sunglasses, she couldn't stand the slightest exposure to light[3] as the intensive care team pumped her full of antibiotics and hoped for the best.

Living with the meningococcus

Like Hib and pneumococcus, the meningococcus passes from throat to throat in respiratory droplets and uses a polysaccharide capsule to hide from the immune system.

We've all had meningococci in our throats for a few weeks at a time, but most of us never notice.[4] It can colonise us at any age, but there are two periods when it's particularly likely. The first is in early childhood, between birth and five years old. The second is in young adulthood, from the mid-teens to the early twenties.[5]

At fifteen, Clair had just entered that second period of high vulnerability. The pain and aversion to light were bad enough, but if her memories of her week in hospital were any clearer, she might remember an aching cold in her hands and feet. It's a common symptom of meningococcal septicaemia, caused by blood leaking from inflamed blood vessels.

Without enough blood to feed the whole body, the circulatory system prioritises the vital organs, like the heart, brain and liver, at the expense of the limbs. Sometimes the internal blood loss is so severe that the tissue in the limbs withers away and dies. Many people with meningococcal septicaemia lose fingers or toes, and an unfortunate few lose whole limbs.[6]

With modern medical treatment, 85–90 per cent of people with severe meningococcal disease survive,[7] but years later, when Clair related her story for the charity Meningitis Now, she would reflect that survival does not mean full recovery. 'When I was finally released, I bounded to school and was hit with a very different reality. My memory had been wiped.'[8]

She struggled to understand things she'd always found straightforward. 'I recall losing consciousness during one of my GCSE exams. I woke up to blood all over my exam paper, and my teacher apologising to me, saying I had no choice but to carry on. It seemed like I was just in this constant haze of struggle, and no one could reach me.'

Now in her early forties, Clair still struggles to concentrate. 'I often start something on the hob and then forget about it until I can smell burning. [I've] even done this whilst sat right next to the cooker! My partner walked in that day and asked me why there was a fire behind me. My memory just erases.'[9]

The Salisbury outbreak

Anton Weichselbaum at the University of Vienna named the meningococcus in 1887, when he isolated it from an unfortunate who had died of meningitis.[10] His description came when new bacterial diseases were being discovered thick and fast, and with tuberculosis, cholera and typhoid still commonplace in Europe, vaccine pioneers like Koch and Pasteur didn't prioritise meningococcus.

The first scientist to take on meningococcal disease was Mervyn Gordon, who made his name by investigating an influenza outbreak in the House of Commons.

In 1905, influenza was thought to be a bacterial disease, but how it spread was still a mystery. Gordon wondered if the solution to that mystery might lie in some of the honourable members' complaints that the air 'lacked freshness'.[11]

He placed agar plates around the empty chamber of the House of Commons, filled his mouth with a bacterium he'd cultured in his laboratory and spent an hour declaiming from *Julius Caesar* and *Henry V*. Sure enough, his bacterium appeared on the agar plates. It was the first demonstration of how a bacterium can be transmitted through the air.

Gordon's experiment established him as an authority on the bacteria of the mouth and throat. A decade later, he was the man the army turned to when meningitis broke out among recruits training on Salisbury Plain. As the days shortened into the first winter of the war that was supposed to end all wars, Gordon was propelled into the Royal Army Medical Corps with the rank of lieutenant-colonel and a brief to do something about it.

With the outbreak spreading into the civilian population of Salisbury itself, Gordon quickly identified meningococcus as the bacterium behind the outbreak. While Spencer Lister was wrestling with the many types of pneumococcus in South Africa, Gordon was much quicker than Lister to recognise that he was dealing with several different serotypes,[12] or groups as they are usually called with the meningococcus.

Gordon and his colleagues applied Wright and Haffkine's isolate, inactivate, inject approach to make a vaccine containing meningococci from four different groups. In February 1915, they rolled out the first vaccine underpinned by a grasp of the different serotypes of a single bacterium. Salisbury's hospitals immediately saw a drop in the number of meningitis patients and by the beginning of the summer, the outbreak was over.[13]

With no unvaccinated control group, it was hardly a robust trial, and we can't be sure it was Gordon's vaccine that ended the outbreak. Like all droplet-borne microbes, meningococcal infections are more common in the winter, so the outbreak may have been coming to a natural end.

The six faces of meningococcal disease

If Gordon was much quicker than Lister to recognise that he was dealing with different types, it was because the meningococcus is not as bewilderingly diverse as the pneumococcus. Meningococcus has thirteen groups, of which only six frequently cause disease. When Gordon identified four types, there was a good chance that he'd discovered the one causing the Salisbury outbreak. His job was much easier than Lister's, which involved dealing with over ninety different types.

The dangerous meningococci are clustered at either end of the alphabet as groups A, B, C, W, X and Y, classified in the same way as the pneumococcus: by the antibodies that bind the capsule polysaccharide.

For decades after the groups were named in the early 1950s,[14] it was assumed that the groups were distinct from each other. That a meningococcus B, for example, was descended from a long line of meningococcus B ancestors and would give rise to a long line of meningococcus B descendants.

The assumption lasted until researchers could look beyond the capsule to the DNA that coded for it. In 1993, a team led by John Swartley of Atlanta's Emory University found that in the West Coast states of the USA, a worrying number of people were being hospitalised by the ET-5 strain, which had a group B capsule.[15]

The following year, patients started arriving in hospitals infected with a meningococcus C. In earlier decades, Swartley's team would have had to assume that the new capsule meant a new bug on the block. By the 1990s, they were able to look beyond the newcomer's capsule to its DNA, which told a different story. It was the same ET-5 strain but with a different capsule. At some point, an ET-5 group B must have colonised the same throat as a different strain with a group C capsule and picked up the DNA coding for that capsule.

Swartley showed how changeable the meningococcus can be, and also that how dangerous a strain is doesn't only depend on its capsule. There were a lot of strains with group B capsules in circulation, but most of them were bouncing from throat to throat without doing any harm. It was only ET-5 that was making people seriously ill in any number.

The ET-5 strain is 'hypervirulent', meaning it is among the minority of meningococci that cause the majority of meningococcal disease.[16]

By then, there had already been many attempts to make vaccines against the meningococcus's capsule polysaccharide. In the late 1960s, meningococcal meningitis once again interfered with men training for war. This time, it was American teenagers drafted into the 'Green Machine' that fought in Vietnam. Vaccinologists at the Walter Reed Army Institute of Research used a more sophisticated approach than Gordon's, using purified polysaccharide from groups A and C, which caused most of the cases.[17]

The US Army's draftees were squarely in the young adult period of vulnerability, and the pure polysaccharide vaccine made sure they didn't succumb to meningitis before the Viet Cong got a shot at them. However, it wasn't going to help with the young childhood period of vulnerability, much of which falls below the age at which children start responding to polysaccharide vaccines. Those young children had to rely on luck and antibiotics – until John Robbins and Rachel Schneerson invented their protein-polysaccharide conjugates.

Evaluating the conjugates

Britain was among the first countries to roll out meningococcal conjugate vaccines, which meant Britain was also the proving ground for their effectiveness.

As a cause of meningitis in children, meningococcus had played second fiddle to Hib, but in the early 1990s, it was still hospitalising more than 2,500 people across Britain every year with meningitis, septicaemia or both at once.[18] For every twenty of those people, six were left with some sort of long-term debilitation[19] like Clair Michna, and two or three weren't recovering at all.[20]

After the success of the Hib conjugate vaccine, there was every reason to expect that what worked with Hib would also work with meningococcus. The problem was how to prove it.

Those 2,500 cases added up to a lot of suffering, but they were so thinly spread that a conventional clinical trial, with a treatment and control group, would need to recruit every child in the country to get a result in a reasonable time period. No one was prepared to bankroll a trial on that scale, so a different approach was required.

That approach involved two stages: first, small-scale trials to confirm that a vaccine was safe and triggered antibodies that reacted to the meningococcal capsule. Second, a larger-scale evaluation on essentially the same principle that Gordon had used in Salisbury: if there were fewer cases after the roll-out, it was probably thanks to the vaccine.

Meningococcus C, which caused most cases in 1990s Britain, was targeted first. Vaccines from three different manufacturers passed the first stage, triggering antibody responses in babies without causing any serious side effects.[21,22,23] The second stage began in 1999, when all British children and teenagers under eighteen years old were vaccinated against meningococcus C.[24]

The meningococcus C conjugate did not disappoint. Within a year of the roll-out, meningococcus C all but disappeared from Britain.[25] Not only did vaccination protect the vaccinees, but there was also a substantial drop in cases among adults too old to have been vaccinated.[26] It appeared that meningococcus, like the pneumococcus, mostly circulated among children, who were the main source of infection for adults.

Less promising was that the protection didn't look like it was going to last. The schedule was for babies to be vaccinated at two, three and four months, which triggered ample antibodies to protect a child through her first year, but those antibodies were waning rapidly by her second birthday.

Experience with the Hib vaccine was showing that with conjugate vaccines, the number of doses in the first few months was less important than having a booster dose in the second year. The same lesson was applied to meningococcus C and, as it became less common in Britain, the need to protect very young children became less pressing. In 2006, the first dose was delayed until one year without leading to an increase in group C cases in babies.[27]

From C to ACWY

With meningococcus C off the scene, it was meningococcus A, B and Y that were most likely to send patients to hospital, but in 2000, hospitals around the world started seeing a worrying rise in the number of cases caused by meningococcus W.

At first, it looked like a single outbreak at the 2000 *hajj*;[28] the annual pilgrimage to Mecca, Saudi Arabia, undertaken by Muslims around the world. Hundreds of thousands of people crowd into makeshift accommodation for what is simultaneously a festival of devotion and a public health nightmare.

Sometime in the 1990s, a hypervirulent strain had switched from a group C to a group W capsule.[29] With both pure polysaccharide and conjugate vaccines available against group C but not group W, there was nothing to stop it spreading around the world.[30] When it found its way into the 2000 *hajj*, meningococcus W suddenly became a priority.

The next generation of conjugate vaccine combined groups A, C, W and Y, and was ready for roll-out by 2015, which proved to be not a moment too soon because the hypervirulent meningococcus W was on the rise.

In the wake of the 2000 *hajj*, Britain saw around 200 cases of group W meningococcal disease, mostly among recently returned pilgrims or people they had been in contact with. However, the outbreak petered out without meningococcus W becoming established in Britain, even as it spread around other parts of the world.[31]

The hypervirulent meningococcus W returned to Britain in 2010,[32] and this time it stayed. Its return wasn't connected with the *hajj* or any particular event, but in a country as globally connected as Britain, it was always going to arrive sooner rather than later.

In 2014, Britain saw 119 cases of the hypervirulent meningococcus W; not a huge total in a country of over 65 million, but it was twice as many cases as in the previous year.[33] The NHS nipped the situation in the bud with an emergency vaccination campaign starting in August 2015. They made the new ACWY vaccine available to all teenagers between fourteen and eighteen, and to anyone under twenty-five going to university.[34]

Cases dropped sharply over the next year,[35] heading off the spread of meningococcus W in Britain. The ACWY vaccine is still scheduled for British fourteen-year-olds, protecting them against four of the six dangerous groups before they reach the vulnerable period of young adulthood.

That leaves groups B and X. Cases of serious meningococcus X disease have never been particularly common, which made meningococcus B the next priority. It's the group most likely to cause meningitis in the under-five danger period,[36] and presents a so-far unique set of difficulties when it comes to vaccine development.

The invention of reverse vaccinology

Conjugate vaccines have been spectacularly successful against encapsulated bacteria, but they fall flat against the meningococcus B that infected Clair Michna.

The human immune system refuses to produce antibodies against the meningococcus B capsule. There's a good reason for that: the group B polysaccharide is so similar to certain molecules on the surface of our brain cells that any antibody that would attack the group B capsule would also attack our brains.[37]

To tackle meningitis B, vaccinologists had to go back to the drawing board.

The polysaccharide capsule protects most of the meningococcus's vulnerable proteins from the immune system but not all of them. It attaches to the throat lining with outer membrane proteins that extend beyond the capsule, leaving them exposed to antibodies.

In the early 1980s, a meningococcus B outbreak in Cuba prompted scientists at Havana's Finlay Institute to exploit that vulnerability. In one of the few conventional trials of a meningococcus vaccine, they assigned children from different schools to receive either a vaccine made from purified outer membrane proteins or a placebo.[38] The vaccine proved effective – but only against the strain causing the outbreak. The diversity of the meningococcus is not limited to the different polysaccharide groups. There is also considerable diversity among different meningococcus B strains: so much that an immune response to one strain's outer membrane proteins rarely protects against other strains.

For once, Cuba's isolation benefited its citizens. The Finlay Institute only had to contend with the one strain that had found its way on to the island. Their approach wouldn't have worked in Cuba's estranged neighbour, the USA, or anywhere else where many different meningococcus B strains were in circulation.[39]

A decade later, a team led by Rino Rappuoli at the Chiron Corporation in Siena, Italy, repeated the Cuban success to counter a single-strain outbreak in New Zealand.[40,41] Rappuoli knew as much about meningococcal vaccines as anyone in the world, having produced one of the first meningococcus C vaccines. However, he later said, 'I came to the conclusion that with the technologies we had at that time, we could not solve meningococcus B.'[42]

To come up with a multi-strain meningococcus B vaccine, Rappuoli needed to come up with a whole new technology. Much of the work was led by Mariagrazia Pizza, who had planned to spend a couple of years gaining experience in the private sector before returning to academia. Thirty years and 150 patents later, she's still there.[43]

Rappuoli and Pizza planned to look beyond the meningococcus's proteins and polysaccharides and into the genes coding for them. The strict definition of a gene is that it's a fragment of genetic material that codes for a single protein. If Pizza could identify a single gene, she could synthesise an identical fragment and slot it into the DNA of a different bacterium, *Escherichia coli*, which would produce it for her. She then purified each protein and injected it into mice.

It was painstaking, repetitive work, but gene by gene and protein by protein, Rappuoli and Pizza identified 350 different meningococcal proteins that triggered mouse lymphocytes to produce antibodies against them.[44] Rappuoli later said, 'We realised we were on top of what we call a goldmine. We knew we were going to make a vaccine. We didn't know exactly how.'[45]

The *how* depended on which of those 350 proteins were exposed to antibodies when they were part of a living meningococcus. There was no point in triggering antibodies against a protein that was shielded by the capsule.

Which, it turned out, was most of them. Their 350 candidates dropped to seven.

Rappuoli and Pizza rejected another three because they varied so much between strains that antibodies produced against the protein of one strain wouldn't recognise the protein of another.

The remaining four became the basis of today's meningococcus B vaccine. As long as an infecting strain carries the genes for at least one of the four proteins in the vaccine, then the vaccine will trigger immune memory that protects against it.

Rappuoli and Pizza had invented more than a vaccine against group B meningococcus. They had also invented reverse vaccinology: a way to take the Pasteur doctrine to a whole new level. Using reverse vaccinology, the 'isolate' stage of the doctrine refers not only to the microbe but to the individual proteins that make up the microbe. Those proteins are then injected into mice, whose immune systems decide which are important.

The meningococcus B vaccine

Having four proteins that looked like good antibody targets still didn't add up to a vaccine, and it would be more than ten years before the meningococcus B vaccine was tested in humans.[46]

By the time the vaccine had been branded as 'Bexsero' and was ready for a general roll-out, Chiron's vaccine division had been passed on to GlaxoSmithKline, taking Rappuoli and Pizza with it.

It was one thing to show the vaccine was safe and triggered antibody production. It was another to show that it was effective, and here, the group B vaccine ran into the same problem that the other vaccines had: no one would fund a large enough trial to test it against a placebo.

Once again, the only way to test it was to roll it out and see whether it lowered the rate of meningococcus B disease. Once again, the first country to try it was Britain.

In September 2015, the NHS rolled out Bexsero with a three-dose schedule: the first two doses at eight and sixteen weeks to protect during the first year, and a booster given to one-year-olds.[47] Combined with the ACWY conjugate, it left British children with more comprehensive protection against meningococcal disease than children anywhere else in the world.

By the end of 2016, the first data on Bexsero's effectiveness was looking hopeful. Among the age group that received the vaccine, there were only half as many cases as in the years before.[48]

One year's data might have been down to Bexsero being effective, or it might have been a quiet year for meningococcus B, but after three years, cases were still low.[49] The verdict was in: Rappuoli and Pizza's reverse vaccinology had delivered an effective vaccine.

Since then, several other countries have rolled out the meningococcus B vaccine, many along with the ACWY conjugate combination. Meningococcal disease is becoming increasingly rare in the high-income countries where most research and roll-outs have taken place,[50] but at the time of writing, meningococcal vaccines have seen far less use in the low-income countries where meningococcus disease is most prevalent.

There's one place in particular where meningococcus has run riot for more than a century. However, thanks to an innovative approach to vaccine development, it is finally being brought under control.

The Meningitis Belt

In 1898, General Sir Herbert Kitchener of the British Army raised the Egyptian flag over the city of Khartoum, ending the Mahdist War and seizing Sudan in the name of Khedive Abbas II of Egypt. Abbas was nominally a vassal of the Ottoman Empire, but Kitchener was there because Egypt was a British protectorate in all but name. Whatever flag Kitchener ran up the pole, his army had brought the British Empire to Khartoum.

At the same time, it probably brought the meningococcus south of the Sahara Desert.[51] There's no evidence of it in the region before the invasion, but it was so common in both Britain and northern Egypt that some of Kitchener's British and Egyptian troops must have been carrying it.

Kitchener didn't linger in Khartoum. He went on to command the British Army in the Anglo-Boer War, where he became an early exponent of the concentration camp, and later he became the face of the original 'Your Country Needs You' First World War recruitment poster.

Meningococcus did not leave with him. It spread across the Sahel, the arid region south of the Sahara. Every few years, meningococcus A would cause an outbreak of meningitis that started in Ethiopia or Somalia and rolled westward across the 'Meningitis Belt',[52] as the region became known, to the Atlantic coast of The Gambia and Senegal. Every outbreak left tens of thousands dead. Even in the years between outbreaks, Sahel residents were ten times more likely to suffer meningococcal disease than anyone anywhere else on earth.[53]

The arrival of antibiotics improved the situation but not by very much. The Sahel nations are among the poorest in the world, and many people can't get to a clinic. A vaccine that could be delivered in a single injection would have made a huge difference, but when conjugate vaccines appeared in the 1990s, they were priced beyond the shoestring budgets of the Sahel health ministries.

In 1996, several Sahel governments approached the WHO for help with their century-long public health crisis. The WHO looked at producing a meningococcus A vaccine for less than a dollar, but their findings were depressing: it was certainly possible for pharmaceutical firms to do so and still make a profit, but none were willing to divert resources away from more profitable ventures.[54]

The wealthier world's meningococcal vaccines were not going to trickle down to the part of the world most ravaged by meningococcal disease. The Sahel needed a vaccine designed to be affordable from the outset, and because Robbins and Schneerson had never patented the technology behind conjugate vaccines, anyone who wanted to give it a try was free to do so.

In 2001, the Bill & Melinda Gates Foundation put up a $70 million grant that turned a problem into an opportunity. A consortium of companies used it not to invent a new technology, but to refine the manufacturing process so it could deliver the existing conjugate vaccine technology at an affordable price. In 2003, the Serum Institute of India could offer a meningococcus A vaccine called MenAfriVac at 50 cents per dose and still make a profit.[55]

'What was viewed by established vaccine companies in Europe or the USA as an opportunity cost, was seen by the developing country manufacturer as an opportunity,'[56] some of the project leaders later wrote.

One of the first countries to embrace the new vaccine was Burkina Faso, which achieved one of the fastest national vaccine roll-outs in history. In ten days of December 2010, all 11 million Burkinabes between one and twenty-nine years old were vaccinated,[57] covering both the early childhood and young adulthood high-risk periods.

The effect was dramatic. Meningococcus A vanished from Burkina Faso almost immediately,[58] and two years later, a survey found only one person carrying meningococcus among nearly 5,000 tested.[59] The same success was repeated in every country that adopted MenAfriVac,[60] and by the end of 2014, 217 million people across the Sahel had been vaccinated.

Conjugate vaccines are technically complex, but MenAfriVac showed they can be made affordable to the poorest parts of the world with a combination of hard science and hard cash – though not that much hard cash. For most vaccine development programmes, you wouldn't expect any change out of $500 million, so MenAfriVac's $70 million (£45 million at 2010 exchange rates[61]) was a steal. When MenAfriVac was rolled out in 2010, £45 million paid for less than a week of British military operations in Afghanistan.[62] I leave it to you to decide which was the more worthwhile endeavour.

Getting rid of meningitis A didn't banish meningococcal disease from the Sahel. By the time MenAfriVac was rolled out, meningitis C had appeared in northern Nigeria and it caused a minor outbreak of its own over the next few years, although it fell short of re-establishing the Meningitis Belt.[63] Nor was the region spared the global rise of meningococcus W.

The meningococcus first arrived in the Meningitis Belt by steamship and route march but now jet engines can carry a colonised throat from one continent to another in a few hours, the meningococci are more mobile than ever. Vaccination against a single group may win a battle, but winning the war needs vaccines that cover multiple groups that are currently only available in the wealthier parts of the world.

Meningococcus vaccines are still relatively new, and there's still a lot we don't know about them. At the time of writing, the first children to be given Bexsero are past the early childhood period of vulnerability, but we've yet to learn whether they'll need boosting before the second danger point of early adulthood.

There's also the problem of meningococcus X, which, of the six dangerous types, is the least likely to cause disease. However, the rare cases it does cause are as serious as those caused by the other five, and there's no guarantee it will stay rare. If a hypervirulent strain switches to group X, it could spread as fast as the hypervirulent meningococcus W did in the 2000s.

At the time of writing, there's reason to place some hope in a new vaccine that combines groups A, C, W, X and Y.[64] Its development was initiated not by the usual suspects of academic or pharmaceutical researchers but by the British government's Department for International Development* in the hope of putting an end to the Meningitis Belt for good. It has proved safe and effective,[65] and it looks likely to be combined with a meningococcus B protein vaccine and rolled out in the Sahel in 2022,[66] bypassing the high-income countries that usually get first dibs on a new vaccine and perhaps becoming the first vaccine to trickle up the world's wealth gradient rather than down.

The possibility of combining all six dangerous types in one vaccine raises the prospect of protecting children around the world against the sort of life-shattering experience that Clair Michna endured.

Today's array of vaccines arrived too late for her. She is still

* Now part of the Foreign, Commonwealth and Development Office.

frustrated by the impairments that meningococcus inflicted on her three decades ago. She told me, 'I'm ... nearly halfway through my life ... it's like, oh damn, I haven't really got much time now ... I'm just like, yeah, let's make the most of the rest of it now.'[67]

Chapter 10

Hepatitis B virus (HBV)

The stories behind the vaccines on the childhood schedule are, by definition, success stories. Unless a vaccine is both safe and effective, it doesn't make the list in the first place. The hepatitis B vaccine is such a success, but it starts with one of the biggest snafus in the history of vaccination. In 1942, the US military accidentally caused the largest ever outbreak of acute hepatitis B by injecting servicemen with contaminated yellow fever vaccine.

Yellow fever had long been the scourge of American soldiers serving in the tropics, but when the USA entered the Second World War, Max Theiler and his team at the Rockefeller Institute were testing a new vaccine against it.[1] Faced with the prospect of seeing American forces once again decimated before they could come to grips with the enemy, the War Department had every recruit injected with the new vaccine before the testing was complete.

After a few months, something was evidently awry. By March 1942, newly minted soldiers and sailors were reporting sick with weakness, vomiting and, most tellingly, the yellow skin, yellow eyes and dark urine of jaundice.[2]

Something was stopping those young men's livers from

regulating the vast array of chemicals that make up the human body. Military doctors knew the signs of liver inflammation, or, to use the medical term, hepatitis. They didn't know what was inflaming those livers, but before long, their attention settled on the yellow fever vaccine. After all, a connection between yellow fever vaccine and hepatitis had already been suggested.

Out of sorts

The suggestion had been made by George Findlay and his Canadian assistant, Frederick MacCallum, at London's Wellcome Institute. In the late 1930s, Africa was 'the white man's grave', and the Colonial Service snapped up a vaccine against one of the diseases that made it so. However, Findlay and MacCallum found a disturbing number of otherwise fit vaccinees who were left 'out of sorts' – an understated way of saying they felt like merry hell – with hepatitis a few months after being vaccinated.[3]

Their findings were echoed by researchers in Brazil,[4] whose government had rolled out the vaccine as soon as they could get their hands on it.

The British and Brazilian observations raised questions about the vaccine, but nobody made much effort to answer them until it put 50,000 American servicemen in hospital and killed around 100.[5] That made the US War Department sit up and pay attention.

Their investigation found that all the hepatitis cases could be traced back to a few production lots of yellow fever vaccine. It looked like the cause was some contaminant in those lots rather than the vaccine itself, but whatever that contaminant was, no one managed to isolate it.

The War Department's scientists fell back on an educated guess as to how those lots were contaminated. The yellow fever vaccine was an attenuated virus cultured in cells nourished with human serum from blood donors.[6] They inferred that a microbe infecting some of the blood donors had found its way into the vaccine. In April 1942, they switched the human serum for animal serum.

There were no new cases after that, but it didn't immediately end the outbreak because once the hepatitis B virus infects someone, the first symptoms may take as long as six months to appear. An infected man has time to reach the front line before it makes him ill. Fighting in Guadalcanal or Tunisia was miserable enough without having to contend with hepatitis. We will never know how many men died in combat because hepatitis slowed them down.

The British War Office had embraced the yellow fever vaccine as enthusiastically as their American counterparts, and while the British military outbreak is not as well documented as the American one, we do know that a lot of British troops contracted hepatitis.[7] Findlay, who was then in West Africa with the Royal Army Medical Corps, saw its effects first-hand. He also noticed that African soldiers, who were not vaccinated against yellow fever, occasionally caught hepatitis from jaundiced British officers. Whatever they were dealing with, it was infectious.[8]

The mystery of the hepatitis virus

With Findlay in West Africa, MacCallum stepped into his mentor's shoes. He led two different research groups throughout the Second World War and still found time to volunteer as a fire watcher and a Home Guardsman.[9]

The mysterious infectious hepatitis was high on MacCallum's priority list, especially as evidence rolled in that the yellow fever vaccine wasn't the only way to catch it. Many hepatitis patients had received a blood transfusion a few weeks earlier,[10] reinforcing the idea that it was an infectious agent carried by blood. MacCallum couldn't see it through a microscope, which pointed to a virus,[11] but every attempt to isolate it drew a blank.

As the war drew to a close, a frustrated tone entered MacCallum's papers on the subject. He probably didn't miss the problem when, in 1947, he took on the task of establishing a viral diagnostic service to support the nascent NHS. MacCallum left one final, critical insight: that he'd spent the last ten years on the trail of not one type of hepatitis but two, which he called hepatitis A and hepatitis B.[12] We now know of five viruses that cause hepatitis, named with the letters A to E, but the hepatitis B that plagued allied soldiers during the Second World War is by far the most common.

Baruch Blumberg finds the Australia antigen

Baruch Blumberg of Philadelphia's Institute for Cancer Research* didn't set out to pick up where MacCallum had left off. Blumberg's interest was in blood transfusion, and in how repeated transfusions might affect the person receiving them. Every healthy person's blood contains the same suite of cells and solutes made up of the same mix of proteins, lipids and carbohydrates. However, the precise structure of those proteins, lipids and carbohydrates varies from one person to another, and Blumberg noticed that transfusions triggered an antibody response in some recipients.

Blumberg set out to map the diversity of blood constituents, which he could do thanks to a post-war spirit of scientific internationalism. Before the Second World War, scientists often exchanged letters and occasionally samples with foreign peers,

---

* Now Fox Chase Cancer Center.

but scientific projects rarely crossed national borders. By the mid-1960s, Blumberg could request samples from collaborators across much of the world – although not from Eastern Europe, the Soviet Union or China. Sixties-style internationalism only went so far.

In a sample from an indigenous Australian, Blumberg and his team found an anomaly: an antibody response to a protein they hadn't seen before. The protein targeted by an antibody is called its 'antigen', so they called the mysterious protein the 'Australia antigen' and went looking for it in other samples.[13]

Among Americans, the Australia antigen turned up in children institutionalised with Down's syndrome, haemophilia patients who received regular blood transfusions and people who had recovered from hepatitis. It was an odd pattern, but odder still was that in Taiwan, it was common in the general population.[14]

Had Blumberg been working in isolation, he probably wouldn't have realised what he was on the trail of. The key insight came from his collaborator, Kazuo Okochi at the University of Tokyo, where the Australia antigen was more common than in America but less common than in Taiwan. Okochi noticed that when donated blood contained the Australia antigen, the people it was donated to often developed hepatitis.[15] More than twenty years after MacCallum had hypothesised the existence of a hepatitis B virus, Blumberg and Okochi had found direct evidence of it.

The many faces of hepatitis B

The hepatitis B virus proved to be a very strange beast. While most viruses have one process of infection, the hepatitis B virus has several.[16]

Most of the servicemen infected during the Second World War got 'acute' hepatitis. The virus infected their liver cells and replicated itself there until it attracted the attention of their immune systems. Once their killer T-cells woke up to what was going on, they purged the infected cells, which got rid of the virus but also damaged their livers, leaving them jaundiced and thoroughly out of sorts. It was deeply unpleasant, but all except an unfortunate few recovered within a year.

Or so they thought.

In nine cases out of ten, they thought correctly. Their hepatitis B infection was gone and they were immune to the virus for the rest of their lives – however short those lives might be once they were fit for duty. The unfortunate tenth would have entered a state of 'chronic' hepatitis in which the virus somehow avoided attracting too much attention from the immune system. They would have suffered regular flare-ups as their immune response waxed and waned. Each flare-up saw killer T-cells destroying virus-infected liver cells, which their bodies replaced with scar tissue. In an unfortunate few, it would have led to liver cancer. For most, it was a slow degradation of the liver in the years and decades after they hung up their uniforms for good.[17]

It was through blood donors carrying that sort of chronic infection that the hepatitis B virus got into the yellow fever vaccine in the first place. Those people had no idea what they were passing on through the vaccines that their blood was used to make.

Massive as the Second World War outbreak had been, hepatitis B remained rare in America because the virus is not particularly infectious. Unless it's transmitted through blood or sexual intercourse, infection requires prolonged close contact, such as in the barracks where Findlay had observed African soldiers being infected by their officers or in the crowded institutions that held American children with Down's syndrome.

When Blumberg identified the Australia antigen, he made it possible for hospitals to test donated blood for it and eliminate it as an unavoidable hazard of blood transfusions.[18] If hepatitis B followed the American pattern of infection throughout the world, Blumberg would have been able to say job done when he was awarded the 1976 Nobel Prize in Physiology or Medicine.

However, his finding that the virus was far more common in Taiwan than in the USA was the first indication of a completely different pattern of infection. In Taiwan, most hepatitis B infections were happening not in adults but babies, and the source of that infection was usually their mothers.

When hepatitis B virus infects a baby, the infection is far more likely to turn chronic than in an infected adult. As that baby becomes a child and then an adult, their killer T-cells keep chipping away at virus-infected liver cells without ever fully purging the virus. It's a slow battle that leaves the liver laced with scar tissue, ultimately leading to cirrhosis and liver cancer. Girls infected as babies usually live long enough to bear children of their own, whom they then infect, sustaining a grim cycle of mother-to-child transmission.

Cirrhosis and liver cancer develop faster in men than in women, and once they knew what they were looking for, researchers found that hepatitis B accounted for one in every five deaths among working-age Taiwanese men.[19]

Once the mother-to-child transmission pattern was identified, researchers found it didn't only happen in Taiwan. The same pattern appeared across much of Asia and Africa. The hepatitis B virus was cutting short hundreds of thousands – if not millions – of lives every year, and nobody had noticed.

Enter Maurice Hilleman

By 1970, researchers could use electron microscopes to visualise the Australia antigen in the blood, and they found it in two distinct configurations.[20] One was as part of the capsid – the protein coat that protects the hepatitis B virus's genetic material when it's between cells – which is why it was later renamed the surface protein. The other was in much smaller spherical structures that contained no genetic material. Those spherical structures were the debris of viral replication, synthesised in an infected cell but never incorporated into a virus's capsid.

Hepatitis B virus continued to be as stubbornly difficult to isolate as it had in MacCallum's time, and it remains difficult to culture in the laboratory. It defied attempts to apply the first stage of the Pasteur doctrine by isolating it, but to Blumberg, those spherical structures suggested a way around the problem. Instead of trying to isolate the virus, perhaps he could isolate the debris and use it to trigger an immune memory that would recognise the identical protein in the viral capsid.

Blumberg's daughter was then at school with the daughter of Maurice Hilleman,[21] head of vaccine research at Merck and the man who, more than any other, drove the USA's mid-twentieth-century viral-vaccine boom. Like Robert Austrian a decade before, Blumberg turned to Hilleman to move his idea from the laboratory to the clinic.

Preparing the vaccine proved to be the easy part. Hilleman's team recruited chronically infected people, filtered those particles out of their blood and ran them through a series of treatments to be sure that no microbe, known or unknown, could sneak into the vaccine along with those surface proteins. As it would turn out, it was just as well he was meticulous about sterilisation.

Hilleman's team showed the vaccine was effective in experimental animals,[22] but when it was ready for large-scale human trials, they encountered the vaccine developer's nemesis: an uninterested funding committee. Hepatitis B might have been a blight across Asia and Africa, but because it remained a rare disease in the USA, Merck didn't see a market for a vaccine.

'The feedback we got was well, you know, this is only going

to be used in poor countries,' Blumberg said, years later. 'That did get me upset.'[23]

The way forward was suggested by Wolf Szmuness, a Polish-born epidemiologist at New York's Columbia University with a history of starting at the bottom and working his way up. His first public health responsibility resulted directly from the Soviet invasion of eastern Poland in 1939: he was imprisoned in a Siberian labour camp and put in charge of sanitation. Szmuness must have impressed someone, because he was released to take charge of epidemiology for the whole region. He was still in the Soviet Union in the 1950s when his wife, Maya, nearly died of hepatitis following a blood transfusion.

It piqued his interest in hepatitis, and when he and Maya emigrated to the USA, he took his interest with him. At first, the only job Szmuness could get was as a laboratory technician. Once again, he must have impressed someone, because five years later, he was a senior epidemiologist and an internationally recognised authority on hepatitis.[24]

Although hepatitis B was rare across the USA as a whole, it was common in certain groups – and one of those groups was New York's often marginalised and persecuted gay community. Szmuness was among the few who took an interest in their health, and when he asked for help testing a vaccine, many gay men were willing to step up.

A phase 3 vaccine trial usually involves tens or hundreds of thousands of volunteers and often years of follow-up. Until a reasonable number of volunteers who received the placebo are infected, there's no way to tell if the vaccine protected the volunteers who got the vaccine. It's what makes vaccine trials so expensive.

On the New York gay scene, hepatitis B was so prevalent that Szmuness's trial recruited a mere 1,083 volunteers, and in eight months, Szmuness conclusively showed the vaccine worked[25] without giving Merck's accountants any reason to suck their teeth.

For Szmuness's volunteers, their hepatitis B problem was already being overtaken by something much worse. Some of Szmuness's fellow epidemiologists were noticing a cluster of unusual infections among gay men that they called acquired immunity deficiency syndrome or, as we now know it, AIDS. While hepatitis B belongs in a list of vaccine success stories, AIDS does not. The virus that causes it, HIV, has been eluding every candidate vaccine thrown at it for the last forty years.

What HIV did not elude was Hilleman's sterilisation technique, which was just as well because some of the blood from which Hilleman was extracting the hepatitis B surface protein must also have contained HIV. If Hilleman had been less thorough, the vaccine would have infected a lot of Szmuness's volunteers with it.[26]

Breaking the mother-to-child transmission cycle

Szmuness had showed that the vaccine protected adults from infection, but it didn't necessarily follow that it would break the mother-to-child transmission cycle in countries like Taiwan. Many babies were being infected by their mother's blood as they were born, so even if they were vaccinated with their first breath of air, there was no way to vaccinate them before they were infected.

On the other hand, the hepatitis B virus takes several weeks to get established in the liver, while a vaccine usually triggers a full-blown immune response within a week or two. Even if the vaccination was slightly later than the infection, it might still be in time to stop the infection from taking hold.

The possibility was tested by a team led by Hilton Whittle at the British government's Medical Research Council research unit in The Gambia, where hepatitis B infection followed the same mother-to-child transmission cycle as in Taiwan.

By the time I arrived at MRC Gambia in 2002, Whittle was known not only for his research achievements but for having nurtured a wheelbarrow-sized tortoise called Perky, who regularly escaped from his garden inside the MRC compound. As head of the infant immunology team, my duties occasionally included retrieving what Whittle referred to as his 'galloping tortoise'.

The unit's infrastructure could be unreliable, and I learned to stockpile any supplies that could get held up in transit and to work around the electricity supply's surges and outages. Trying as I sometimes found it, Whittle had to contend with much worse when he headed The Gambia's first hepatitis B vaccine trials in the early 1980s. It was the beginning of a project that would last for decades, helmed by Whittle and his colleague, Maimuna Mendy, who cut her scientific teeth by processing thousands of blood samples from the hepatitis B study in between the regular power outages.

Whittle and Mendy showed that vaccinating newborn babies massively cut the number who grew up to carry the hepatitis B virus. They couldn't stop them from getting infected during birth, and some developed acute hepatitis, but being vaccinated made them far more likely to recover.[27] Better still, the immunity lasted. A decade and a half later, the children who had been vaccinated at birth were still immune.[28]

The vaccine had broken the mother-to-child transmission cycle.

A vaccine for the world

The New York and Gambian trials were promising, but there was a problem: the idea behind vaccination was to eliminate chronic infection, but without chronically infected people from whom to isolate surface protein, there would be no vaccine.

Hilleman's team broke the cycle with the brand-new technology of genetic engineering. They inserted the virus's surface protein gene into yeast cells, which then produced an endless supply of it.[29]

Culturing yeast was a lot cheaper than finding donors and sterilising their blood products. Whittle and Mendy's trial had been criticised for testing a vaccine that, at $60 per dose, was never going to be affordable in a low-income country like The Gambia. Hilleman's engineered yeast, on the other hand, produced vaccines at $1 per dose.[30]

Taiwan was one of the first countries to embrace the yeast-derived vaccine, giving it to all children from the late 1980s. Because babies infected with chronic hepatitis may live well into adulthood before developing cirrhosis or cancer, it was nearly thirty years before the programme could be evaluated, but when it was, the results were clear. Vaccination had reduced deaths from liver disease by more than a hundredfold.[31]

By then, Taiwan was not alone. The 1990s and 2000s saw many more countries add hepatitis B to their childhood vaccine schedules.[32]

In Britain, the pattern of infection was similar to the USA in that it has never established a mother-to-child transmission cycle. Although the WHO recommended that all babies around the world should be vaccinated,[33] the NHS maintained that routine hepatitis B vaccination would not be cost-effective as late as 2011,[34] especially as there were now treatments that could suppress chronic hepatitis if not completely cure it.[35]

However, with around 340,000 chronically infected people in Britain,[36] and not all of them aware of it, there was a steady trickle of new infections. The nudge that changed the NHS's policy[37] was GlaxoSmithKline's Infanrix '6-in-1' vaccine, which combines the hepatitis B surface antigen with vaccines against diphtheria, tetanus, whooping cough, polio and Hib in a single injection. It was only slightly more expensive than the '5-in-1' vaccine already in use, and its safety was well-established because it was already widely used around the world.[38]

Infanrix was added to the childhood vaccination schedule in 2017,[39] bringing Britain in line with the WHO's recommendations.

The legacy of Baruch Blumberg

Humanity's victories over infectious diseases are usually won by the hard work of many different scientists approaching the disease from different angles. Baruch Blumberg is one of the very few scientists who led the charge from discovering an infectious agent to developing the vaccine.

Blumberg was never immodest enough to put it that way, but when he spoke of the tears of a Senegalese surgeon explaining how 'for forty years he has been operating on people with primary cancer of the liver and it had been of no value', or of an Italian physician describing how he no longer had to advise chronically infected women not to have children, he added that it was 'a rare pleasure for a basic medical scientist to witness such a wholesome outcome to their research'.[40]

Many scientists are drawn to medical research because we hope to feel that pleasure, but few of us earn it as comprehensively as Blumberg did.

In 2016, the WHO set 2030 as the deadline for global eradication of hepatitis B. That was over-optimistic[41] even before the

COVID-19 pandemic disrupted global vaccination programmes, but it doesn't detract from the success of the vaccine in breaking the once endless cycle of mother-to-child transmission. By 2017, the WHO estimated that the vaccine had prevented over 14 million chronic hepatitis B cases.[42] Blumberg's legacy was summed up by his colleague, Jonathan Chernoff: 'Barry prevented more cancer deaths than any person who's ever lived.'[43]

Chapter 11

Polio

John Prestwich took his last autonomous breath the week of his seventeenth birthday.[1]

He'd always wanted to go to sea, and as a deckhand on a merchant ship docked in Corpus Christi, Texas, he was living the life he'd dreamed of. That morning, he woke up and couldn't raise his head off his pillow. His shipmates called an ambulance, but before they got him to the hospital, Prestwich stopped breathing. The medics rocked him back and forth on the stretcher, which before mouth-to-mouth resuscitation was the approved method of forcing air into inactive lungs.

He regained consciousness to what he described as 'something in front of me and this swishing noise'. That swishing noise was the piston doing his breathing for him.

His body was encased in a sealed cylinder. As the piston raised and lowered the pressure within it, air was pulled in and out of his lungs.

John Prestwich was inside an iron lung.

He wasn't alone. He was in a row of mechanical cylinders, each with a head protruding from one end. It's hard to imagine a more horrific awakening.

Like everyone else in those cylinders, Prestwich's spinal cord had been attacked by the poliovirus. It had severed the link between his brain and everything below his neck, including the muscles he used to breathe.

Prestwich would not leave his iron lung for the next seven years, the first two of which he spent in Corpus Christi, and the next five in London's Royal Free Hospital. After that, he started to use a cuirass ventilator strapped across his chest, allowing him to sit in a wheelchair.

Prestwich was determined to live as full a life as was possible for a man who couldn't breathe. On one occasion, his friends wheeled him out of the Royal Free and all the way to the top of the Eiffel Tower. He later married the love of his life, Maggie Biffen, and they lived for thirty-five years in their own home.

Nevertheless, from that day in 1955 to his death in 2006, his every breath was taken for him by a machine.

How clean water gave us polio

The disease that paralysed Prestwich is a product of cleanliness.

The late nineteenth and early twentieth centuries saw the spread of possibly the single most important public health innovation ever invented: the closed sewer. Separating drinking water from waste water freed cities from what London half-jokingly called 'King Cholera'[2] and his allies, such as typhus. The nineteenth-century sewage pioneers couldn't know they were also fatally changing the pattern of poliovirus infection.

Poliovirus usually infects through the faecal-oral route. It's a nauseatingly literal description of the cycle that sees polio getting into the mouth and down to infect the cells lining the intestines, then finding its way out in the faeces and from there into another mouth, usually through the water supply.

Before the closed sewer, polio was so rife that most babies were infected before their first birthday.[3] At that age, their mother's antibodies protected them from serious disease until their own lymphocytes recognised the poliovirus and retained a memory of it.

Sanitation reduced poliovirus exposure, but it couldn't completely prevent it. As Prestwich found out, reducing exposure did not prevent infection, but it did delay it until childhood or early adulthood – long after maternal antibodies had waned.

When poliovirus infected Prestwich, the odds were on his side. In around 199 infections out of 200, poliovirus remained in the intestine and caused nothing worse than a minor fever.[4] Prestwich was the unlucky one. The poliovirus found its way out of his intestine and into his spinal cord, where it caused the paralytic disease called poliomyelitis. How much damage it did once it got there varied from one victim to another.

Many poliomyelitis victims made at least a partial recovery, although many were still left depending on crutches or wheelchairs. Others spent the rest of their lives dependent on iron lungs.

In describing polio in the past tense, I am allowing myself a degree of optimism. Our hospitals no longer have wards packed with swishing iron lungs, and there are very few places in the world where children must roll the dice with polio.

Polio has been beaten back despite today's doctors having the same number of anti-polio treatments as the doctors who treated Prestwich in 1955: none. Its retreat is entirely down to infections being prevented by two vaccines developed in the mid-twentieth century.

The first steps of the March of Dimes

The tale of the two vaccines is often told as a fable of heroic ingenuity and international cooperation vanquishing a scourge on humanity. It was all of that, but it is also a cautionary tale of blind alleys and blunders, and of what happens when decisions about public health are warped by political pressure.

When people limping, crutching or using wheelchairs after poliomyelitis were an everyday sight, those unfortunates were called simply 'polios'. The story of those two vaccines began with the most famous polio of them all, Franklin Delano Roosevelt.

For the young man who would become the USA's longest-serving president, political dalliances were interludes in his playboy lifestyle rather than preparation for a career. Play came to a crashing halt when, at thirty-nine years old, he was abruptly paralysed from the waist down. His doctors diagnosed polio and, although a recent re-evaluation suggests that his illness was more likely to have been an autoimmune condition called Guillain-Barré syndrome,[5] Roosevelt believed himself a polio until the day he died.

He spent years trying to walk again and failing before he redirected his energies against polio itself. In 1927, Roosevelt and his friend and lawyer, Basil O'Connor, started fundraising to support polios and to pay for research on the disease that defined them.

Between Roosevelt's high-society contacts and O'Connor's capable directorship, the dollars rolled in. Roosevelt took the cause with him when he entered politics two years later, beginning his meteoric rise to the presidency, a post he occupied from 1933 until his death in 1945.

O'Connor's fundraising operation rose with Roosevelt. In 1938, it adopted the slogan that would define it: the March of Dimes. It was a play on both the *March of Time* cinema newsreels and the catchphrase of the Great Depression, 'Brother, can you spare a dime?'[6] The March of Dimes rebranded the operation, taking the emphasis away from the wealthy donors of Roosevelt's social set and placing it on ordinary Americans, who donated what little they could spare. If America was going to war with polio, the heroes of that war were not Rockefellers or Carnegies but the cattleman, the housewife and the machinist. The people who lived in fear of their own children being struck down by poliomyelitis.

The March of Dimes became one of the USA's largest medical research funders, making a polio vaccine the number-one prize for virology research. It proved to be a mixed blessing.

A blessing because it drove research that massively expanded understanding of the poliovirus and by extension, of viruses in general. Mixed because some researchers focused more on the reputation that a polio vaccine would make than on the many pitfalls that lay on the way to it.

The first to blunder into one of those pitfalls was John Kolmer, who tried to attenuate wild-type poliovirus into a vaccine strain using a technique we might generously call hocus-pocus.* Five dead children later, Kolmer's reputation was in tatters, and other polio researchers were applying a healthy dose of caution to their approach.

Through most of the 1940s, polio researchers concentrated on learning what they were up against. A key discovery was that they were dealing with not one poliovirus but three, now known as types I, II and III. Type I is far more likely to escape the intestine and infect the spinal cord than types II or III,[7] which might explain why the late 1940s saw a dramatic jump in poliomyelitis cases across Europe and North America. The plot on page 187 shows that in 1947, England and Wales saw five times as many cases as in the previous year,[8] and although no subsequent year would be as bad, the annual polio outbreaks continued to be far worse than they had been before.

The most likely explanation is that the Second World War's mass troop movements introduced the more dangerous type I

---

* See Chapter 3.

poliovirus to regions that had previously only seen types II and III.[9] However, we can't be sure, because nobody was documenting what types were found where before the late 1940s.

Whatever the reason, the rise in cases renewed the pressure for a vaccine but, while researchers could isolate it, they found poliovirus difficult to culture in the laboratory. Droves of rats, rabbits and monkeys were sacrificed so researchers could infect their spinal cords with poliovirus, but none managed to culture it reliably.

Knowing what we now know, that's not surprising. They were using spinal cords because poliomyelitis is caused by infection of the spinal cord. Nobody had noticed that most poliovirus infections do not cause poliomyelitis, which is why they didn't realise its main site of infection was not the spinal cord but the intestine.

For as long as everyone was fiddling with spinal cords, progress toward a vaccine was going nowhere.

The Enders-Weller-Robbins technique

John Enders was a man of contradictions. His experience as a First World War flying instructor had left him with a lifelong fear of flying. He started his academic career with a degree in English literature and ended it hailed as 'the father of modern vaccines'.[10] While other virologists bombarded O'Connor with requests for funding for bigger laboratories and more staff, Enders preferred to keep his team at Harvard small.

By the late 1940s, those members included Thomas Weller and Frederick Robbins, who were working on culturing the chickenpox virus on various types of cells from stillborn babies. Enders suggested that while they had the cells, they might as well try poliovirus with them. It was a shot in the dark. Like everyone else, they assumed that poliovirus needed nerve cells to replicate, but they had the cells and they had the virus, so why not give it a try?

To the surprise of all three, poliovirus proved easier to culture in several different cell types than in the nerve cells that everyone had been using.[11] They tried cells recovered from the intestinal wall, and once again, the poliovirus took.

Showing that poliovirus primarily infects the intestines rather than the nervous system won Enders a Nobel Prize, which, characteristically, he insisted on sharing with Robbins and Weller.[12] More practically, the Enders-Weller-Robbins technique allowed vaccinologists to culture poliovirus in the bulk quantities needed to produce a vaccine.

The next question was how to turn the wild-type into a vaccine. With the prize now in sight, the next few years saw competition raging not only between individuals but between the two schools of thought that had permeated vaccinology since the beginning of the twentieth century: those who wanted to attenuate the virus and those who wanted to inactivate it.

The two approaches were later described as 'strangling a parrot or teaching it to talk'.[13] When Enders and his team published their technique, most vaccinologists were committed parrot-stranglers. They isolated pathogens, killed them, called them vaccines and injected them. But then, most vaccinologists were working on bacteria, not viruses.

The only routinely used viral vaccine was against yellow fever, and it had been made by attenuating the virulent wild-type into a mild vaccine strain.[14] If attenuation worked with one virus, the parrot-teachers argued, wasn't that the best place to start with another?

Jonas Salk didn't agree. He had cut his virological teeth at the University of Michigan where, as we'll see in Chapter 17, he worked on influenza vaccines that he made by inactivation. When he moved from working on influenza to working on polio, he took his parrot-strangling approach with him.

The Salk inactivated polio vaccine

Most scientists are, by nature, backroom boys. Their names ring no bells outside their field, and even the larger egos rarely seek recognition beyond their professional peers.

Jonas Salk was an exception. He was more comfortable in front of the press's cameras than in his laboratory, where, ironically enough, he often persuaded the press he was most at home by borrowing someone else's white coat for his frequent photo ops. He left the painstaking process of parrot-strangling – or rather, culturing poliovirus, inactivating it and testing it – to Julius Youngner, the head of his laboratory team, whom Salk rarely acknowledged.[15]

The media might have connived in Salk's self-portrayal as a lone prodigy but O'Connor was not taken in. When Salk announced that he had developed a vaccine that should be rolled out across the USA, O'Connor insisted that it was tested by someone with a reputation to protect instead of a reputation to build. The man he approached was Salk's former mentor, Thomas Francis, who was still at the University of Michigan.

In 1954, clinical trials were still considered optional, especially with diseases as thinly spread as polio. As visible as polios made the disease, there was still no way to detect the large majority of infections that were confined to the intestine. To compare poliomyelitis rates between vaccinated and unvaccinated groups of children, Francis was going to need a lot of children.

A lot of children was what Francis got: around a million and a half by the time he'd finished recruiting. Undeterred by the sheer scale of the trial, Francis applied the complex double-blind, placebo-controlled approach recently pioneered by the British Medical Research Council's whooping cough vaccine trials. It was – and still is – the most rigorous way to test a vaccine, but it's never before or since been applied on such an enormous scale.

Francis and his team spent a year recruiting, injecting and following up. As they pored over their reams of data, anticipation across America was building to a fever pitch. Francis announced the results on 12 April 1955, the tenth anniversary of Roosevelt's death, to hundreds of reporters packed into Rackham Hall in Ann Arbor, Michigan.

Francis's announcement was broadcast live in cinemas across America, and audiences quickly realised that, unlike Salk, Francis was no showman. He droned on about the technical details of vaccine preparation and testing while the nation hung on his every word in case it was the word that answered the only question anyone cared about: did the vaccine work? When he said that it was effective in 65–85 per cent of the children who received it, America rejoiced. The victory of the March of Dimes was announced over factory tannoy systems while church bells and air-raid sirens sounded the nation's jubilation. The cattleman, the housewife and the machinist had defeated polio.

The celebration was premature. With it came political pressure, which, combined with the scant consideration given to scaling up manufacture, set the stage for a disastrous blunder.

The Cutter Incident

America wanted to get Salk's vaccine into children as soon as possible. Pharmaceutical companies rushed to production with hastily issued government licences but neither the facilities nor the expertise to safely handle poliovirus.

What happened next was tragic and entirely avoidable: large numbers of children were injected with poliovirus that had not been properly inactivated. The 'Cutter Incident',[16] named for the

Cutter Laboratories* whose botched batches paralysed fifty-one children and killed five, remains one of the worst pharmaceutical disasters in history.

The Cutter's staff knew they weren't completely inactivating the virus going into their vaccines, and had even discussed their difficulties with Youngner, who was horrified that they hadn't halted production to sort out these issues. Youngner reported the problem to Salk, who, never a man to concern himself with inconvenient details, did not pass the information on to the authorities who could have acted on it.

The Cutter vaccine had also failed safety tests at the government's National Laboratory for Biologics Control. The Cutter Incident was exactly what those tests had been implemented to prevent, but when the failures were reported, concerns from the unglamorous discipline of quality control were crushed under the political pressure to follow up on Francis's announcement.[17]

Even in the year of the Cutter Incident, Salk's inactivated vaccine prevented more poliomyelitis cases than it caused.[18] Nevertheless, it threw a bucket of cold water over national enthusiasm and uptake was less than it might have been.

In Britain, the government contracted Glaxo† to make a version of the inactivated vaccine, using the technique that Salk and Youngner had developed with different strains of the three polioviruses.[19] In 1956, the Ministry of Health made it available to children across the country, but Britain was still somewhat recalcitrant about vaccines and uptake was initially slow. A turning point came in 1959, courtesy of Britain's national religion: football.

Jeff Hall epitomised youthful vigour. He was a right-back for Birmingham City and occasional England captain. When he

---

* The Cutter Laboratories are now defunct, having been bought out by Bayer in 1974.
† Now GlaxoSmithKline.

developed poliomyelitis a couple of days after an energetic ninety minutes against Portsmouth, it made polio feel real even to people who knew no polios themselves. Hall died two weeks later, leading many football clubs to publicly organise vaccinations for their players. For neither the first nor the last time, Britons followed where professional footballers led.

The polio parrot learns to talk

By the late 1950s, Salk's inactivated vaccine was being rolled out around the world. The parrot-stranglers appeared to have won the day, but not everyone had given up on teaching it to talk.

The inactivated vaccine's 65–85 per cent effectiveness was impressive, but it wasn't going to eliminate polio. Moreover, the spectre of the Cutter Incident had never been fully exorcised, even though there were no more cases of poorly inactivated vaccines causing poliomyelitis. The parrot-teachers argued that because an attenuated vaccine would not involve the virulent wild-type, it would be inherently safer because it required no inactivation process for someone to make a mess of.

One of attenuation's leading proponents was the Polish-born Albert Sabin at the University of Cincinnati. By 1954, he had vaccine strains of all three types that were so attenuated, they didn't infect nerve cells at all. To confirm they were safe in humans, he first tested them on convicted prisoners. Drafting prisoners into clinical trials is now considered grossly unethical, but in 1950s America, prisoners were considered an expendable resource for medical progress.

When no prisoners showed any ill effects, Sabin's next test was equally characteristic of the mid-twentieth-century vaccinology. As he later put it, 'Because I could not ask other parents for permission to perform the necessary studies … if I did not believe that the accumulated data were sufficient to warrant studies on my own family, the next phase ... involved detailed studies on my own wife and children, their three playmates, and their ... parents.'[20]

He was following what was then called the 'golden rule' of medical research: don't do anything to your volunteers that you're not willing to do to yourself. The corollary was that before you ask parents to volunteer their children, do whatever you have in mind to your own.

There are good reasons why the golden rule has gone the way of prison trials. Some sixty years later, Sabin's eldest daughter, Deborah, spoke of what the golden rule had meant to her: 'There aren't many people out there who grow up as human guinea pigs. Whose parents are injecting them with things, or giving them things orally, that you have no idea what they're going to do.'[21]

Today's ethical frameworks are designed to protect insti-tutionalised children or prisoners from being coerced into 'volunteering' for medical research. They also relieve the pressure on scientists to demonstrate their confidence in a vaccine's safety by using their own children.

Vaccines across the Iron Curtain

Unlike the inactivated vaccine, Sabin's attenuated vaccine is not injected. Because it used a live virus, it was introduced into the mouth and left to find its way to the intestine in the same way as the wild-type. The route of entry led to it being called the oral polio vaccine, although generations of children remember it simply as the vaccine that came in a sugar cube.

By the time Sabin's attenuated vaccine was ready, it was too late to test it in the USA. No one was going to withhold the well-established inactivated vaccine to take a chance on an unproven vaccine or a placebo.

A solution presented itself in 1956, when the Soviet Union's leading polio researcher, Mikhail Chumakov, visited the USA. Sabin shared his views and his vaccine with Chumakov and started a lasting collaboration.

In 1950s America, collaborating across the Iron Curtain could be a risky business, especially for a man who had been born on the wrong side of it. Sabin risked career-ending censure for un-American activities, but in the event, his gamble paid off.

Chumakov didn't carry out any sort of trial but simply rolled it out. When polio rates fell,[22] he concluded the vaccine was effective and extended the roll-out across the Soviet Union and its Eastern European allies.

By 1960, which country used which vaccine was defined by geopolitical alignment. The USA and its allies used the inactivated vaccine, while the Soviet Bloc used the attenuated vaccine. If anyone had done a proper trial of the attenuated vaccine, it would have revealed what eventually emerged out of years of epidemiological studies: the oral vaccine was more effective, with infections vanishingly rare in children who had completed a course of three doses.

Because the oral vaccine strain infects in the same way as wild-type poliovirus, it triggers a stronger immune response in the intestine, where it's most needed.[23] The better effectiveness led the USA to switch from the inactivated to the oral vaccine in 1961,[24] and Britain followed in 1962.[25]

It looked like the parrot-teachers had triumphed – until it emerged that when Chumakov and Sabin had skipped systematic trials, they had missed the attenuated vaccine's dark side.

Prolonged culture had selected for mutations that adapted the virus to replicating fast in culture rather than infecting a human being. The problem is that once it infects a human's intestine, the selection is reversed and vaccine strains occasionally revert to something similar to the wild poliovirus. The closer they get to their original state, the more dangerous they become.

In the vast majority of cases, the reverted strain does no harm and the immune system clears it after a few days, but as early as 1962, it was recognised that for every million or more doses given,[26] a reverted vaccine strain can cause one case of poliomyelitis.[27] As rare as one in more than a million is, vaccines are not supposed to cause paralytic disease at all. It wasn't until 2000 that anyone found that even if a vaccinee shows no ill effects, a mutated vaccine can infect other people and cause an outbreak of vaccine-derived poliovirus.[28]

Lessons learned from the Cutter Incident prevented it from happening again, and indeed have dramatically improved quality control in the production of all vaccines. The inactivated vaccine remains extremely safe, while, contrary to the early arguments in its favour, the oral vaccine is not. Nevertheless, during the 1950s, 1960s and 1970s, the dangers from the oral vaccine were far less than the dangers of the wild-type poliovirus, and as one country after the other initiated vaccine campaigns, the number of children developing poliomyelitis tumbled.

Endgame

In 1960, Czechoslovakia became the first country to eradicate polio, showing that polio might be a problem that could be solved once and for all. In 1962, Cuba proved the point when it became the first country to mount a systematic polio eradication campaign and succeeded within a few months.[29]

Several others followed suit, and in 1988, polio became the only human disease since smallpox to be targeted for worldwide eradication. By international agreement, the Global Polio Eradication Initiative, or GPEI, was inaugurated to completely eradicate polio from the world by the turn of the millennium.[30]

Twelve years was an incredibly ambitious timeframe, and,

viewed from a world in which children still get poliomyelitis two decades after the deadline, one that's easy to disparage. However, the GPEI's achievements in those twelve years were enormous. The number of cases around the world dropped a hundredfold and the last case of type II poliovirus was seen in 1999.[31] Polio eradication entered what epidemiologists call the endgame, meaning that poliovirus was reduced to a few pockets out of which it was particularly difficult to prise it.

Those pockets continued to shrink and in 2012, type III followed type II into history. At the time of writing, only one pocket of type I remains. Its last stronghold is the mountainous region straddling the border between Afghanistan and Pakistan. In 2011, polio got a helping hand from an unlikely ally: the CIA.

Following the assassination of Osama bin Laden, Pakistani intelligence uncovered a plot that reads as if it were dreamed up by a Bond villain.[32] The CIA believed they had tracked bin Laden into a compound in the city of Abbottabad, but they needed to confirm he was where they thought he was. With the connivance of a regional health official, they organised a campaign to vaccinate children against hepatitis B. They then tested the DNA left on the needles, and when they found children related to bin Laden, they sent in the men in black helicopters to kill him.

The backlash was predictable. Islamist militias came to see anyone involved in vaccination programmes as potential CIA informants and by 2014, thirty healthcare workers had been murdered.[33] Despite the dangers, the heroic efforts of health-care workers on both sides of the border keep polio teetering on the brink of eradication. Some years have seen fewer than fifty cases recorded, but the type I poliovirus has proved frustratingly tenacious. Not only does it cling on in its border stronghold, but several times, an infected individual has inadvertently carried it further afield and caused a flare-up in a part of the world where vaccination had been interrupted.

Those flare-ups show us that for as long as poliovirus is circulating anywhere in the world, it can turn up anywhere else. As long as there is a risk of an infected traveller reintroducing it, children need to be protected by vaccination.

Most countries now use the safer, if less effective, inactivated vaccine, because even if some vaccinated children are not protected, there are few enough of them to make it vanishingly unlikely that they will be infected by those occasional infected travellers. In Britain, the switch was made in 2004, and since 2017, the inactivated vaccine has been given as part of the Infanrix '6-in-1' vaccine, combined with the diphtheria, tetanus, whooping cough, Hib and hepatitis B vaccines.

There is reason to hope that the checkmate of full eradication will come in the next few years. In 2013, Vincent Racaniello, a leading polio virologist, described polio as 'truly a virus with a brilliant past, but no future',[34] and as long as vaccination continues worldwide, that will remain true.

The top plot on the opposite page shows the percentage of children vaccinated against polio by their second birthday. The middle plot shows the number of poliomyelitis cases. The bottom panel shows the number of deaths attributed to polio.

All three plots show data from the beginning of systematic records until 2020. Vaccine coverage data is from England and Wales until 1977 and from England only from 1978 onward.[35, 36] Reports of cases and deaths are from England and Wales.[37]

Children vaccinated by their second birthday

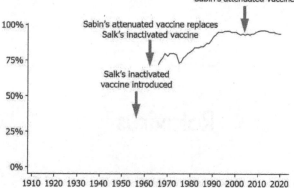

Polio cases

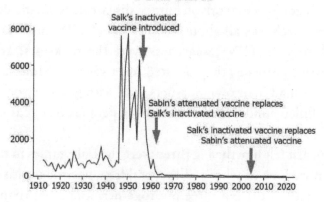

Polio deaths

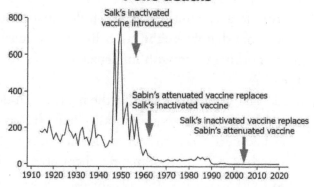

Chapter 12

Rotavirus

When I left zoology to work on human disease in 2002, infectious disease research was all about the 'big three': HIV, malaria and tuberculosis. The HIV researchers were the rockstars, armed with massive grants as they quested for a vaccine. Malaria and tuberculosis had their own pursuers, and with good reason. The big three killed hundreds of thousands of people every year – and still do.[1]

At times, it felt like the big three were the only games in town, but when we look at what's killing children, gastroenteritis kills more than all of the big three put together[2] and more than any other disease except pneumonia.

Gastroenteritis is a catch-all term for inflammation of the stomach or intestines that we might call bellyache, stomach flu – even though it's nothing to do with influenza viruses – or, more viscerally, the shits.

Diarrhoea doesn't grab headlines like the big three. It doesn't spark exciting debates about sexual morality like HIV or invite donations for bed-nets that protect children from malaria-carrying mosquitoes. Children squirting themselves to death is not a subject most of us care to contemplate, but fortunately, some strong-stomached scientists do contemplate it so the rest of us don't have to.

Few parents would be surprised to learn that a lot of microbes can cause diarrhoea in young children. There are many reasons why what goes in one end comes out the other with an unpredictable consistency, but rotavirus stands out as the most likely cause of diarrhoea bad enough to send a child to hospital or worse.

Rotavirus is also one of the most spectacular successes of twenty-first-century vaccinology, but it's a success that's received so little attention that even as an infectious disease immunologist, I was only vaguely aware of it until I started researching this book.

The Mexico City study

It's a lucky child anywhere in the world who makes it to their fifth birthday without being infected with rotavirus at least once, and a very unusual child who hasn't had several infections by then.[3] For most of us, rotavirus caused yet another passing bout of diarrhoea we inflicted on our parents, but sometimes, the diarrhoea dehydrates a child so badly that he needs to be hospitalised.

To understand how and why rotavirus makes some children so ill, we need to understand how it behaves in the large majority of mild cases. The only way to do that is through studying a lot of babies' faeces, which is what Raúl Velázquez of Mexico City's Instituto Nacional de la Nutrición did.[4]

Velázquez's team recruited 200 babies at birth and collected a stool sample every week for two years.[5] This sort of 'prospective cohort' study depends as much on getting the logistics right as the science. The right sample needs to be collected from the right child at the right time and processed in the laboratory before it deteriorates. Field workers ask after the children with regular questionnaires, giving answers that need to be collated with laboratory data so all the different pieces of information can be related to the right child at the right age. It's complex, it's expensive, and we can only guess at the collective sigh of relief that Velázquez's team must have released when the last child started their terrible twos.

It also collects information that can't be collected in any other way.

Velázquez's Mexico City study showed some children picking up rotavirus before they were a week old, which wasn't altogether a bad thing. They were still young enough to be protected by their mothers' antibodies,[6] and that wasn't the only help they got from their mothers. Breast milk is suffused with antibodies that flow through the gut, neutralising viruses before they have a chance to latch on to a baby's cells.[7]

The maternal antibodies that protect against rotavirus don't last long. A third of the babies were infected before they were six months old.[8] By their first birthday, rotavirus had caught up with two-thirds. Hardly any had escaped by the time they bade a final *adiós* to the study field workers at two years.

An infection of the small intestine

How rotavirus infected them is a question that has still been only partially answered. We know it's transmitted by the same faecal-oral route as polio, with viruses that come out in one child's faeces finding their way into another's mouth.

However, we also know that the faecal-oral route is not the whole story.

Like other faecal-oral viruses, rotavirus is extremely resilient outside the body. It can survive on the skin for more than an hour, and is very easily transferred between hands and surfaces.[9]

Someone changing a child's nappy can't help spreading any virus around, and if there's one thing that babies and toddlers can be relied on to do, it's to stuff anything grabbable into their mouths.

Good hygiene usually gives some protection against faecal-oral pathogens, but it doesn't help much against rotavirus,[10] which suggests it has an alternative way in. That route is probably through airborne droplets created when a rotavirus-infected child vomits. The evidence for droplet-borne infection is indirect, inferred from most rotavirus infections in Britain and the USA happening during the winter.[11] That's not a pattern we see with other faecal-oral infections, which happen all year round, but it's typical of droplet-borne viruses like influenza.

What we know for sure is that once rotavirus gets into a child's mouth, it follows everything else he swallows down his throat, through his stomach and into his small intestine, where it infects a type of cell called the mature villous cell.[12] Other viruses, like polio and measles, do their worst when they escape their initial infection site to go rampaging around the body. Rotavirus doesn't do that. It stays in those mature villous cells, raising the question of how a virus that's so fastidious about its location can be so destructive.

The answer lies in rotavirus having a trick we see more often in bacteria than viruses: it produces a toxin. The NSP4 toxin forces the cells lining the intestine to draw water from the child's body into the intestine.[13] Diarrhoea is mostly water, which is what makes it so disgustingly liquid.

Having primed the pump, NSP4 pulls the handle by triggering intestinal spasms that cause diarrhoea and vomiting.[14] The fluids that come out of one or both ends are packed full of rotavirus, and the more copiously they're projected into the outside world, the more likely they are to find someone else to infect.

The NSP4 toxin is why rotavirus can cause such dangerous

dehydration. A small child needs water for his metabolic processes, not for firing viruses at other small children.

Velázquez's team found that the first time rotavirus infected a
child, that child had a fifty-fifty chance of getting through that
infection with no diarrhoea at all. Among the unlucky half, the
diarrhoea ranged from the sort of mild bout that every baby suffers now and again to illness bad enough to be classed as severe.

Velázquez didn't record how many of the 200 children were
hospitalised, but it's almost certain that some would have
been. Rotavirus hospitalises one child in fifty before their fifth
birthday.[15]

There's no medication that targets rotavirus directly, so all a
hospital can do is keep a child hydrated. It's a simple procedure,
and is usually all it takes to support him through the week or so
that the rotavirus infection takes to run its course.

Rotavirus does its worst where there's no hospital to go to. In
many parts of the world, parents can only wait and hope that
their child doesn't turn out to be that one in fifty. If they draw
the short straw and rotavirus reduces their child to a feverish,
diarrhoeal wreck, all they can do is hope for the best. They may
get lucky and see their child pull through.

They may not.

As recently as the mid-2000s, rotavirus was killing one in
every 300 children born anywhere in the world before their fifth
birthday.[16] There are a lot of short straws to draw.

Remembering one strain but infected by many

While rotavirus is replicating in the intestinal lining, the
immune response attacks it from both sides at once. Killer
T-cells work their way in to destroy infected cells before they

have a chance to release new virus. Antibodies are secreted into the mucus lining the inside of the intestine to neutralise viruses trying to find their way out. The infection doesn't last long under the onslaught, which is why even severe cases rarely last longer than a week.

The immune memory is now primed and the T-cells and antibodies remain on patrol. The antibodies that attacked rotavirus on its way out remain in place to block any more from coming in, and if they get past the antibodies, the T-cells kill any infected cells before the infection can get established.

Unfortunately, the T-cells and antibodies are only completely effective against the rotavirus strain that activated them in the first place. When we talk about rotavirus, we're not talking about a single virus that leaves us with lifelong immunity, like mumps or measles. We're talking about a lot of related strains.

Exactly how many is a moving target thanks to a particular trick of the rotavirus. While most viruses have all their genes on a single strand of DNA or RNA, rotavirus's twelve genes are split between eleven separate RNA strands. When two different rotaviruses infect and replicate in the same cell, the genes mix and match so that each progeny virus has some genes from one of the two ancestral strains and some from the other. This 'reassortment' is as close as viruses ever come to sex, which is fundamentally a way of mixing up the genes of two individuals.

We inherit genes from our mothers and our fathers, giving us features of both, but in a combination that makes each of us unique. As with us, so with a reassorted rotavirus. If that new virus is unique enough, it will be only partially recognised by the immune memory triggered by either of its ancestral strains.

In the Mexico City study, Velázquez found that children infected once would encounter a different strain and be infected again. And again. And again. Most were infected at least twice in their first two years. A few were infected as many as five times.

Every infection expanded the children's repertoire of immune memory, but the repertoire is never complete. Even adults pick up the occasional rotavirus infection, often while caring for their children's gastroenteritis.[17] However, rotavirus only occasionally makes adults seriously ill. Serious gastroenteritis in adults is far more likely to be caused by norovirus, the notorious 'winter vomiting bug'.[18]

The good news is that while immune memory to one rotavirus strain can't stop another from infecting, it can mitigate the severity of that infection. Velázquez found that most severe cases were during the first infection and some during the second. After that, the children's immune memories limited the damage to a few days of liquid in the nappy.[19]

For vaccinologists, the seriously ill children were the reason to pay attention to rotavirus, but the many who got through their first infection unscathed suggested a way forward because their immune memory was as robust as those who had been seriously ill.

Their first infection had acted as we would want a vaccine to act.

It suggested the possibility of tweaking the wild-type into a strain that could be trusted never to make a child seriously ill but always to trigger immune memory. It was a solid theory. The difficult part was putting it into practice.

The discovery of rotavirus

In the mid-twentieth century, the prevailing view was that gastroenteritis was caused by bacteria. If hospital laboratories didn't always find a bacterium in the stool samples of their gastroenteritis patients, they didn't expect a perfect hit rate. The culprit would be one among many species of bacteria shot out of someone's gut, and bacteria species can be hard to tell apart by peering down a microscope.

Sometimes a whole outbreak went undiagnosed. One such mystery was a wave of upchucking that swept through a school in Norwalk, Ohio, in 1968. No one found out what caused it until three years later, when Robert Chanock and Albert Kapikian at the National Institutes of Health dug some samples out of a laboratory freezer to try a new technique called immune electron microscopy. They found them packed full of a virus that no one had seen before, which they called norovirus after Norwalk.[20]

Many medical scientists started wondering how many cases of viral gastroenteritis had been written off to non-existent bacteria. One of them was Ruth Bishop at Melbourne's Royal Children's Hospital, which, like any hospital that treated children, saw a lot of severe diarrhoea. Bishop followed Chanock and Kapikian's approach of using immune electron microscopy, and sure enough, she found another new virus.[21]

When scientists started looking for Bishop's virus, it turned up in intestines all over the world – and not all of them were human. At the East Birmingham Hospital, medical researchers compared notes with their veterinary colleagues and found they were dealing with a similar problem. Bishop's virus didn't only cause diarrhoea in children; it also caused it in cattle.[22]

The Birmingham team coined the name 'rotavirus', because they thought its capsid looked like the spokes of a wheel, the Latin word for which is 'rota'.

Some researchers were looking for viruses in intestinal maladies other than gastroenteritis. Tasuke Konno of Tohoku School of Medicine in Sendai, Japan, led the first study that looked at a rare condition called intussusception.

The intestines are encased in a tube of muscle that wafts food along with a series of rhythmic waves. It's not something we usually spare much thought for – unless it goes wrong. One way it can go wrong is if the rhythmic contractions become so unco-ordinated that instead of wafting food along the intestine, they fold part of the intestine into another. That's intussusception. It doesn't happen often, but when it does, it's usually in children under two years old.[23]

Konno wanted to know what caused it, and, like everyone else interested in intestinal problems in the late 1970s, he looked for viruses. He found that more than a third of babies and toddlers hospitalised with intussusception were infected with rotavirus.[24]

His discovery would return to haunt the quest for a rotavirus vaccine.

The RotaShield story: in Edward Jenner's footsteps

In the mid-1980s, that quest was started by Chanock and Kapikian, the discoverers of norovirus. They knew that different rotaviruses infected many different mammal species, and they knew those rotaviruses rarely transmitted from one species to another. Mouse rotaviruses stuck to mice, cattle rotaviruses stuck to cattle and human rotaviruses stuck to humans.

Chanock and Kapikian took their inspiration from Edward Jenner, the grandfather of vaccination. Jenner had found that the immune response to cowpox protected humans against the related smallpox, so perhaps the immune response to a cow rotavirus would protect humans against the related human rotaviruses. When they tried it, their results were disappointing. Their experimental vaccines worked reasonably well in some trials but not at all in others.[25]

Chanock and Kapikian went back to the drawing board. They had known that human rotavirus made children ill but left them immune to it. Now they knew an animal rotavirus that didn't make children ill wouldn't trigger immunity that protected against a human rotavirus. Putting those two facts together, they reasoned that they needed a safe animal rotavirus carrying a component of the human rotavirus for the immune system to react to.

Today, a vaccinologist can turn to well-established gene-editing techniques. Chanock and Kapikian had to improvise. They used rotavirus's reassortment trick against it, infecting cells with a monkey rotavirus and, at the same time, with a human rotavirus. The progeny viruses that came out of the infected cells contained various combinations of genes from the human and monkey rotaviruses, including the one they were looking for: eleven genes from the harmless monkey rotavirus and one from the human rotavirus.

They repeated the trick with four different human rotavirus strains to produce a cocktail of four different vaccine strains, each made up of four identical monkey rotaviruses carrying one gene from a different human rotavirus. They hoped that when they dripped their vaccine cocktail into a child's mouth, all four strains would find their way down to the small intestine and infect the mature villous cells in the same way as a wild-type human rotavirus. The difference was that the monkey rotavirus would be so far out of its element that a child's immune system would stamp it out before it could do any damage, but would retain a memory of proteins from four human rotavirus strains. It wouldn't completely protect them against every strain they'd encounter, but, Chanock and Kapikian hoped, it would spare them anything worse than mild diarrhoea.

They were effectively using the monkey rotavirus as a viral vector for the human rotavirus protein, using the principle that would later underpin the Oxford/AZ COVID-19 vaccine. However, the terminology had yet to be coined, and they called their strategy 'modified Jennerian'.

Chanock and Kapikian's early trials caught the attention of the pharmaceutical giant Wyeth-Ayerst, who funded phase 3 trials in the USA and Finland. They showed the vaccine protected children against diarrhoea and, more importantly, against the sort of severe diarrhoea that would put an American or Finnish child in hospital and a child in a less fortunate part of the world in an early grave. In 1999, the US government's Advisory Committee on Immunization Practices (ACIP) recommended that children across the USA should be given the vaccine virus that was now called RotaShield.[26] You can't involve a pharmaceutical firm without getting some corporate branding.

There was just one fly in the ointment: intussusception.

The RotaShield story: first hopes dashed

Tasuke Konno had shown that human rotaviruses occasionally cause intussusception. What nobody knew was whether the monkey rotavirus in RotaShield could cause it.

During the RotaShield trials, only five of 10,054 children given RotaShield developed intussusception. That was about the normal rate in American children,[27] so there was no reason to think the vaccine was causing intussusception. It would have been strange if the rate was any lower.

The problem was that only one of the 4,633 children in the placebo group developed intussusception, which *was* lower than the normal rate and *was* strange – although not that strange, because intussusception is so rare. It would only have needed one more child to develop intussusception and two in 4,633 wouldn't look different to five in 10,054. This is why clinical trials need to be so large: even with data from nearly 15,000 children, not enough had developed intussusception to give a clear result.

The lack of a clear result was reassuring. If RotaShield caused intussusception in even one child in a thousand, it would have jumped out as being twice the normal rate.

The ACIP concluded that the trials provided no evidence that RotaShield caused intussusception, but added the caveat that 'postvaccination surveillance for occurrence of rare side effects is important'.[28]

The RotaShield roll-out began in October 1998. By July 1999, fifteen cases of intussusception had been reported.[29] All fifteen recovered, and, in themselves, fifteen reports didn't prove that RotaShield was causing the intussusception. RotaShield wasn't the only cause of intussusception, and among the tens of thousands of children who had received it, those fifteen reports didn't add up to an unusually large number.

On the other hand, the ACIP had warned that intussusception reports should be taken seriously. RotaShield vaccination was suspended[30] and the CDC commissioned two different studies to take a closer look. One study compared the intussusception rate in vaccinated and unvaccinated children. They reviewed the records of 460,000 children, of whom 56,000 had been given RotaShield, giving them a lot more to work with than the clinical trials of RotaShield had given the ACIP. The results were clear: RotaShield nearly tripled the chance of intussusception.[31]

Another team approached the question from the other end. They dug through the records of children hospitalised with intussusception to see whether they were more likely to have received RotaShield than children of the same age born in the same hospital. Once again, the association was clear. Children with intussusception were twice as likely to have received RotaShield as their peers who had not.[32]

That was the end of RotaShield.

RotaShield would have saved thousands of children from severe diarrhoea for every case of intussusception, but severe dehydrating diarrhoea is a much less serious condition than intussusception.[33]

RotaShield still had its advocates, most of whom had never seen American children as its main beneficiaries. They had wanted it for where there was no hospital bed and friendly nurse to rehydrate a baby with severe diarrhoea. They wanted it rolled out where children with severe diarrhoea had to take their chances.

There was a flip side to their argument. Where there is no hospital capable of treating severe diarrhoea, there's certainly no hospital capable of treating intussusception. Charles Weijer, an ethicist at Dalhousie University in Halifax, Canada, estimated that with no hospital treatment, RotaShield would save between 160 and 213 children for every child it killed.[34]

It was the same logic that, a few decades earlier, had underpinned the continued use of the oral polio vaccine in the USA after it was known to occasionally cause poliomyelitis. At the dawn of the new millennium, the ethic of the greater good proved to be too brutally utilitarian. The medical maxim of 'first, do no harm' was now the watchword.

The ethical arguments puttered on for several years, but with Wyeth no longer making RotaShield, their outcome was moot.

A new generation of rotavirus vaccines

RotaShield left more than an ethical debate behind it. It also left two practical lessons: that a vaccine against rotavirus was possible, but that any new vaccine needed to be tested with a lot more than 15,000 recruits to confirm whether or not it caused intussusception.[35]

In 2006, two new rotavirus vaccines were presented in the pages of the *New England Journal of Medicine*, one of the world's foremost medical journals. Both had proved effective at protecting children against rotavirus, and both had been tested on four times as many volunteers as RotaShield had. Neither showed any sign of causing intussusception.

One of those vaccines followed the 'modified Jennerian' approach that Chanock and Kapikian had pioneered with RotaShield. Merck's RotaTeq[36] was based on a rotavirus isolated from a calf – making it more literally Jennerian than RotaShield – reassorted to express human rotavirus genes. Each vial of vaccine contained five different variants, each with a gene from a different human rotavirus strain.[37]

The vaccine currently used in Britain is GlaxoSmithKline's Rotarix, based on a virus that emerged from the rear end of a small child in 1989. At the time, David Bernstein and Richard Ward of Cincinnati Children's Medical Center were trialling one of the early 'Jennerian' rotavirus vaccines. They saw the same thing that Velázquez found in Mexico City: infection with wild-type rotavirus protected against serious illness in later infections and it did so a lot better than the vaccine they were testing.[38]

They isolated one of those wild-type viruses and, while Chanock and Kapikian were reassorting human and animal rotaviruses, Bernstein and Ward opted for the more traditional approach of attenuation. They cultured their rotavirus into submission on monkey kidney cells until they had a strain that caused no ill effects in adult volunteers.[39] When it didn't harm the adults, they tested it in young children. It didn't make them ill, and over the next two years, the vaccinated children handled their inevitable rotavirus infections far better than children who had received a placebo.[40]

Bernstein and Ward's virus had come so far from that anonymous child that it was now a vaccine strain. It was time to bring in the big guns – or rather, the deep pockets.

GlaxoSmithKline had funded Ward and Bernstein's small-scale trials, but now they had a vaccine, they threw their full weight behind it. They passaged it through several more cultures of monkey kidney cells before they ran trials in twelve countries. There was no sign of intussusception or any other serious side effects, but it did protect children from severe diarrhoea.[41] GlaxoSmithKline rebranded the vaccine virus Rotarix, and it joined RotaTeq in being rolled out around the world.

Rotavirus today

In 2013, Britain chose Rotarix over RotaTeq because GlaxoSmithKline offered a better price in response to the NHS's tender.[42] Britain joined an increasing number of countries to vaccinate children against rotavirus and, at the same time, to worry about rotavirus vaccines causing intussusception. As large as the trials that tested both vaccines were, they couldn't have picked up a side effect that was too rare to appear more than once or twice among the 60,000 children in those trials.

In 1998, it took the CDC only a few months to identify the one case in 10,000 caused by RotaShield. A decade and a half since RotaTeq and Rotarix were rolled out, neither the CDC nor their various counterparts around the world have found any sign of either RotaTeq or Rotarix causing intussusception.

On the contrary, they actively prevent it. Researchers scrutinising hospital records from across England found that as Rotarix protected children from severe diarrhoea, so it protected them from intussusception caused by rotavirus.[43]

RotaTeq and Rotarix's most spectacular successes have been in low-income countries where many parents can't get their children to hospitals. Between 2000 and 2013, rotavirus deaths around the world halved[44] even though RotaTeq and Rotarix had yet to reach all the countries where they were most needed. Since then, more and more countries have been incorporating rotavirus vaccination into their childhood schedule, and it's a safe bet that the next review will reveal an even greater fall in rotavirus deaths.

The defanging of rotavirus is one of those good-news stories that rarely gets reported. Before the vaccines were available, the half-million children it killed every year[45] was too abstract a figure to warrant more than a brief mention on a quiet news day. When the story became a quarter of a million children *not* dying, there was always a minor politician who couldn't keep his trousers on or a B-list celebrity having a Twitter meltdown that was deemed more newsworthy.

But those quarter of a million children get to go on living.

Chapter 13

Measles

Roald Dahl has enthralled generations of children with the word-mangling antics of *The BFG*, but few notice the story behind the two-word dedication: 'For Olivia'. Olivia's story was short, simple and contained none of Dahl's trademark humour:

> Olivia, my eldest daughter, caught measles when she was seven years old ... one morning, when she was well on the road to recovery, I was sitting on her bed showing her how to fashion little animals out of coloured pipe-cleaners, and when it came to her turn to make one herself, I noticed that her fingers and her mind were not working together and she couldn't do anything.
>
> 'Are you feeling all right?' I asked her.
>
> 'I feel all sleepy,' she said.
>
> In an hour, she was unconscious. In twelve hours she was dead.[1]

In the words of actress Patricia Neal, Olivia's mother and Dahl's wife, 'Roald came back from the hospital and he cried. Oh, he cried.'[2]

Olivia's parents speak for generations of parents whose children have been killed or disabled by a virus nastier than any of Dahl's child-munching villains.

Measles infection: fever, rash and immune amnesia

Two things make measles so nasty: it's extremely good at passing from one person to another, and it spreads throughout the body.

A child like Olivia catches measles in the same way she might catch a common cold: someone who already has measles breathes out virus-laden droplets, which she then breathes in. Like a cold virus, measles infects cells in the sinuses or the back of the throat. Unlike a cold virus, it doesn't stay there.[3] It hijacks the lymphocytes of the immune system and rides them through the bloodstream to every corner of the child's body.

While measles is spreading, the child appears to be perfectly healthy. She goes to school and plays with friends, with nothing to show that every time she breathes out, she exhales a cloud of measles-laden droplets.

She'll stay healthy for a week or two,[4] which is much longer than with most viruses, and is one reason why measles is one of the most infectious microbes around. The average person infected with measles can infect five times as many people as the average person infected with influenza.[5] In one case, an American teenager infected sixty-nine people at her school and on the buses she took there.[6] In another, an athlete at the 1991 International Special Olympics infected twenty-five people simply by being in the same stadium.[7] In both of those cases, the one infected person probably passed measles on to every non-immune person who came anywhere near them.

The first an infected child or her parents know of the measles infection is when she develops a runny nose and a cough. Her parents might think she's catching a cold, but worse is to come. A couple of days later, she is running a high fever and a rash flares up across her whole body.

She and her parents may think this is the measles virus getting started, but in fact, the rash is caused by her immune system calling time's up. Her lymphocytes have been adapting to the invading virus since it first infected her and, after a week or two, her killer T-cells are ready to kill the cells it's replicating in.

Unfortunately for the child, that's a lot of cells throughout her body. The skin rash is the visible manifestation of the purging taking place in every organ.

It may not look like it, but the lymphocytes have the upper hand from the moment the rash appears. They're already stopping the virus from completing its reproduction, so she's no longer breathing it out and can no longer spread the disease. That's unlikely to be much consolation for the two or three days it takes her immune system to finish the job, and her body will take longer than that to repair the damage.

There are no antiviral medicines that work on measles, so treatment options fall into the category of supportive: keeping her alive and as comfortable as possible until her immune system fights off the virus. In most cases, that would mean syrups that her parents can buy over the counter, which bring down her pain and fever. In a severe case, it might mean an intensive care unit's ventilator helping her to breathe. Hospitals can now offer supportive treatment so good that even if a child becomes critically ill with measles, she'll probably survive it. In modern Britain, measles only kills around one in every thousand children who catch it,[8] although it remains a painful and traumatic experience for that child and her parents.

For most children, the road to recovery begins when the rash and fever ease off. Olivia Dahl was not so lucky. The measles virus got into her brain and caused a rare, extremely serious complication called encephalitis. If it isn't fatal, measles encephalitis can cause permanent brain damage.[9]

Because the measles virus attacks the immune system's lymphocytes, it can open the door to the infections that those lymphocytes would normally protect against. Children with measles often develop pneumonia, but the infection is usually a bacterium or virus other than measles itself.[10]

Measles also destroys lymphocytes that carry the immune memory of past infections and vaccinations. The 'immune amnesia' caused by measles strips a child of some of that immune memory, leaving her vulnerable to infections she's already fought off once.

Among the generations of children who were defenceless against measles, we have no idea how many survived it only to be killed by an infection they were immune to before their bout of measles. All we know is that it's a lot.[11]

The measles of David Edmonston

Part of Olivia Dahl's tragedy is that after centuries of unavoidable deaths from measles, hers was among the last. When she died in 1962, the measles vaccine was well on the way to being widely available.

It was a product of the flurry of research into viral vaccines that swept American universities in the mid-twentieth century. While the March of Dimes had funded the development of a whole new set of techniques in virology and after the Second World War, the US government's funding bodies started to look beyond infections that interfered with military operations and began to support research into diseases of children.

One of the leaders of the virus boom was John Enders at Harvard, the man who first cultured the poliovirus. He recruited a physician called Thomas Peebles to work on measles, which is how, in 1954, Peebles found himself taking throat swabs and blood samples from eleven-year-old David Edmonston.

He was one of several boys in the infirmary of Boston's elite Fay Boarding School. They had been put there by a measles outbreak, which drew Peebles in search of measles virus to isolate. David was so ill that he wasn't fully aware of what was going on around him. Years later, he told a journalist, 'It was pretty nasty, and I was pretty much out of it the whole time.'[12]

If any of the sick boys were less out of it than David, they were probably more impressed by Peebles having been a decorated navy bomber pilot than by his hopes of putting an end to measles. Peebles chose David as one of his subjects because his rash had appeared in the last twenty-four hours, which he thought meant David's infection was at its height. It wasn't yet known that the rash indicates that measles is on its last legs.

Peebles got no virus from the throat swabs – it was too late in the course of David's infection for that – but there was still some measles floating around his bloodstream. That was all Peebles needed. He only needed to isolate measles virus once to have a strain he could attenuate into a vaccine. As long as the virus kept replicating, it would keep mutating, and a lucky few of those mutants would be better suited to laboratory culture than the human being they had come from.

If, that is, Peebles could keep the virus supplied with cells in which to replicate. In 1954, the science of laboratory cell culture was in its infancy. Today's virologists can order from a range of different cell types out of a catalogue and download instructions on how to keep them alive. Peebles had to work with whatever cells he and Enders could get their hands on. Initially, they succeeded in infecting human kidney cells, and when the supply of kidneys dried up, they switched it to cells from placentas discarded from a maternity ward.[13]

They may not have realised that they were succeeding without having a consistent supply of one cell type for the same reason that measles is such a nasty infection in the first place. It's able to spread through the body because it can infect many different types of cells, which makes it a lot less fussy about the cells it replicates in than many other viruses.

Preparing fresh cells for culture and passaging small samples of measles virus into them every few days was painstaking work that would be lost if any fungi or bacteria got into the cultures. Like most lead scientists, Peebles and Enders left it to their technicians, but unlike most lead scientists of their day, they acknowledged Ann Holloway and Yinette Chang[14] when they eventually published their work.

The breakthrough came after the twenty-eighth passage, when the measles virus started replicating in chicken embryo cells. When Peebles had first isolated the virus from David's blood, it had refused to do that. Holloway and Chang were now passaging a virus fundamentally different to the virus that infects human beings. Not so different that the immune system could distinguish it from the wild-type, but different enough that it wouldn't be able to make a child ill. At least, that was what Peebles hoped.

His hope was only partially realised. The 'Edmonston B' strain caused fevers and rashes in more than half the children into whom it was injected.[15] The US government reasoned this was better than a natural infection, which would cause a worse disease in nearly all the children it infected. They licensed the first measles vaccine in 1963 and began mass vaccination in 1967.[16]

In Britain, the NHS was less enthusiastic. The vaccine was licensed but was not included in the childhood vaccination schedule, and few parents opted to give it to their children.

Meanwhile, American scientists had not finished with the Edmonston strain. Peebles and Enders had been happy to give samples to anyone who asked, and Anton Schwarz and Maurice

Hilleman, who worked for the competing pharmaceutical companies of Pitman-Moore and Merck respectively, had both taken up the offer. Their teams spent years passing the measles virus from one tube of chicken embryo cells to another, pushing it further and further from its human-adapted ancestors.

Schwarz and Hilleman produced very similar vaccine strains that were rolled out in Britain, the USA and several other countries in 1968. Their vaccine strains are still used in most of the world's measles vaccines. Most of the children they are given to don't react at all, although, like all vaccines, they sometimes cause mild side effects. For every twenty children vaccinated, between one and three develop a mild fever or a rash, though they fully recover within three days.[17] A measles vaccine strain is still a strain of the measles virus. More importantly, the vaccine strains do not cause immune amnesia.[18]

The plots on pages 213–14 show that in Britain, cases and deaths began to fall soon after the vaccine was introduced. Uptake was relatively slow, but it increased steadily and, by 1983, 60 per cent of children had been vaccinated by the time they were two years old. In 1988, by which time uptake was over 75 per cent, the NHS replaced the single-dose vaccine with the MMR, combining measles, mumps and rubella in a single injection. By the early 1990s, uptake was over 90 per cent and cases started to fall more rapidly.

At present, there are two versions of the MMR used in Britain under the brand names of Priorix and M-M-RVAXPRO, produced by GlaxoSmithKline and Merck respectively, both of which can trace their ancestry directly back to a fever-ridden boy in a boarding school infirmary in 1954.

Peebles didn't forget David Edmonston, who is the source of nearly all the measles vaccine used around the world. He returned to thank David for the most auspicious case of measles in history. 'They offered me a steak dinner,' Edmonston later recalled, 'but I didn't care for steak.'[19]

Timing the vaccination

It would take longer to work out the ideal age at which to give the vaccine.

Initially, children were vaccinated at birth, but throughout the 1970s, measles outbreaks continued among vaccinated children. It turned out that the antibodies children were receiving from their mothers were killing the vaccine strain before the children had a chance to react to it.[20]

There was a simple solution: delay the vaccination until children are one year old, when there are not enough maternal antibodies to get in the way. The catch is that maternal antibodies usually wane after a few months, leaving a window of vulnerability between the disappearance of the maternal antibodies and the vaccination. To make matters worse, children infected in the first year are particularly vulnerable to the more severe manifestations of the disease.[21]

Fortunately, the measles vaccine is among the most effective ever developed; two doses give lifelong protection in around 99 per cent of children.[22]

In Britain and many other countries, the current regime is for the first dose at one year and the second at three years and four months, in case some maternal antibodies had lingered on at one year.

Those two doses not only prevent a child from becoming ill with measles, but prevent measles from infecting at all, which stops measles from using an infected person as a Trojan horse to infect babies who have not yet been vaccinated. If nineteen out of every twenty people in a population are immune to measles, it's unlikely to be able to get a foothold, and the unvaccinated twentieth should be safe from ever coming into contact with someone who might infect them.[23]

The beginning of the end for measles?

That blood sample that Thomas Peebles took from David Edmonston may ultimately prove to be the beginning of the end for the measles virus – albeit a very drawn-out end. The measles vaccine is now distributed around the world, and if every child is immunised, measles will have no one left to infect and will die out.

While the world's medical establishments were trying to get the vaccine distributed as widely as possible, the measles vaccine became a bugbear for the world's antivaccine movement. It was first driven to prominence in 1998, when a now struck-off doctor called Andrew Wakefield made the fraudulent claim that the MMR vaccine can cause autism. It does not, and Chapter 21 will cover how we know that, but it was widely reported at the time and the claim is still repeated occasionally despite the conclusive evidence disproving it. It put off enough British parents that uptake of the vaccine fell to a low of 80 per cent in 2003,[24] leaving enough babies unprotected that measles returned to infect several thousand children during the 2010s, killing fourteen of them.[25]

Despite the antivaccine movement, measles has been on the back foot for most of the twenty-first century. While a few parents, mostly in Britain and the USA, were backing away from the measles vaccine, UNICEF was making it available in low-income countries whose governments need assistance in procuring vaccines. Around the world, the estimated number of children dying of measles fell from 540,000 in 2000 to 142,000 in 2018, meaning that the vaccine saved 23 million lives in those eighteen years.[26]

However, with a virus as infectious as measles, it only takes a few vulnerable children to establish an outbreak. That happened in several countries in 2017, and started a slow but steady rise in the number of cases that lasted until 2018.[27] It remains to be seen if this is the beginning of a resurgence or simply a blip.

As long as measles exists anywhere in the world, it remains a threat to unvaccinated children everywhere.

The top plot on page 214 shows the percentage of children vaccinated against measles by their second birthday. The middle plot shows the number of measles cases reported. The bottom plot shows the number of deaths attributed to measles.

All plots are from the beginning of systematic records until 2020. Vaccine coverage data is from England and Wales until 1977 and from England only from 1978 onwards,[28,29] with a gap between 1988 and 1990 due to ambiguous data during the transition from single-dose measles vaccine to MMR. Reports of cases and deaths are from England and Wales.[30]

Children vaccinated by their second birthday

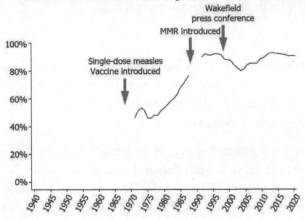

Measles cases

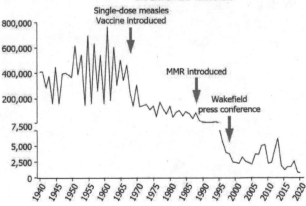

Measles deaths

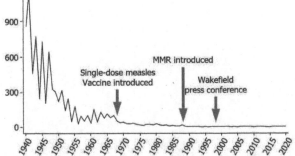

Chapter 14

Mumps

Did you ever notice that Elastigirl speaks through the side of her mouth? That's because the flexible superhero of the *Incredibles* animated films is voiced by Holly Hunter, who has been deaf in one ear since a bout of mumps when she was nine years old. Her asymmetric hearing gave her an asymmetric way of speaking that Pixar's animators worked into Elastigirl's delivery of Hunter's characteristic growl.

Mumps outlasted most of the infections that were once a childhood rite of passage. Parents were lovingly comparing their children's swollen faces to hamsters or chipmunks long after measles and German measles were vaccinated into painful memories.

On parotitis and grimaces

The two parotid glands take up a space that runs from just in front of the ears down to the back of the lower jaw. Most of the time, they secrete saliva without drawing attention to themselves. When mumps virus gets into them, they swell up to take up a lot more space. Parotitis, to give the swelling its medical term, distorts the face so much that it gives mumps its name. A *mump* is an old English word for a grimace.

The mumps virus is in the same family as measles and, like measles, it spreads through the droplets in an infected child's exhalations. As viral infections of the throat go, mumps develops relatively slowly. It spends ten days or more spreading through the parotid glands before it appears in the saliva and the child becomes infectious.

She won't know that, because she still has another week before she starts feeling unwell.[1] That's a whole week to breathe mumps virus all over her classmates, playmates, siblings and anyone else who comes near her. That week is one reason why mumps is twice or three times as infectious as influenza.[2] That's only half as infectious as measles,[3] but it's enough to make mumps one of the more infectious viruses around.

If she's lucky, her immune system will quietly see off the infection without her ever knowing she's had it. That happens in around a third of cases, although being a girl improves her odds. Mumps is nastier in men and boys, while women and girls have a better chance of never developing symptoms at all.[4]

If she's lucky enough to have one of those asymptomatic infections, she'll get to watch the faces of everyone she infected swell up while feeling blessed in having got away with it. More likely, she'll spend a few days in bed with a painful parotitis and fever, failing to see the humour in being called a hamster or a chipmunk.

For most children, that's as bad as it gets. The swelling subsides after a few days, and she'll fully recover, now immune to mumps for the rest of her life.

For an unfortunate few, it can get a lot worse than that.

It's not uncommon for mumps to get into the meninges: the membranes around the brain and spinal cord. Mumps meningitis is unpleasant, but it's rarely a life-threatening emergency like meningitis caused by bacteria like Hib, pneumococcus and meningococcus. Most children recover after a few days of high fevers and vomiting.

Mumps does its worst when it doesn't stop at the meninges. The first account of what happens if it gets into the brain itself was by a physician called Robert Hamilton, who described his treatment of mumps patients in King's Lynn, Norfolk, between 1758 and 1769. One of his patients was a twenty-two-year-old man who 'was seized with a most frantic delirium, the nervous system was shattered with strong convulsions, and he died raving mad the third day after'.[5]

It reads like mumps had caused encephalitis, an infection and inflammation of the brain. There was nothing Hamilton could do to help him. He'd already concluded that letting blood and administering laxatives did nothing to treat the more commonplace swellings of mumps. Hamilton did insist that raising blisters on the parotitis swellings cured his patients, though if he'd paid more attention to what happened in anyone he didn't treat, he would have noticed that the swelling resolved by itself. His patients were recovering despite his administrations, not because of them, thanks to their immune systems clearing the virus before it got into their brains. That delirious, convulsing twenty-two-year-old was not so lucky.

Three centuries later, we now know that blistering only makes a miserable patient even more miserable, but that's as far as mumps treatment has progressed. There is still no drug that stops the mumps virus from replicating. Even in a modern hospital, all doctors can do is treat the symptoms and hope the patient's immune system gets on top of the infection.

In most cases, it does. Only one child in a thousand develops encephalitis, and among those unlucky few, all but around 1.5 per cent recover[6] – mostly. The brain is the last place that anyone wants a battle between their lymphocytes and a virus, because even if the lymphocytes win, they're likely to do some damage in the process. That damage is most likely to be to the nerve cells that process sound. It's not uncommon for mumps to leave a child deaf in one or both ears: not because of damage to the ear itself, but because her ears are no longer connected to the rest of her brain. The deafness is usually temporary, but some, like Holly Hunter, never recover. Before the vaccine was available, mumps was the most common reason for children to become deaf.[7]

When mumps was as inevitable as death and taxes, it was best to get it out of the way before puberty. In adult women, mumps often causes painful swellings of the breasts and ovaries, respectively called 'mastitis' and 'oophoritis'. In adult men, it can cause 'orchitis': a medical term reminiscent of the delicate beauty of an orchid that actually refers to an extremely painful swelling of the testicles. It can lower a man's fertility and occasionally leaves him completely sterile.[8]

The trail of mumps virus led from King's Lynn to Tennessee

Nearly two centuries after Hamilton tormented his patients, science got properly on the trail of the mumps virus with the new techniques – and casual disregard for the people they were used on – that characterised early twentieth-century virology. Claud Johnson and Ernest Goodpasture of Vanderbilt University in Nashville, Tennessee, fitted right in.

Johnson and Goodpasture took an interest in mumps in 1933 when they found that the saliva from a parotitic medical student caused parotitis in monkeys even after they'd passed it through a Chamberland filter.* With electron microscopes still a decade in the future, that remained the working definition of a virus.

---

* See Chapter 2.

They confirmed their filtered saliva contained mumps virus by passing filtered saliva from parotitic monkeys to healthy monkeys. It caused parotitis every time.[9]

They evidently didn't consider monkeys sufficient to prove the point, because their next move was to return their invisible agent to its original organism: human beings. Specifically, children who had not had mumps and so would not be immune to whatever it was they were passing between their monkeys.

A modern research oversight committee would have something to say about that, but in 1933, there was no one to say no. Johnson and Goodpasture killed the fourteenth generation of monkeys they had infected and ground their mumps-ridden parotid glands into an emulsion. They found their children in what they called Johnson's 'home-community', saying he was 'was intimately known by those whose consent was obtained'. Intimately known or not, it's hard to believe that parents would have let him spray infected monkey glands into their children's mouths if they'd known what he was up to. Whatever he told them, that's what he and Goodpasture did to thirteen children.

Nine children developed mumps, confirming that Johnson and Goodpasture had indeed isolated the mumps virus. How Johnson was later regarded in the community where he was 'intimately known' is not on record.

The first attempt: killed mumps vaccines

Johnson and Goodpasture had isolated the mumps virus, but to properly study it, scientists needed a way to culture it in their laboratories. In the 1930s, scientists knew that viruses replicated in living cells, but they weren't very good at keeping cells alive in their laboratories.

Before Goodpasture started spraying mumps around, he'd

developed a technique using cells that came with a built-in culture system: the cells of a chicken embryo inside an egg. All he had to do was keep the egg warm and the embryo cells would live, divide and thrive, ready to receive any virus he injected them with.[10,11]

It was a simple technique that became a mainstay of early virology, but it was only ever a partial solution to the problem of isolating human viruses. Human viruses are adapted to human cells, not chicken cells. Nevertheless, Goodpasture found that several human viruses did replicate in chicken embryos, and mumps turned out to be one of them.

Goodpasture invented the technique of virus culture in chicken eggs and co-discovered the mumps virus, but he didn't put the two together. Among those who did was John Enders, for whom mumps was an early success on his trajectory to becoming America's virus-tamer general.

Mumps proved much easier to work with than an older and more experienced Enders would later find polio and measles to be. When he injected mumps virus into an egg, it started replicating straight away. Enders could sustain it in his laboratory by regularly harvesting it from one egg and injecting it into another. With each 'passage', he checked that he was actually passaging virus by testing it on monkeys. He noticed that the more times he'd passaged the virus, the less severe the parotitis it caused. His mumps virus was becoming attenuated.

As we've seen, virology in mid-twentieth-century America was driven by a buccaneering spirit, with researchers eagerly injecting their concoctions into themselves, their children and anyone else they could get their hands on to see what would happen. When Johnson and Goodpasture deliberately infected healthy children with mumps, they were doing nothing out of the ordinary. Enders, however, was not a buccaneer by nature. He was never comfortable with deliberately infecting children, which might be why he didn't present his attenuated mumps virus as a possible vaccine strain.

Instead, he opted for an inactivated vaccine that wouldn't give a child mumps if it turned out to be less attenuated than he thought.

His inactivated vaccine was certainly safe, but it didn't work very well. Some of Enders's colleagues, who didn't share his qualms, tested it by giving it to children and then spraying wild-type mumps virus into their mouths, and also into the mouths of children whom they hadn't vaccinated. The vaccine protected some of the children to whom it was given, but too many developed parotitis for it to be called effective.

In 1946, Enders published his work on mumps[12] and moved on to polio and measles, which were then higher priorities. He had established two principles that would underpin future mumps research: repeated passages in chicken embryos attenuated it, and a killed-virus vaccine wasn't going to work.

It would be nearly twenty years before those principles were put into practice.

Jeryl Lynn Hilleman's sore throat

On 30 March 1963, five-year-old Jeryl Lynn Hilleman woke her father to tell him she had a sore throat. Her mother had recently died, making it a distressing enough time for her without falling ill in the middle of the night.

Jeryl Lynn's father's first reaction was that of a typical father. He comforted her and tucked her back into bed. Maurice Hilleman, however, was not a typical father. By then, he was entrenched as the head of Merck, Sharpe and Dohme's vaccine division, from where he would take the hepatitis B and pneumococcus vaccines from university laboratories to clinics around the world. His involvement with the mumps vaccine began at a much more seminal stage.

Hilleman left Jeryl Lynn in the care of his housekeeper and drove to his laboratory to pick up some swabs. He returned home, woke up Jeryl Lynn to swab her throat,[13] then drove back to put the samples in his lab freezer and flew off to a conference of the Pan American Health Organization the next day.[14]

Mumps hadn't been high on Hilleman's to-do list, and if he'd wanted to get hold of mumps virus to work on, there were plenty of chipmunk-faced children for him to get it from. Something about Jeryl Lynn waking him up that night must have pushed mumps up his priorities, because when he got back from his conference, he set his team to attenuating Jeryl Lynn's mumps virus using Enders's technique of repeated passages through chicken embryos.

After twelve passages, they tried the vaccine in two institutions for children then called 'mentally retarded'.[15] This is where their buccaneering spirit led Hilleman and his contemporaries into territory that makes for very uncomfortable reading today.

We have a lot to thank men like Hilleman for. One headline writer called him 'the man who saved your life',[16] and for many of us – and we have no way to know which of us – that was no exaggeration. Nevertheless, the research organisations that celebrate him and his contemporaries now impose ethical oversight to make sure nobody saves lives in the same way again.

Recruiting institutionalised children is the sort of thing that oversight committees are there to stop. In the mid-1960s, it was a common practice and, from a purely practical perspective, institutions are the perfect place to test a vaccine. When a virus like mumps got into an institution, which it inevitably did every few years, every child would catch it. Because every child was constantly monitored, there were clear records on all children who had been given a vaccine or a placebo.

Perhaps most uncomfortably, getting an institution's director to agree to a trial involving every child under their care was a lot easier than asking every child's parents individually.

Before condemning the vaccine buccaneers too harshly, we

should remember that they were following the medical ethics of their time. Most tried their vaccines on themselves and often their own children first, which, while less than ideal parenting, is not what someone indifferent to the suffering of their research subjects would do.

Moreover, Hilleman's team were not doing anything to those children that nature didn't. If the vaccine worked, then at least some of the institutionalised children would grow up without ever catching mumps. If the vaccine proved less attenuated than they hoped, the worst that would happen was that it caused a disease they were going to get sooner or later anyway.

That's what happened to a quarter of the vaccinated children, in whom Hilleman's first mumps vaccine caused parotitis. It was far from attenuated enough to be called a vaccine strain, but a quarter with parotitis was less than the two thirds that a natural outbreak would have caused. Hilleman was on the right track.

They tried again after the seventeenth passage,[17] and this time they saw what they were hoping to see. None of the children developed parotitis and none had any virus in their saliva. The virus they were now calling the Jeryl Lynn strain was so well adapted to chicken embryos that it could make children neither ill nor infectious. What it could do, Hilleman confirmed, was trigger antibodies that neutralised the wild-type mumps virus.[18]

Hilleman's next trial was on a much larger scale, recruiting children from regular schools where mumps outbreaks took place every few years. As luck would have it, there was a mumps outbreak within a few months of the beginning of the trial, so Hilleman had his answer more quickly than he could have expected: the attenuated Jeryl Lynn strain was an extremely effective vaccine. Around half the unvaccinated children developed mumps, while only one in fifty of the vaccinated children did.[19]

The Jeryl Lynn vaccine was licensed in 1967, only four years after her fateful sore throat. Jeryl Lynn Hilleman, who is now a successful businesswoman,[20] has consistently refused any credit. 'All I did,' she said, some fifty years later, 'was get sick at the right time, with the right virus, with the right father.'[21]

The not-quite-attenuated Urabe strain

Many of Hilleman's vaccines were adopted around the world as soon as they hit the market, but his mumps vaccine received a lukewarm response. Mumps was still among the less serious childhood diseases, and few governments regarded the occasional case of encephalitis as a national priority.

Britain wasn't unusual in only introducing the mumps vaccine when it was combined with measles and rubella in the MMR vaccine,[22] more as a peripheral benefit of vaccinating against rubella than as a priority in itself.[23]

By then, Hilleman's was one of several mumps vaccines available. Merck held the patent for the Jeryl Lynn strain, but once Hilleman showed how to attenuate wild-type mumps into a vaccine strain, several other pharmaceutical firms made their own vaccine strains. One was the Biken Institute in Osaka, Japan, whose Urabe strain accounted for around one in five MMR doses given to British children in the late 1980s and early 1990s.

At the same time, Canadian epidemiologists picked up the first hint that all was not well with the mumps vaccine; a worrying number of children were turning up with a condition called aseptic meningitis soon after they received the MMR:[24] 'aseptic' meaning that there were no bacteria associated with it, which was a strong hint that whatever was causing the meningitis was a virus. It looked exactly like the sort of meningitis caused by wild-type mumps.

That didn't prove that the mumps vaccine was causing the meningitis. Aseptic meningitis remained very rare, and when doctors see a child with a rare condition, they're likely to look at the child's recent past for an explanation. If a child turned up in a hospital soon after receiving the MMR, the doctors were likely to blame the MMR. If they hadn't had a recent MMR, doctors would have to look elsewhere for a cause.

However, it was also possible that there was a downside to the mumps virus having been so easy to isolate. It hadn't been like measles, which had needed so many passages before it infected chicken embryos that the vaccine strain differed fundamentally from the wild-type. Mumps had taken to chicken embryos straight away, which might mean that the mumps vaccine strain hadn't come as far from the wild-type as the measles vaccine strain had needed to.

A team at Gunma University School of Medicine, Japan, looked into whether there really was a problem with the Urabe strain. They had to cast a very wide net to find enough cases to work with, monitoring admissions to twenty-four hospitals over eight months. They found thirty-six children admitted with aseptic meningitis, and, in the spinal fluid of thirty of those children, they found the Urabe mumps vaccine strain.[25] That couldn't be a coincidence.

All of the children fully recovered, meaning that meningitis caused by the Urabe strain was manageable as well as rare. Epidemiologists at the British Public Health Laboratory Service would later calculate how rare: there was one case for every 12,400 doses given,[26] which is far less than the one-in-1,000 caused by the wild-type.[27] However, vaccines are not supposed to cause meningitis at all, and the Urabe strain was withdrawn around the world.

Most countries replaced it with the Jeryl Lynn strain, which remains the most widely used mumps vaccine in the world. Since 1992, it has been the only mumps vaccine used in Britain.[28]

The Urabe strain's misbehaviour focused the attention of the world's public health agencies on aseptic meningitis cases, but after three decades of scrutiny, no aseptic meningitis has ever been associated with the Jeryl Lynn strain.[29]

In Britain alone, more than a million and a half doses of the Jeryl Lynn strain have been given without once causing aseptic meningitis.[30]

That's as close as you'll ever hear an epidemiologist come to saying that something doesn't happen. The Jeryl Lynn strain is as safe as anyone is ever likely to be able to prove.

Mumps today: eradication remains elusive

Thanks to the Jeryl Lynn strain, new parents no longer expect parotitis to puff up their children's faces. By the 2000s, mumps looked to be going the way of measles, but in the late 2010s, it started to reappear.

The new outbreaks were not among children, but among people in their late teens and early twenties. It's not the first time that mumps changed its pattern. In eighteenth-century Norfolk, Robert Hamilton had described mumps as an affliction of young men between puberty and thirty years old, but he never saw it in any girl above the age of ten.[31] Quite how those young men had made it to puberty without catching mumps from their sisters remains a mystery.

A later shift was reported by the US military, who found that mumps swept through army training camps during the First World War but not the Second,[32] implying that mumps had become a ubiquitous childhood disease between the wars.

Now it's back as a rare disease of young adults.

When it first reappeared, Public Health England* attributed the new outbreaks to the 'Wakefield cohorts':[33] babies born in the

---

* Now the UK Health Security Agency.

late 1990s and early 2000s whose parents opted not to have them vaccinated because of Andrew Wakefield's fraudulent claim that the mumps-containing MMR vaccine causes autism.

The epidemiologist's catchphrase is 'It's a bit more complicated than that,' and so it proved when NHS Scotland's epidemiologists showed that it wasn't only unvaccinated people who were catching it.[34] Focusing on a 2017–18 outbreak in Lothian, they found 324 cases of mumps. One in ten of the sufferers had never been vaccinated, which was a much higher proportion than in Britain as a whole. It appeared that the Wakefield cohorts were indeed highly vulnerable to mumps. However, 90 per cent of the sufferers had received at least one dose of MMR and fully three quarters had received both prescribed childhood doses.

That didn't show the mumps vaccine to be ineffective. Lothian contains Edinburgh's four universities, so those 324 must have been a tiny proportion of the young adults exposed to mumps.

The Lothian study echoed reports of outbreaks in the USA[35] and the Netherlands.[36] Mumps can't infect most vaccinated people, but it can infect enough to cause the occasional outbreak.

In both the American and Dutch outbreaks, vaccinated men who were unlucky enough to develop parotitis were a lot less likely to develop orchitis than unvaccinated men. Even where vaccination fails to protect a throat, it usually protects testicles.

It would be useful to know if vaccination also cuts the risk of other complications like meningitis and oophoritis, but because the recent outbreaks are so small, there simply weren't enough of those rarer complications to tell.

That the Jeryl Lynn mumps vaccine can't eradicate mumps is disappointing, but it has protected millions of people. A vaccinated child has a very strong chance of living out their whole life without ever experiencing mumps, and if a man has a breakthrough infection, vaccination is likely to protect him from orchitis. Good news for hearing and testicles everywhere.

Chapter 15

Rubella

Three Sydney housewives met in an ophthalmologist's waiting room. That's not the beginning of a medical school joke. It was what led to the discovery that rubella – or, as a Sydney housewife probably called it in 1941, German measles – could be a lot nastier than anyone had realised.

They were there because their children, all about a year old, had been born with cataracts; opaque patches of the lenses in their eyes that partially or completely obscure vision. As the housewives talked, they realised that all three had caught German measles in the first few weeks of their pregnancies.

When one of the women took her child in to see the ophthalmologist, she asked him the question they had been mulling over: could German measles have caused their children's cataracts?

She probably didn't know she was asking a radical question. In the 1940s, most doctors explained babies born with disabilities by invoking genetics, which, before anyone had made the connection between genes and DNA, was little more than handwaving.

The ophthalmologist she was asking, Norman Gregg, was

not most doctors. In an era when many doctors preferred their patients to be billed but not heard, Gregg had a reputation for being approachable,[1] which is probably why the housewife felt able to put her question to him.

With only the coincidence of the three similar cases to go on, Gregg couldn't answer immediately. All three women had caught German measles during a large outbreak that infected a lot of young women, some of whom were pregnant. On the other hand, it was unusual for a baby to be born with cataracts, and when Gregg examined the three children in question, their cataracts didn't quite look like any of the types described in his textbooks.[2]

Gregg wrote to his fellow ophthalmologists to ask if they were seeing anything similar. Their replies convinced him that something strange was afoot. All over Australia, babies were being born with cataracts, and more than half of them also had heart defects. Tellingly, nearly all their mothers had had German measles in the first two months of their pregnancies.

Gregg had enough data to publish a case series; a report on several patients with a similar condition. Like any good case series, it raised more questions than it answered. He only had data on babies whose cataracts had landed them in front of ophthalmologists, so he had no idea how many pregnant women caught German measles and gave birth to perfectly healthy babies. Nor did he know how many babies with cataracts and heart defects had been born to mothers whose pregnancies were unmarred by German measles.

He did, however, show a pattern strange enough to warrant further investigation, and when epidemiologists investigated, they found that those three housewives and Gregg had indeed noticed something that everyone else had missed. German measles in the first two months of pregnancy often caused the baby to be born with what became known as congenital rubella syndrome.[3] Congenital because they were born with it. Syndrome meaning a range of conditions that occurred in various combinations.

It was time for a re-evaluation of German measles.

Rötheln, German measles or rubella?

Before Gregg got on the case, German measles had been regarded as one of the less serious illnesses that children coughed, sweated and vomited their way through. It would make a child thoroughly miserable with a sore throat, fever and rash, but rarely for more than a few days.[4]

It was the rash that gave it its two English names. A lot of the early study of childhood diseases revolved around discerning one type of rash from another and, in the nineteenth century, some German physicians noticed a type of rash that looked a bit like measles and a bit like scarlet fever, but wasn't an angry enough shade of red to be either.[5] They called it *Rötheln*, meaning 'reddening'.

In 1866, a British Army surgeon called Henry Veale raised a very British objection to that name. Describing an outbreak in the Presidency of Bombay,* he declared: '*Rötheln* is harsh and foreign to our ears.'[6] He suggested that 'rubella' which is Latinesque, if not quite Latin, for 'little red' would be rarefied enough for his countrymen's auditory senses. Rubella remains the medical term, although it's often called 'German measles', recognising the German surgeons who first described it.

The rubella virus behaves in a very similar way to the mumps virus, although they are unrelated. It's about as infectious as mumps and, like mumps, it spreads through the droplets that an

---

* Now split between India and Pakistan.

infected person breathes out and an uninfected person breathes in. Like mumps, that infected person is likely to be walking around infecting people for a couple of weeks before they know they're ill. Like mumps, there are no drugs that stop the virus from replicating, so it's left to the immune system to see off the virus, after which it retains lifelong immune memory.[7]

Another similarity is that the rubella virus often finds its way into the nervous system, usually without doing any serious damage. However, around one in 6,000 rubella infections progresses to encephalitis, and around one in five rubella encephalitis cases are fatal.[8]

Rubella was usually classed as a childhood disease because before vaccination, it was so commonplace that few people made it to puberty without being infected. However, a significant number of people somehow avoided it until young adulthood, which, for women, meant their childbearing years.

1965 was a bad year for American babies

Not every boy is excited at the prospect of a younger sibling, but Billy Stonebreaker, a twelve-year-old Californian, certainly was. 'I'll take care of him, I promise,'[9] he told his mother, Dolores, when he asked for a kid brother.

Then two things happened in quick succession. Dolores fell pregnant. And Billy caught rubella.

Billy recovered as quickly as most boys do, but not before he gave it to Dolores. This was 1965, the year in which Martin Luther King marched from Selma to Montgomery, the Rolling Stones couldn't get no satisfaction and America was in the throes of a major rubella epidemic. By then, congenital rubella syndrome was well enough understood that Dolores's doctor could tell her there was a strong chance that her child would be seriously mentally or physically disabled.

Among mothers infected in the first two months of pregnancy, nine out of ten give birth to babies with congenital rubella syndrome. The later in the pregnancy the infection happens, the lower the risk. By the second trimester (weeks fourteen to twenty-six), the risk is down to three out of ten.[10] Dolores Stonebreaker's dilemma was that until her baby was born, there was no way to know how the syndrome would manifest, how serious it would be, or even if the virus had crossed the placenta to infect the foetus at all. She had to play the odds with the child she dearly wanted.

The Stonebreakers weren't wealthy. They couldn't afford to care for a disabled child so Dolores opted for an abortion.

We know her story because it was chronicled in a photographic essay in *Life* magazine. One photo captured the agonising moment when Dolores told Billy that he wouldn't be getting his kid brother after all. Dolores's comforting arm can't stem Billy's tears as Dolores herself turns away from the camera. Another shot captured the conflicting emotions on Dolores's face in the abortion clinic's waiting room.[11]

The abortion revealed that rubella had already killed her unborn child, and Dolores would have miscarried sooner rather than later. Dolores Stonebreaker was only one among thousands of American women whom rubella forced into making the same choice.

The National Communicable Disease Center* estimated that 20,000 children with congenital rubella syndrome were born in 1965, and 5,000 pregnancies were terminated.[12] 'Estimated' might be overstating the precision of the calculation. There was no nationwide registry of cases, and the supposed 5,000 terminations

---

* Now the Centers for Disease Control and Prevention (CDC).

look more like the product of cigarette packet scribblings than of sound epidemiology. However, it was never disputed that a lot of babies were born with congenital rubella syndrome, and a lot of pregnancies were terminated through fear of it.

America's rubella babies of 1965 were extensively researched as they grew into children. It's largely thanks to them that we now know that congenital rubella syndrome encompasses far more than cataracts and heart defects. It could leave a child blind, deaf or both. It could leave them diabetic. It could damage a developing brain, leading to conditions ranging from fairly mild behavioural disorders to intellectual disabilities that would never allow them to live independently.[13]

A child psychiatrist called Stella Chess noticed some of them showed a particular set of behaviours. Those children formed stronger emotional bonds with objects than with people, showed repetitive actions like rocking back and forth, and were greatly upset when someone rearranged the furniture.[14]

Chess recognised the signs of autism, a condition for which the causes are still less than clear. It is now thought to arise out of a combination of genetic factors and external triggers,[15] and Chess identified congenital rubella syndrome as the strongest external trigger yet identified.

The 1965 epidemic kicked rubella up the priority list. Rubella usually hit the USA every few years, and vaccinologists were now confident enough to believe they might have a vaccine ready before the next epidemic – if they moved fast.

Stanley Plotkin's virus in Leonard Hayflick's cells

When Stanley Plotkin was fifteen years old, he read a novel called *Arrowsmith* by Sinclair Lewis. The eponymous Martin

Arrowsmith is distracted from his calling by a couple of marriages before he joins other like-minded men in a monastic commitment to science. The novel inspired the young Plotkin,[16] who was yet to learn that the true enemy of a scientist's focus is not their spouse but the funding committee.

As a young doctor, Plotkin took a research post at Philadelphia's Wistar Institute, where he worked on anthrax and polio before rubella caught his attention. When he arranged a stint at London's Great Ormond Street Hospital, the Wistar's director promised him a laboratory to continue his studies in when he came back.[17]

At about the same time, Paul Parkman's team at the US Army's Walter Reed Research Institute published a technique for culturing rubella virus in monkey kidney cells.[18] It solved a problem that had hampered rubella research up to that point: unlike mumps, rubella does not reliably replicate in chicken embryos.

Plotkin arrived in London in the summer of 1962, which, given his interest in rubella, was perfectly timed. A rubella outbreak was sweeping Europe, and Parkman's technique gave him a brand-new tool to bring to the study of it.

While he learned to work with rubella in the laboratory, Plotkin was also confronting it in the clinic. Many of his patients were women facing the same dilemma that Dolores Stonebreaker would face three years later: whether to terminate a pregnancy that they very much wanted or to have a child who might be so disabled that they couldn't care for it.

By 1965, Plotkin was back in the Wistar and ensconced in his promised laboratory. That was when he saw a way to put an end to congenital rubella syndrome for good.

By then, the business of culturing viruses in cultured cells was, if still not quite science, at least closer to art than witchcraft. It had come a long way in the decade since Enders and Peebles had started trying to conjure a measles vaccine strain. Progress had been led by Leonard Hayflick, a cell biologist at the Wistar who had taken on the unglamorous task of establishing some principles behind cell biology.[19]

Hayflick's work led him to establish the WI-38 cell line from an aborted foetus. He'd been able to keep his cells alive and culture them predictably, and he'd worked out how long he could culture them for before they started to show signs of ageing.[20]

Plotkin was among the first to recognise how Hayflick's work would revolutionise laboratory cell culture. The problem with the Parkman process, which Plotkin had used in London, was that monkey kidney cells didn't last long after they were removed from the monkey and placed in culture medium. They might divide once or twice, but it wasn't long before they lost the shine of a living cell under a microscope and took on the dull lethargy that precedes a cultured cell's death.

Hayflick's WI-38 cells replaced the need for a constant supply of monkeys and gave Plotkin an unending supply of identical cells. As they were foetal cells, they were exactly the type of cell that rubella virus infects and replicates in.

Plotkin's breakthrough came from Foetus 27, which is the only name it was ever given. All we know about Foetus 27's mother is that she was twenty-five years old and eight weeks into her pregnancy when she broke out with the dreaded rubella rash.[21] We can only guess how painful the decision to terminate her pregnancy must have been. That rash may have been the worst thing ever to happen to her, but it has been a boon for expectant mothers ever since.

But first, Plotkin had to tame the virulent wild-type rubella virus he isolated from Foetus 27 into a mild vaccine strain. He used the established technique of serial passage: culturing it in one batch of cells, harvesting the replicated virus and inoculating another.

Plotkin added another element to the attenuation process,

which was to lower the temperature. Human cells are usually cultured at around thirty-seven degrees Celsius, at the high end of normal human body temperature, but Plotkin habituated some of his RA27/3 cultures to a chilly thirty degrees. The idea was that as well as adapting the vaccine strain to replicating fast in culture instead of dodging an immune response, he was also adapting it to replicating in a much colder environment than that in which it would encounter the immune system. The more disadvantages he could heap on the virus, the more likely the immune system would be to stamp it out before it made anyone ill.

Every passage increased the weight of those disadvantages, but Plotkin couldn't know how many passages he would need. The only way to gauge its attenuation was to give it to children.

Like Maurice Hilleman when he was testing the mumps vaccine, Plotkin found the children he needed in institutions for the 'mentally retarded' for much the same reasons. Rubella swept through these institutions as often as mumps.

Plotkin tested many different variants of his RA27/3 strain, meticulously recording how the number of passages and the temperature at which it had been cultured affected the German measles it caused.[22]

It would bring foam to the mouths of a modern oversight committee, but in the event, none of the children suffered more than they would have done with wild-type rubella, and most suffered less. Further, Plotkin's approach worked. The more time RA27/3 spent in Hayflick's cells, the less serious the German measles it caused. Equally importantly, it retained the ability to trigger substantial levels of antibodies, which was the best measure Plotkin had of whether it left them immune to the wild-type.

Passage by passage, RA27/3 was looking less like a pathogen and more like a vaccine.

The Philadelphia rubella race

Plotkin wasn't the only scientist racing the next outbreak. A few miles away, Maurice Hilleman's team at Merck were working with Paul Parkman, now at the government's Division of Biologics Standards.* Parkman, like everyone else who didn't have the benefit of working with Hayflick, was still doing things the old-fashioned way of regularly killing monkeys for their kidney cells. He could keep rubella virus in monkey kidney cells but his virus was not becoming attenuated.

Hilleman revisited the problem of culturing the virus in eggs and found that, although it disliked chicken embryos, it replicated well in duck embryos and became attenuated as it did so. By the late 1960s, Hilleman's team were testing their HPV-77 strain on institutionalised children in the same way as Plotkin.[23] Between Merck, the Wistar and the University of Pennsylvania, there can't have been many institutionalised children in 1960s Philadelphia who didn't end up in a vaccine trial.

Plotkin's RA27/3[24] and Parkman and Hilleman's HPV-77[25] both arrived at the point of being attenuated enough to be called vaccine strains in 1969, and they were both used to contain an outbreak in Taiwan.[26]

The next outbreak in the USA was expected imminently. If policymakers wanted to beat rubella to the punch, they needed to roll out a vaccine within a year or two – and that meant they had to decide which one.

Much of the debate came down to Hayflick's newfangled human cell culture system. It was opposed by Albert Sabin, whose success with his attenuated polio vaccine had made him one of

---

* Later transferred to the Food and Drug Administration and renamed the Center for Biologics Evaluation and Research.

the most influential scientists in the USA. He argued that because Hayflick's WI-38 cells originated from a human, they might contain a human virus that would find its way into a vaccine.[27]

Plotkin countered that he and Hayflick had been working with WI-38 cells for long enough that they would know about any stray viruses they carried. On the other hand, no one knew where all the monkeys and ducks used to culture HPV-77 had been. If monkey and duck cells could host a human virus like rubella, it followed that they might carry duck or monkey viruses that could infect a human. With new animals needed all the time, there was no way to know what might be sneaking into a vaccine vial.

Today, Plotkin's argument sounds like common sense. It's one reason why modern vaccine production uses well-characterised cell lines instead of an ongoing harvest of monkey cells. Another reason is that monkeys are expensive and nobody enjoys killing them for their kidney cells. However, in 1969, harvesting cells from freshly killed monkeys was a tried and tested technology while human cell lines were not.

Plotkin's arguments were received more sympathetically outside the USA, beyond the sway of Sabin's influence.[28] His RA27/3 was adopted by two of the world's biggest pharmaceutical companies, the Institut Mérieux in France and Burroughs Wellcome in Britain.

In the USA, Sabin's objections ensured that only Parkman and Hilleman's HPV-77 was licensed.

Maurice Hilleman's one-shot dream

The licensing of HPV-77 opened the door to what Hilleman called the 'culmination of a long-term dream that it might be possible, one day, to develop a vaccine that would protect against [measles, mumps and rubella] in a single shot'.[29]

In turning his dream into a plan, Hilleman couldn't assume that a child would handle three attenuated viruses as easily as he handled one at a time. He needed to be sure that the triple-whammy wouldn't overwhelm a child's immune system, either making him seriously ill or leaving him unable to develop lasting immune memory to all three.

When Hilleman's team tried it, the triple vaccine worked as well as they could have hoped. The adverse events caused by the MMR, as they called it, were no worse than if the three vaccine strains were injected separately,[30] and it induced antibodies against all three.[31]

Merck's MMR was licensed in 1971, which looked like the end of the road for Plotkin's RA27/3. It was only a matter of time before the convenience of the single-shot MMR, containing Hilleman's HPV-77, elbowed RA27/3 out of the market.

But Plotkin wasn't done.

Dorothy Horstmann is a pain in the ass

Several researchers compared the two rubella vaccines and they all found the same result: RA27/3 was simply better. It was more likely to induce an antibody response, and it protected more children against German measles.

Plotkin summarised the various studies in a 1973 paper that acknowledged the market dominance of HPV-77. In his opening paragraph, Plotkin admitted that 'another rubella vaccine strain may seem like Marshal Ney at Waterloo, arriving after the battle is over'.[32]

Likening himself to a man who was late for a defeat was perhaps not the best way to open an argument, even if Plotkin had named the right marshal. It was Grouchy, not Ney, who missed Waterloo.

Plotkin wasn't the only one to take the field on behalf of RA27/3. One study that showed RA27/3 to be superior to HPV-77 was led by Dorothy Horstmann, an authority on childhood diseases who didn't leave her results to speak for themselves.[33]

Horstmann didn't carry enough influence to change vaccine policy, but Hilleman did, so Horstmann determined to influence Hilleman. She phoned him to put her case, but Hilleman hadn't achieved his influence by being easy to persuade. He wasn't going to change his view after one phone call. However, Horstmann wouldn't have been the first woman to be appointed professor at Yale Medical School if she were the type to leave it at one phone call.

Hilleman can't have wanted to admit to HPV-77's short-comings, but he took Horstmann's calls and listened to her arguments. Eventually, he called her a pain in the ass and admit-ted that she had a point.[34] Not long after that, he called Plotkin out of the blue and asked if Merck could try his RA27/3 strain.

With Merck's resources to draw from, Hilleman was able to compare the two vaccines on a scale of which Horstmann and Plotkin could only have dreamed. The results were conclusive. Plotkin's RA27/3 induced antibodies in more children than HPV-77 – and it induced more of them.[35] Plotkin's Waterloo-based argument was comprehensively validated by the man he was arguing against.

The end of the road turned out to be not for RA27/3 but for HPV-77. With most of the manufacturers outside America already using RA27/3 and now Merck using it in the MMR, it became the most widely used rubella vaccine strain in the world – and remains so.

Who to vaccinate and when?

By 1980, the question of which vaccine strain to use was settled, but the question of how best to use it was not. Plotkin and Hilleman's priority had always been to prevent congenital rubella syndrome, but they couldn't vaccinate a foetus. Moreover, protecting young children from rubella might not have been their starting point, but that didn't mean it wasn't worth doing. Vaccination could spare children a week of being ill, and at least some of those children would endure that week while their mothers were pregnant with a foetus vulnerable to congenital rubella syndrome.

In the USA, the rubella vaccine was given to children as soon as it was rolled out. Cases of German measles started falling immediately and the feared early 1970s outbreak never materialised.

The British strategy was different. In 1970, rubella vaccination was introduced for schoolgirls aged eleven to fourteen, and in 1972, for women of childbearing age who weren't already immune.[36] It was never going to eliminate rubella, but it wasn't intended to. The aim was to prevent congenital rubella syndrome, not to prevent rubella in children. As long as women were immune before they got pregnant, their foetuses would be protected.

Through the 1970s, the number of cases was lower than estimates for the 1960s,[37] but those estimates weren't reliable. A national registry of congenital rubella syndrome was only established in 1971 and reporting wasn't mandatory until 1988.

The data was good enough to show that during an outbreak in 1978–9, the number of babies born with congenital rubella syndrome jumped. It happened again in 1983[38] while the number of cases in America remained low.[39] Those jumps showed the British approach wasn't working. Too many women were falling through gaps in the system and becoming pregnant while still vulnerable to rubella.[40]

The 1980s saw most European countries adopt the MMR, which made the question of when to give the rubella vaccine moot.[41] To protect against measles, the MMR needs to be given before a child's first birthday.

Britain was a late adopter of the MMR, but in 1987, the JCVI agreed that after seventeen years of targeting schoolgirls had failed to get rid of congenital rubella, it was time to try adding rubella to the early childhood schedule. If a mumps vaccine came with it, so much the better.[42] The NHS introduced the MMR for one-year-olds in 1988, and added the second dose in 1994.[43]

The plot on page 243 shows how dramatic the effect was. In 1988, the year the MMR was rolled out and the year a national registry of cases was established, there were nearly 25,000 cases across England. By 1991, there were fewer than 10,000. Cases continued to fall, with 1998 being the last year with over 1,000 cases. The effect of the second dose kicked in around then, driving cases even lower. The last year with 1,000 cases was 2010.

More important than how many people get German measles, the number of cases of congenital rubella syndrome in Britain has been in single figures since the early 1990s.[44]

Britain had become one of many countries in which expectant mothers no longer need to fear German measles thanks to Plotkin's persistence, Hilleman's open mind, Horstmann being a pain in the ass and a small gift from the anonymous mother of Foetus 27.

Children vaccinated by their second birthday

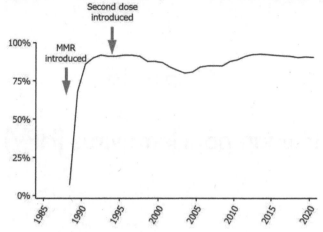

Rubella cases

The top plot shows the percentage of children receiving the MMR by their second birthday from its introduction in 1988 to 2020. The bottom plot shows the number of rubella cases reported from the beginning of systematic records until 2020.

Vaccine coverage data is from England only.[45,46] Reports of cases and deaths are from England and Wales.[47]

Chapter 16

Human papillomavirus (HPV)

In 1842, when most doctors simply treated patients, sometimes to their benefit and sometimes not, Domenico Rigoni-Stern was counting them. The science of epidemiology was but a twinkle in the eye of a few visionaries like Rigoni-Stern, a professor of clinical medicine in Padua, so if his landmark paper on who died of what cancer contained a couple of rookie errors, it's hard to blame him.

Rigoni-Stern observed that uterine cancer was more common than breast cancer in married women, but among nuns, the reverse was true: breast cancer was more common than uterine.[1]

His first rookie error was in his characterisation of 'uterine cancer', which did not distinguish the uterus, otherwise called the womb, from the cervix – the narrow neck between the uterus and the vagina. We now know that cancer arises far more often in the cervix than the uterus, so many cancers that Rigoni-Stern called uterine would have been cervical. In 1842, understanding of the female anatomy was as primitive as epidemiology.

Rookie error number two was to assume the overall cancer rate was the same in nuns as in married women. Had he checked, he would almost certainly have found that married women were more likely to develop cancers than nuns, and that most of the discrepancy lay in married women being far more likely to get 'uterine' cancer. It would have been a strong indication that cervical cancer was sexually transmitted.

Assuming that nuns were as likely to get cancer as married women sent Rigoni-Stern down a blind alley. He concluded that breast cancer was somehow replacing 'uterine' cancer among nuns, and wondered if being a nun might be bad for the breasts. 'Could it be their habits are too tight?' he speculated. 'Or, perhaps, the long-sustained, bent position assumed while saying prayers with forearms resting on knees and compressing the breasts.'[2]

His suggestion that praying causes breast cancer appears absurd today, but in fact, he was on to something. Rigoni-Stern was one of the first to associate cancer with lifestyle and to back the association up with data, even if he had no framework for interpreting that data. It's easy to snigger at his misinterpretation, but he was well ahead of his time. It would be more than a century before anyone understood why married women were more likely to get cervical cancer than celibate nuns.

No one was going to connect sexually transmitted infection and cancer until it occurred to someone that an infection might cause cancer at all. A cancer results from a cell dividing uncontrollably and attacking the body from the inside. An infection invades the body from the outside. They appeared to be fundamentally different types of disease.

Rotkin's personal question and a cancerous mouse

A century after Rigoni-Stern, the idea that cervical cancer might have something to do with sex was beginning to take hold.

In 1967, I. D. Rotkin of the Kaiser Foundation Research Institute in Oakland published an exhaustive comparison of the sex lives of Californian women who did and did not develop cervical cancer. He found that cervical cancer had nothing to do with their favoured sexual position, what they thought of during sex or which of twenty-one listed items they used to masturbate. He did, however, conclude that cervical cancer was more common among women who 'experienced first coitus on the ground [than] in a hotel or motel'.[3] We can only imagine the conversations involved in gathering his data.

Some years earlier, Sarah Stewart and Bernice Eddy, respectively at the US National Cancer Institute and Division of Biologics Standards, both in Bethesda, Maryland, had discovered a virus that caused cancer in mice.[4] Stewart and Eddy opened the door to a whole new field of research on cancer-causing viruses, but at the time, their discovery was seen as an interesting phenomenon of no great significance to human disease. If Rotkin was aware of it, he didn't associate it with cervical cancer.

While Rotkin's questions must have seemed strange to the women he put them to, their answers revealed that the single most important risk factor was the number of sexual partners, which pointed the finger at a sexually transmitted infection.

Rotkin missed it.

He was more interested in cervical cancer being associated with 'first coitus' on the ground rather than in a hotel, which is an association that remains a mystery.

Rigoni-Stern misinterpreted his observations because he didn't have a framework with which to interpret them. Rotkin misinterpreted his because he had a misleading framework that put cancers in one box and infections in another.

The jackalope introduces the papillomaviruses

The path to the correct framework began when an American trapper noticed something strange about a rabbit. We don't know who the trapper was, but in around 1930, stories of horned rabbits on the Iowa prairies reached Richard Shope at the Rockefeller Institute.

If Shope believed he was on the trail of the fabled jackalope, he would have been disappointed to find the 'horns' were merely large warts. When he ground up a wart and passed it through a Chamberland filter, he found he could induce the same warts in another rabbit. He concluded the warts were caused by a virus, and because the medical term for a wart is a papilloma, he called the invisible agent he'd discovered a papillomavirus.

In the following decades, many more papillomaviruses were found causing warts in many different mammal species. In the early 1970s, papillomaviruses of humans attracted the attention of Harald zur Hausen, who was seeking the cause of cervical cancer at the University of Freiburg. Zur Hausen was convinced there was a virus involved, and his prime suspect was herpes simplex-2, which causes genital warts. His logic was that if a virus can cause the abnormal growth of a wart, it might also cause the abnormal growth of a cancer. His team scrutinised cervical cancer samples, but whatever they tried, they could find no herpes simplex-2 in them.

They changed tack when they heard anecdotal reports of genital warts caused not by herpes simplex-2 but by papillomaviruses. When they started looking for papillomaviruses in cervical cancer, they found them.[5] Lots of them.[6]

In 1983, zur Hausen's team finally explained the oddity that Rigoni-Stern had noted in 1842. The overwhelming majority of cervical cancers are caused by the human papillomavirus, usually abbreviated to HPV, and HPV is sexually transmitted. No wonder Rigoni-Stern found more cervical cancer in married women than nuns.

The explanation had needed whole branches of science to be invented, and depended on work by Stewart, Eddy and Shope, who, at the time, had no idea if or how their work would matter to human health.

Once zur Hausen showed that the third commonest cancer in women[7] was caused by an infection, it followed that the cancer could be prevented by preventing the infection. The question was how.

The self-assembling building blocks

When Ian Frazer was a boy in Edinburgh, he and some friends thought it would be fun to dig a tunnel in a nearby quarry. However, digging is hard work, and they tired of the game after shifting a few rocks.[8]

When Jian Zhou was a boy, hard work was not optional. The Cultural Revolution saw him packed off to work on a farm and later assigned to hauling 50kg (110lb) packages around a knitting factory.[9]

The two men met in 1989, when their parallel work on HPV led them both to sabbaticals at Cambridge University. They hit it off immediately. Frazer was interested in the immune response, while Zhou wanted to understand how it turned a normal, healthy cell into a cancer.[10]

When Frazer returned to his laboratory in Brisbane's University of Queensland, he persuaded Zhou to join him to work on the structure of HPV's capsid.

Like all viruses, HPV is much simpler when it's between

cells than when it's inside them. In transit, it's a strand of DNA encased in a capsid made of only two types of protein, called L1 and L2. The capsid protects the DNA, and when it encounters a potential target cell, it attaches to that cell and inserts the DNA into it. Stripped of its capsid and inside the target cell, HPV initiates the complex set of processes involved in replicating itself without tipping off the immune system about what it's up to.[11]

Frazer and Zhou concentrated their attention on capsid protein L1. Using samples shared by zur Hausen, Zhou worked out how to engineer the yeast cells to produce L1.

The L1 proteins then pulled a trick that Zhou hadn't been expecting. They assembled themselves into a structure essentially similar to HPV's capsid.[12] Frazer later said, 'It was a bit like throwing a pile of building bricks into the corner and them building themselves into the Eiffel Tower.'[13]

Zhou's synthetic L1 proteins had formed a virus-like particle: a structure similar enough to the capsid for the immune system to see it as identical to the real thing, but without the genetic material it needed to infect anyone's cells. Frazer and Zhou had been trying to understand the basic biology of the virus, but they ended up with something they could use as a vaccine.

So far, HPV research had epitomised modern medical research at its best. Gone were the days of culturing viruses on whatever cells came to hand or dunking them in formalin and crossing fingers. Zhou and Frazer's vaccine was born of stripping the virus down to its component parts and building what they needed out of them. It had been an international effort, with the vaccine being made by Scottish and Chinese scientists who'd met in England, working in Australia and using samples shared by colleagues in Germany.

As Zhou and Frazer worked to turn their research product into a functional vaccine, a less wholesome aspect of modern medical research reared its head; they became embroiled in a four-way legal battle over who had been the first to synthesise the L1 protein.[14] The decision eventually went to Zhou and Frazer, but Zhou did not live to see it. In 1999, in his early forties, he died after a short illness.

The many faces of HPV

While Zhou and Frazer were working on the vaccine, zur Hausen's team were developing a better understanding of HPV itself. They found that HPV is not a single virus. It's an ocean of diversity with many different 'types'.[15]

All HPV types infect the cells of the epithelium, which forms the envelope between the human body and the outside world. There are different types of epithelium, including the skin, the linings of the airways and digestive system, and, most importantly when we're talking about papillomaviruses, the interior of the reproductive organs.

Some HPV types, like 1, 2 and 4, gravitate towards the skin of the feet, where they cause verrucas, which are annoying but not dangerous. Types 6 and 11 prefer the epithelium inside the throat or the genitals, where they cause more painful warts but rarely turn cancerous. The really nasty ones are types 16 and 18, which cause most HPV-related cancers, and, for reasons that remain unknown, are particularly likely to cause them in the cervix.

Ethel-Michele de Villiers, a longstanding member of zur Hausen's team and later his wife, found that the differences that defined the types lay in the same L1 capsid protein that Frazer and Zhou were using as a vaccine. This meant that vaccinating someone with L1 would only protect against the type of HPV that particular version of L1 was drawn from. An L1-based vaccine is never going to protect against all of the ninety types identified so far.[16]

Fortunately, it doesn't need to. Most HPV types come and go without our noticing. A vaccine effective against types 16 and 18 is enough to protect against the vast majority of HPV-related cancers.

The life and death of Jade Goody

Jade Goody was south London's answer to Kim Kardashian. She shot to fame on *Big Brother*, the show that brought reality TV into the mainstream, and was one of the few reality TV stars to turn five minutes of fame into enduring celebrity. She lived her life on camera, playing up the stereotype of a Bermondsey girl who thought Cambridge was 'abroad'.[17] She inspired love in some, hate in others and bemusement in many, but in the early 2000s, nearly everyone in Britain had heard of her.

Goody's story changed from farce to tragedy when she was diagnosed with cervical cancer.

For most people, a cancer diagnosis is an intensely private affair, but privacy was not Goody's way. In August 2008, she received her diagnosis on camera while filming for the Indian reality show *Bigg Boss*. She shared her unfiltered emotions with the whole world as treatment after treatment failed to cure her. She shared her hysterectomy, her chemotherapy-induced vomiting and her wedding, at which she walked proudly bald down the aisle[18] a month before she died in March 2009. She was twenty-seven years old.

Goody was unlucky. Most HPV infections resolve without causing cancer, and even the nastier types 16 and 18 usually clear within a year without the infected person noticing. They're so common that more than half the people in the world have an HPV infection at some time in their lives.[19] One study found that a third of women studying at the University of Washington were infected in their first year.[20]

Part of the reason it's so common is that HPV does not need intercourse to transmit. It can also be transmitted by skin contact, so while condoms make transmission less likely,[21] they're not as definitive a barrier as with other sexually transmitted infections like HIV.

Quite why HPV-related cancers are more likely to start in the cervix than anywhere else remains a mystery. The HPV must infect the vagina before it can reach the cervix, and it usually reaches the vagina through an infected penis. While HPV does sometimes cause vaginal and penile cancers, they're far less common than cervical.[22]

An infection may take ten or twenty years to develop into a cancer,[23] which is why the NHS offers a screening every few years. The infection causes a visible lesion for some years before turning into full-blown cancer, and removing that lesion is such a minor procedure that it doesn't even need a general anaesthetic.

The earlier a cervical cancer is identified, the less aggressive the treatment needed, and the more likely it is to be successful. It may involve surgery to remove some of the damaged tissue, with or without radiotherapy or chemotherapy.[24] Jade Goody's cancer wasn't identified until it had metastasised to other parts of her body, so her doctors threw everything they had at it. Cervical cancer treatment is successful more often than not,[25] but as Goody showed us all on live television, there are no guarantees.

Gardasil comes to Britain

The year 2008 was HPV's moment in the headlines. It was the year Goody was diagnosed, the year zur Hausen received the Nobel Prize for nailing down its association with cervical cancer, and the year that the HPV vaccine was rolled out in many countries, including Britain.

The roll-out was the culmination of a prolonged and painstaking journey from Frazer and Zhou's synthesis of the L1 protein to a safe and effective vaccine. Two versions were produced by different pharmaceutical firms: GlaxoSmithKline's Cervarix, which the NHS rolled out in 2008, covers types 16 and 18, which are the types most likely to cause cancers. In 2012, the NHS switched to Merck's Gardasil, which also covers types 6 and 11, which cause genital warts.[26] At the time of writing, the NHS is poised for another change, this time to Merck's Gardasil-9, which contains nine different types and will become the standard HPV vaccine from 2022.[27]

The HPV vaccine is given to pre-teens and teenagers for two reasons. The first is that it triggers antibodies that bind the capsid, which are very effective in closing the door to HPV entering the body, but they can't root it out of a cell that it's already infected. Once it's got into one cell, HPV can replicate and cross into neighbouring cells without ever being exposed to antibodies patrolling the epithelium's surface. When planning a vaccination schedule, that means the best time to vaccinate a woman is while she's still a girl who has yet to take an interest in sex. If the University of Washington study is any indication, HPV infection can come about very soon after a woman becomes sexually active. The young women in that study had been young girls only a few years earlier, and, had a vaccine been available at the time, that would have been the moment to protect them.

The second reason for vaccinating girls rather than women is that the vaccine is more effective if it's given at the earlier age. Two doses before puberty trigger a similar antibody response to three doses given after puberty.[28] Giving it early uses a phenomenon that nature has gifted us.

'The thing we should be doing'

The HPV vaccine roll-out didn't only trigger antibodies to protect women from HPV. It also triggered a lot of people to feel squeamish about the idea of vaccinating pre-pubescent girls against a sexually transmitted infection. The director of the Newcastle-based Christian Institute objected that: 'It's basically a sex jab, encouraging the view that girls can be sexually available ... the thing we should be doing is trying to stop kids being sexually active.'[29]

When Shona Hilton and Emily Smith of the British Medical Research Council's Social and Public Health Sciences Unit asked teenage girls what they thought, they probably weren't surprised that none of them found it sexy. Playground rumour had it that each of the three jabs would be more painful than the last, and some of the boys, who were not then vaccinated against HPV, were enjoying the situation a little too much. One thirteen-year-old girl said that they'd gleefully told her, 'we'd get it in your bum, in your cervix'.[30]

Hardly the stuff of playground seduction. Researchers in the USA looked for, and failed to find, any evidence that teenage girls vaccinated against HPV were more sexually active than those who weren't.[31] The HPV vaccine never became the 'sex jab' that the Christian Institute feared.

Columnist Anne Karpf raised a more secular concern: 'Could it cause fertility problems or birth defects?'[32]

It was a concern shared by many parents. If a vaccine prevented cancer in the female reproductive system, the reasoning went, perhaps it was doing something where no parent of a pre-teen daughter wants to think about anything happening.

Nearly two decades later, the vaccine has been around long enough that women who received it as girls are starting to have children, and we can comfortably repudiate Karpf's concern: it does not cause birth defects.[33] Not that there was never a reason to expect it to. The immune response to an HPV vaccine is similar to that triggered by any other injected vaccine. The immune system responds to it by secreting antibodies into all the body fluids, including the blood, the saliva and the mucus coating the digestive tract and the reproductive system.

A vaccine can't tell the immune system that poliovirus will infect through the intestine, that measles infects through the respiratory tract, and that HPV types 16 and 18 really need to be kept away from the cervix. Antibodies induced by all of those vaccines are secreted in all of those parts of the body. It just happens that with HPV, it matters that the antibodies are in the vagina and the cervix.

Vaccinating boys

When the NHS rolled out the HPV vaccine, they took the view that extending the programme to boys would not be cost-effective, partly because the major impact of HPV is through cervical cancer and partly because vaccinating one gender would be enough to stop most sexual transmission.

It was a controversial view.[34] Vaccinating men would cut off the source of most infections to women and also benefit them directly. HPV causes cancers of the mouth, throat, anus and penis. In recent years, HPV-related mouth cancers in particular have been on the rise, and while they remain nowhere near as common as cervical cancer, they are more common in men.[35] Unlike cervical cancer, other HPV-related cancers cannot be detected by the sort of screening programme that catches cervical lesions while they're still precancerous.

In 2008, the girls-only approach placed Britain in line with most countries that had introduced HPV vaccination, although not all of them. The USA started vaccinating boys in 2011 and Australia in 2013.

In 2015, the NHS recognised that depending on vaccinated women to interrupt transmission was no help to gay men. Vaccination was introduced for gay men attending genito-urinary or HIV clinics – but if they were there in the first place, it was usually because they had already caught a sexually transmitted infection. This approach missed the point that the best time to vaccinate someone is *before* they become sexually active.

In 2019, the NHS finally extended HPV vaccination to boys. It will save many men from cancer in the coming years, as well as keeping them from transmitting HPV to women who have not been vaccinated.

The present and future of HPV

At the time of writing, it is too early to assess how many people have been saved from cancer by the HPV vaccine.

To understand why, let's consider a hypothetical woman. Because she's hypothetical, we can know something we couldn't if she were real: if she hadn't been vaccinated against HPV in 2008, when she was thirteen, her fourth serious boyfriend would infect her with HPV in 2023, when she'd be twenty-eight. She'd skip a couple of cervical screenings, so she wouldn't know she was among the unlucky minority in whom HPV causes cancer. Worse, her progression would be unusually fast, and her HPV infection would only take five years to cause full-blown cervical cancer.

Fortunately for our hypothetical woman, her 2008 vaccination prevents any of this from happening. The point of her story is that it shows why HPV vaccination hasn't had a chance to dramatically affect cervical cancer rates: her cancer wouldn't have appeared on the NHS records until 2028 – or, had it progressed at a more normal rate, until the 2030s or even 2040s.

A decade after the British roll-out, we can only see its effect on women who would have been infected much younger than our hypothetical woman and whose cancers would have developed unusually quickly, but we still can see that the vaccine roll-out is already having an effect. Among girls vaccinated at sixteen to eighteen years old, it has prevented one out of every three cervical cancers, but its effect has been far greater among girls vaccinated aged twelve to thirteen, among whom it has prevented more than four out of every five.[36]

The vaccination programme is already beginning to take effect. The effect we can anticipate was calculated by an international team of epidemiologists in 2016, who showed that if four out of five girls were vaccinated over seventy years, those seventy years would see cervical cancer become a very rare condition.[37]

The timeframe of seventy years was based on the time between the first young girls being vaccinated and the last pre-vaccination women dying of old age. It raises the question of what would happen if the vaccine was extended to women, or to both men and women, who missed the vaccination programme at the time it was rolled out. Many of them may, like our hypothetical woman, be exposed many years after they would have been vaccinated, and so could be protected by a catch-up campaign. At the time of writing, there is no good estimate of how many people would benefit.

The NHS's approach to HPV vaccination may see more refinement in the coming years, but we can be confident that there will be more women alive and healthy who would have developed cervical cancer without the vaccine. We will never know who they are.

Chapter 17

Influenza

Lucy didn't look like a woman who struggles to stand for more than a few minutes at a time. When we Zoomed during the November 2020 lockdown, she looked like the fitness instructor she'd been before influenza knocked her flat two and a half years earlier. The main thing she remembers is 'horrendous exhaustion'[1] as influenza affected her heart function so badly that tachycardia sent her to A&E five times. She never fully recovered, hence her difficulty in standing.

Since then, Lucy has been probed and scanned with a frequency familiar to anyone burdened with a condition that defies treatment. Her heart muscle proved as healthy as her doctors expected in a fitness instructor. Whatever damage influenza had done, it wasn't to Lucy's heart itself but to the nervous system that controls it.

It left her in no condition to return to her gym. She had found some work as a photography model, although she'd had to stop taking bookings a few months earlier. The last thing she needed was COVID-19 on top of the damage done by influenza, so she learned her way around a camera and became her own photographer. Lucy, I realised as we spoke, is not someone who allows her infirmities to define her.

'I'm kind of getting to the point now where I'm going to have to accept that whatever these things have done to me, it's what I have now,' she told me. 'Even if we got to the bottom of why ... I don't think it's going to change anything.'

Seasonal influenza

Lucy's life was changed, possibly forever, by seasonal influenza. It's a catch-all term for several strains of the influenza virus that sweep through the Northern Hemisphere every winter. For the overwhelming majority of people, seasonal flu is a sniffle no different to any of the other 200 or so[2] common cold virus strains in circulation at any given time. Influenza viruses cause around one in ten of the colds we get,[3] and, contrary to what's often believed, are rarely any worse than the other nine.

We tend to refer to anything that sets us coughing and sneezing as a cold until it's bad enough that we need time off work, when it becomes the flu. However, symptoms are not a reliable guide to diagnosing the virus causing them.

The reason seasonal influenza is treated more seriously than other cold viruses is that it's much more likely to cause something worse than a cold. Lucy's case is just one example of the ways influenza can damage the nervous system. It can cause a chronic fatigue syndrome that lasts for months or years,[4] it can invade the brain and cause fatal or permanently disabling encephalitis,[5] or it can cause complications[6] so obscure that Lucy has spent years bouncing between specialists who try to make enough sense of them to help her manage them.

The worst effects of seasonal influenza are most likely to happen to babies, the elderly and adults who are vulnerable for one reason or another. Lucy falls into the latter category since an undiagnosed illness twenty years earlier, when she was seventeen, debilitated her for months and left her with chronic fatigue. Instead of going to university as she'd planned, she spent her early twenties learning to manage her fatigue with the graded exercise that became her gateway to becoming a fitness instructor. Like many people with chronic illnesses, Lucy built a life around her impairments that did not leave her as an invalid.

Until seasonal flu took it all away from her.

And seasonal flu isn't even the worst type of influenza.

Pandemic influenza

The most devastating pandemic of modern times started in a pig, found its way to a soldier and went on to infect the world.

In March 1918, the soldier was at Camp Funston, a training camp centred on Fort Riley, Kansas, where the US Army turned Midwestern farmhands and schoolboys into the doughboys who fought in the trenches of France. Army life may not have agreed with him, because someone, possibly an irritated sergeant, had detailed him to clean Camp Funston's pigpens. He became the first documented case of the new influenza virus, but only just.[7] It swept through Camp Funston like the proverbial dose of salts, and filled the infirmary with writhing and wheezing men.

By then, the new influenza had already infected a lot of pigs. It spread through pigs as fast as through humans, and the 25,000 men based at Camp Funston[8] got through a lot of pork. We'll never be certain where the new influenza arose, although an outbreak in Kansas's Haskell County the previous month makes it the most likely location.[9]

Wherever it started, the new influenza spread across America and then the world, even though, as viruses go, influenza is not particularly infectious. Once it's outside the body, it only survives for a few hours,[10] and human skin kills it within minutes.[11]

Influenza needs people to be packed close together so it can be breathed out – or, even better, sneezed out – by one person and breathed in by another while it's still viable.

Fortunately for influenza, most people now live in cities,[12] where it has ample opportunity to pass from one person to another. Schools, open-plan offices and public transport might have been designed to influenza's requirements, and in 1918, the same was true of military barracks and the troopships crisscrossing the world.

In a world at war, neither side wanted to advertise how many of their soldiers were in no condition to hold up a rifle. The pandemic wasn't openly reported until it spread from under the blanket of censorship into neutral Spain, which got it called the 'Spanish flu'. The name stuck, despite the pandemic's Jayhawk origins.

The Spanish flu virus infected the cells lining its victims' throats and spread down the lining of their windpipes. So far, so like seasonal influenza. The difference was that its victims had experienced seasonal influenza before, so they had some immune memory of it. They had nothing to protect them from this new strain, however, which did far more damage before their lymphocytes mobilised against it. All around the world, hospitals and field dressing stations filled up with feverish, wheezing sufferers.

Most of them recovered. The first wave of Spanish flu was debilitating while it lasted but rarely fatal. The worst was yet to come.

In August, by which time the soldiers who had sweated and coughed through Spanish flu in Camp Funston were sweating and coughing through the shellfire and poison gas of the Western Front, Spanish flu returned in a more aggressive form. This time, no one could take recovery for granted. It inflamed its victims' lungs to cause an often-lethal pneumonia, although more died of bacterial infections of the damaged lung tissue.

By the time the war ended in November, the second wave of the virus had passed, but a few months later, it was back. The third wave tore through countries devastated by the First World War and countries that remained peacefully neutral alike.

Medical historians still debate how many people the three waves of Spanish flu killed. Systematic record keeping by nationwide public health agencies lay in the future, and many governments were more interested in downplaying the situation than understanding it. Estimates vary between 50 and 100 million deaths,[13] which would be two or three out of every hundred people who caught it.[14]

When the number of deaths is so high that it's impossible to conceptualise, we know we are talking about a monumental tragedy.

The ducks of doom

When COVID-19 hit us, we at least knew the nature of our enemy. A hundred years earlier, our ancestors knew the disease plaguing them was called influenza, but what influenza *was* remained a matter for debate.

Plagues and pandemics were nothing new. The term 'influenza' comes from fourteenth-century Florence, when astrologers believed plagues to be *ex influenza colesti*.*[15] In 1918, Richard Pfeiffer's mistaken conclusion that it was caused by the *Haemophilus influenzae* bacterium, covered in Chapter 7, was still the prevailing wisdom. Over a century later, we not only know that influenza is a virus but we know enough about it to piece together what probably happened in that Kansas pig where Spanish influenza began.

---

* Under celestial influence.

If we trace a human influenza virus's ancestry back far enough, we'll end up in the intestine of a water bird.[16] Influenza rarely harms ducks and geese, but when it infects a flock, their faeces can build up a lot of influenza virus in a small area.

Influenza virus straight out of a duck is no danger to a human being. To infect a cell, a virus needs to bind to a molecule on that cell's surface, and, in influenza's case, that molecule is sialic acid. However, the sialic acid of the cells of a bird's digestive system is very different to the sialic acid of human throat cells. Bird influenza very rarely infects humans, and human influenza very rarely infects birds.

However, both human and bird influenzas can infect pigs.[17] The 'Spanish' influenza probably originated on a Kansas small-holding where a farmhand caught seasonal flu at the same time as his chickens were infected by a passing duck. When the farmhand and a chicken infected a pig, the two influenza viruses bound to its cells and injected their genes.

So far, so typical.

Unfortunately, influenza shares the same reassortment trick as rotavirus. Its genes are on separate strands of RNA, so when two different influenza viruses infect the same cell, their genes mix and match to produce progeny viruses that mix characteristics of both original strains. One of those progeny viruses must have carried away a combination of genes that made it enough of a human influenza to infect human cells, but enough of a bird influenza that it wasn't recognised by immune memory from previous human influenza infections.

Pigs fared no better. The new virus swept through American pig farms, including those that supplied Camp Funston, which became its bridgehead into infecting humans.

It was neither the first nor the last 'pandemic' strain of influenza. Most medical historians agree that the first recorded pandemic probably caused by influenza was in 1580, which is more a reflection of the available records than any lack of pandemics before then. There have been two or three every century since then,[18] which have followed much the same pattern as Spanish flu. They start with a nasty first wave, they're followed by an even nastier second and sometimes a third wave, then they fade away. At least, that was how it seemed at the time. In fact, the virus was still out there, but it had lost its virulence. The Spanish influenza virus remained in circulation as a seasonal influenza for decades after the pandemic ended in 1919.

Fortuitous flu in Mill Hill

Spanish flu was a human disaster that killed more people than the First World War. It was also the event that set science on the path to answering the question of what influenza actually was.

The answer could only be found when someone challenged the orthodoxy that it was caused by *Haemophilus*, or Pfeiffer's bacillus as it was still called. As Pfeiffer was one of Robert Koch's team in Berlin, there's a certain inevitability to the challenge having arisen from the Institut Pasteur in Paris. Charles Nicolle and Charles Lebailly found the infectious agent passed through a Chamberland filter,[19] which sparked off a decade and a half of debate about whether influenza was a viral or bacterial disease.

During the Spanish flu pandemic, the man who would resolve the debate was a private in the Royal Army Medical Corps, caught up in a more acrimonious Franco-German dispute than those between Koch and Pasteur had ever been. Wilson Smith was the son of a Lancashire draper who'd died when he was ten years old, leaving his mother to run the shop and raise her four children. It wasn't an auspicious start to life at a time when, even more than now, class was destiny. Mrs Smith must have been an extraordinary woman; all three of her sons grew up to have distinguished academic careers and her daughter became an oratorio singer.[20]

When Smith left the army, he trained in medicine and became interested in research. He took a job as research assistant to Patrick Playfair Laidlaw at the newly built National Institute for Medical Research (NIMR) in Mill Hill Village, which is still just about resisting being engulfed by London's northern suburbs.

By 1933, Laidlaw and his team were at the forefront of the embryonic field of virology, which perfectly placed them to seize the opportunity offered by a particularly bad winter for seasonal influenza. The coughs and sneezes reverberating around London caught up with another of Laidlaw's assistants, Christopher Andrewes. While Smith had been on the Western Front, Andrewes had been a naval surgeon, often to be seen sitting on a depth charge and poring over a medical textbook.[21]

When the flu-benighted Andrewes dragged himself into work, Smith persuaded him to gargle saline solution.[22] He filtered out any bacteria and squirted it up the noses of a few ferrets, who became as flu-benighted as Andrewes. Smith collected samples from those ferrets, filtered them and used them to give another batch of ferrets influenza.

After more than forty years of debate, Smith not only proved influenza was a virus, but isolated it and kept it replicating in Laidlaw's Mill Hill laboratory.

Smith, Andrewes and Laidlaw were not men given to blowing their own trumpets, but we can hope that Andrewes felt well enough to join his colleagues for a celebratory drink before it all went pear-shaped. An outbreak of distemper swept through the NIMR's ferrets and Smith lost the animals he was using to maintain the influenza virus.[23]

Not long after that, seasonal influenza caught up with Smith himself. Seeing opportunity in his malady, he isolated the virus from himself and used it to infect more ferrets.[24] The NIMR team was back in business.

The first influenza vaccines

Smith and his colleagues had succeeded in isolating the influenza virus, but passaging it between cages of ferrets involved a lot of work to produce very little virus. The next breakthrough was finding a better way to maintain it.

At Melbourne's Walter and Eliza Hall Institute, Frank MacFarlane Burnet found that the influenza virus would replicate in chicken embryo cells.[25] He chose his approach because chicken eggs were the only way to keep cells alive in the laboratory at the time. He couldn't know that chicken embryos were in fact the ideal culture system for influenza, because he didn't know that human influenza virus is only one step removed from its chicken-infecting progenitor.

Burnet showed how to produce influenza virus in large enough quantities to produce a vaccine. It was an early success in a distinguished career during which he would earn a knighthood that gained him the nickname 'Sir Mac'.

The year after he published his findings, the USA entered the Second World War, with Spanish influenza far from forgotten. Even if no new pandemic arose, seasonal influenza plagued military bases every winter and not even the most foul-mouthed drill sergeant could mould men into soldiers while they were confined to bed.

The man tasked with solving the influenza problem was Thomas Francis at the University of Michigan in Ann Arbor, who put most of the research in the hands of a gifted and very confident New Yorker called Jonas Salk. As we saw in Chapter

11, Francis and Salk later became famous as the men behind the inactivated polio vaccine, but during the war years, they cut their teeth on influenza.

They isolated influenza virus from someone with seasonal flu, cultured it using Burnet's chicken egg system, inactivated it with formalin and injected it into the latest draft of recruits. While it didn't completely put an end to seasonal flu in training camps, it did shorten their sick parades – but not for long.

Salk and Francis's vaccines quickly lost their effectiveness. A killed-virus vaccine was reasonably effective if they used it in the same year they isolated the virus, but if they used it on the following year's batch of trainees, it protected far fewer of them. They had to isolate a new virus every spring to produce enough virus for the following winter flu season.[26]

Francis and Salk had run into the reason why, however many times we catch seasonal influenza, we never become fully immune to it: the wild-type is constantly mutating. It's a very different adversary to measles, rubella and polio, which are so stable that vaccines produced decades ago still give lifelong immunity to the wild-type circulating today.

Influenza is a moving target for vaccinologists and our immune systems alike. The differences between this year's seasonal influenza and next year's are not as stark as the differences between seasonal influenza strains and a brand-new 'pandemic strain' – that's why seasonal influenza is not as dangerous – but seasonal influenzas still make us ill even though we spend our lives building a repertoire of immunity to them.

That doesn't make seasonal influenza trivial. It kills around 7,000 people in Britain in a typical year,[27] and, as Lucy's experience shows, it can permanently damage the nervous system of the people who survive it. Those severe manifestations are very rare, but when everybody is infected repeatedly, they add up to more fatalities than any other infectious disease in high-income countries[28] before COVID-19 came along, and an unknown number of permanent impairments.

Salk and Francis found that the problem of influenza is almost the opposite of the problem posed by most other viruses.

With measles, mumps, rubella and polio, the problem was to find a way to culture the wild-type virus and attenuate it into a vaccine strain. With influenza, getting from the wild-type to the vaccine was the easy part. It replicated in chicken embryos and there was no need to attenuate it, because simply killing it and injecting it triggered a perfectly good immune response.

The problem was keeping up with the wild-type virus's mutations.

No single vaccine strain could ever give lifelong immunity to influenza. There would need to be an ongoing vaccine development programme, which required two things Salk and Francis did not have.

First, they needed to know what wild-type was in circulation, so they would know when their vaccine became obsolete and a new isolate was needed. Second, they needed to be able to culture those isolates fast enough to vaccinate millions of people before the wild-type mutated and made the vaccine obsolete.

The Global Influenza Surveillance and Response System

The end of the Second World War saw a fleeting moment of cooperation between the major powers left standing, and out of that cooperation came the Global Influenza Surveillance and Response System (GISRS). Its primary task was to quickly identify pandemic strains when they emerge, but the only way to do that was to monitor the circulating seasonal influenza viruses.

The GISRS's first director was Christopher Andrewes, the

man who'd provided the first influenza virus to be isolated. In his middle years, he'd become a modest eccentric with a usually unkempt shock of white hair: so modest that he often declined to share authorship of any paper in which he hadn't directly contributed to the research, an almost unheard-of degree of self-effacement among senior researchers. His friends and colleagues soon discovered his tendency to lose things: usually his suit immediately before any important occasion, but in later life it was as likely to be his false teeth.[29]

Andrewes was an easy man to get on with, and he built collaborations with scientists across twenty-five countries by 1952. The GISRS is now a truly global monitoring system, with scientists keeping an eye on influenza in 122 different countries.[30]

The GISRS fulfilled its primary mandate in 1957, when it warned the world that a new pandemic strain had appeared. It happened again in 1968, and although there was no way to stop the pandemics dubbed respectively 'Asian' and 'Hong Kong' flu, GISRS could at least warn the world's governments to prepare for them.[31] By the time GISRS detected 'swine flu' in 2009, it had become technically possible to produce vaccines on a useful timescale. In the event, the 2009 pandemic strain proved no more dangerous than seasonal influenza,[32] probably because it happened to be similar enough to seasonal influenza strains already in circulation that most people had some immunity to it.[33]

GISRS also monitors seasonal influenza, allowing scientists to check which isolates reflect the current wild-type and which have been left behind by its mutations.

It fulfils the first of the requirements identified by Salk and Francis. The second, a way to produce a useful quantity of vaccine before the wild-type's mutations leave an isolate behind, was the brainchild of Edwin Kilbourne at New York's Mount Sinai School of Medicine.

Edwin Kilbourne, master of viruses and doggerel

Kilbourne's colleagues knew him for doggerel that, in the words of the man who handed him one of his many awards, trod 'a very fine line between hilarity and outright libel'. His *Mating of a Flasher*[34] described the mating habits of fireflies, involving flickering males attracting females:

> Who somehow find they can't ignore
> The boy next door's spermatophore.

Kilbourne's virology has endured longer than his poetry.

His problem was that, while human influenza viruses replicate in chicken embryo cells, they do it slowly. His solution lay with one of the first influenza viruses to be isolated. It had come from a patient in Puerto Rico in 1934,[35] and after more than twenty years of being passaged from one chicken embryo to another, it had adapted to chicken embryo cells so well that it replicated in them much faster than an influenza virus isolated directly from a human. It was also useless as a vaccine because it no longer bore any resemblance to the seasonal strains in circulation.

Kilbourne's insight was based on influenza's trick of reassorting genes when two different influenza viruses infect the same cell. He injected an egg with the fast-replicating Puerto Rican strain and a recently isolated seasonal influenza strain and let nature do the rest. The reassorted progeny viruses that emerged from the egg combined the genes of their ancestors in various combinations, including the combination Kilbourne wanted: one that retained the high-speed replication of the Puerto Rican strain but carried enough genes from the current seasonal influenza strain to trigger an immune response that protected against it.[36]

By the late 1960s, Kilbourne was able to take the new isolates that GISRS identified in the spring, reassort their genes with his Puerto Rican master strain and culture the progeny into enough virus for a mass-vaccination campaign by winter. His approach is still used to produce most of the 'inactivated' influenza vaccines routinely given to adults.

Kilbourne's process was later refined further, and today, the inactivated vaccines that arrive in GP surgeries and high-street pharmacies every autumn are 'split', meaning that they only contain the two proteins from the seasonal influenza that vary most from one season to the next. Fast-replicating master strains like Kilbourne's Puerto Rican isolate remain essential for producing those proteins, but nothing from the master strain makes it into the vaccine. Removing the master strain's proteins maximises the differences between each year's vaccines and triggers a better immune response. It also reduces the side effects, like mild fevers and sore arms, that vaccines sometimes cause.[37]

How a Cold War collaboration gave us attenuated influenza vaccines

When Thomas Francis wowed America by announcing the success of Salk's inactivated polio vaccine, some of the coveted seats in Ann Arbor's Rackham Hall were allocated to his postgraduate students. For the Syrian-born Hunein Maassab, it was a pivotal moment. He determined to make a similar mark on the world,[38] and he spent the next fifty years doing so.

Maassab got his starting point from the work of Galina Alexandrovna of Leningrad's* Institute for Experimental

_____

* Now St Petersburg.

Medicine. She was attenuating wild-type influenza isolates into vaccine strains by culturing them in eggs incubated at progressively lower temperatures. When she'd got them replicating at twenty-five degrees Celsius, plunging them into the human body left them overheated and easy meat for the immune system.

Alexandrovna's strains were safe and triggered immune memory, but her attenuation process took so long that by the time her vaccine strain was ready, the wild-type strain had mutated beyond the point where her vaccine strain would protect against it.

Maassab combined her approach with Kilbourne's. First, he used Alexandrovna's technique to adapt two strains[39] to low temperatures. When he'd got them so well adapted that they replicated rapidly enough to act as a master strain, he followed Kilbourne by infecting cells with them and the current seasonal strain at the same time. The two viruses produced reassorted progeny strains as they had for Kilbourne, allowing Maassab to select a strain as similar as possible to the wild-type while retaining the fast replication of the master strain.

He now had two rapidly replicating attenuated vaccine strains that triggered an immune response to the current seasonal influenza virus. He needed two, because, by the late 1960s, it was recognised that the ever-changing human influenzas fell into two broad categories labelled A and B. Influenza A is the nastier of the two because it mutates faster. All the pandemic strains we know about are influenza A strains, and its seasonal influenza tends to be more serious than that caused by influenza B. Nevertheless, influenza B was already recognised as unpleasant enough to be worth vaccinating against.[40]

Because the master strains were attenuated, Maassab's vaccine was not injected like Kilbourne's, but sprayed up the noses of volunteers. As he hoped, they proved too attenuated to make anyone ill, but they did trigger an immune response that was effective against the seasonal strain.[41]

In 1982, Maassab and Alexandrovna co-authored a paper that described their parallel research.[42] Influenza was an enemy that even superpowers threatening each other with nuclear annihilation would cooperate against.

The vagaries of vaccine development being what they are, Maassab's 'live attenuated' vaccine did not immediately attract the attention of a pharmaceutical firm that could bring it to market. The first attenuated vaccines to be widely used were Alexandrovna's, rolled out across the Soviet Union in 1987.[43] It wouldn't be until 2003 that Maassab's strains followed them in the USA, by which time they had been taken on by MedImmune, and branded FluMist in the USA and Fluenz in Europe.

Maassab's mark was finally made after he retired. There must have been times when he wondered if his vaccine would ever see the light of day, but Maassab had never taken setbacks to heart.

'You have to be smart, that goes without saying,' his friend, Rashid Bashshur, said of him, 'but I think his unique characteristic was perseverance. Scientific discovery doesn't come easy. It's easy to give up, but he would just never give up.'[44]

In presenting the world with an attenuated vaccine, Alexandrovna and Maassab raised the question of how it compared with Kilbourne's inactivated vaccine. The answer turned out to be less than straightforward. In children, the attenuated vaccine triggers a stronger immune response, but in adults, it's the inactivated vaccine that works better.[45]

The difference lies in the fact that the less of the vaccine the immune system remembers, the more likely it is to extend its memory to the parts it hasn't encountered before.

When a child who has never had influenza before receives the live attenuated vaccine, the immune system responds as it would any other infection. It clears the virus and retains a memory for when it sees something similar.

Seasonal influenza is so common that by the time a child grows up, their immune system will have seen something similar several times, either through infection with seasonal flu or through vaccine viruses based on the same master strains. If the immune system can clear the vaccine virus by reactivating the memory of a master strain it has seen repeatedly, it may not expand its memory to encompass the components of the seasonal strain.

That's where splitting the inactivated vaccine comes in. It presents the proteins to which the response is needed without diluting them with master strain proteins that the immune system has got blasé about. This means it's much more likely to be recognised as something new, which makes it more effective in adults.[46]

Influenza vaccination today

Go to any British pharmacy or GP in September or October and you'll be assailed with leaflets and posters about this year's flu vaccine campaign. Those vaccines are the culmination of an international effort that pulls together the global surveillance built by Andrewes and the vaccine production techniques pioneered by Kilbourne, Alexandrovna and Maassab.

In January every year, the WHO issues recommendations for each year's influenza vaccines, giving the manufacturers time to prepare and test the vaccines for a roll-out in September, just ahead of the Northern Hemisphere's winter flu season. They issue another set of guidelines in October, which sets the same process in motion in time for the Southern Hemisphere winter.[47]

Most years, the recommendation is for two or three strains of influenza A and one of influenza B. Those strains are incorporated into a cocktail of attenuated vaccine strains given to children and for the inactivated split vaccine for adults.

Since 2013, the JCVI has recommended that children should be vaccinated every autumn from the ages of two to seventeen,[48] sparing them any nasty bouts of influenza during the winter flu season while building a repertoire of immune memory to a range of influenza strains. It's left to the NHS to interpret the guidelines and in some years, the older children in that range are not offered a vaccine unless they have underlying conditions that make them particularly vulnerable.

Some of the vaccine strains are changed every year, but annual vaccinations enable a child to take their first steps into adulthood with an immune memory of twenty to thirty strains. Left to nature, the same person might have been infected by around half that number, so the regular vaccination equips them far better to live with seasonal influenza.

At the time of writing, the NHS only makes the inactivated vaccine available to adults classed as 'high-risk' for becoming seriously ill. The definition of high-risk is fairly broad, covering pregnant women, everyone over sixty-five and anyone with a long list of underlying conditions.[49]

If you're not on the list, there's no need to be left out, as most pharmacies offer a walk-in service. It's simply a question of whether it's worth £20 a year to avoid a cold.

What vaccination cannot do

When I saunter into my local pharmacy every September and saunter out a few minutes later, I can't see the infrastructure of surveillance and manufacture underpinning the tingling in my arm. Impressive as that infrastructure is, it's never going to send influenza the way of polio and measles. As long as it takes nine months for the WHO's recommendations to be translated into a vaccine on a pharmacy's shelves, the vaccine is going to be nine months behind seasonal influenza's mutations.

That was what caught Lucy out. She'd had the latest vaccine, but between the WHO recommendations of early 2017 and the vaccine roll-out that autumn, one of the seasonal influenza strains mutated into something very different to what the vaccine had been based on.[50] That year's vaccination was less than half as effective as usual,[51] and when she inhaled a seasonal influenza virus, it dodged her accumulated immune memory to damage her nervous system.

The limitations of the seasonal influenza vaccine are not an argument against taking it. Even if it can't stop every infection, the vaccine does protect us against some strains and makes a nasty flu a bit less nasty.[52]

If my neighbour threw an egg at me every time I left my home, I'd never go out without my umbrella. If my neighbour got the occasional egg around the umbrella, I'd still take it, because I'd get egg on my face a lot less often with it than without it. I'd certainly fork out £20 a year if that was how long it took my umbrella to wear out. Even if influenza only causes a nasty cold, that's a lot worse than a smack in the face with an egg.

Chapter 18

COVID-19

Zheng-Li Shi was at a conference in Shanghai when her director called her and ordered, 'Drop whatever you are doing and deal with it now.'[1]

'It' was a pneumonia outbreak filling the hospitals of Wuhan, the largest city in central China. As head of the Wuhan Institute of Virology's emerging infectious diseases department, it was Shi's job to find out what was causing the outbreak. On 30 December 2019, neither Shi nor her director could have known how perfectly suited she was. She had spent the last decade and a half working on the coronavirus family and, as she quickly established, it was a coronavirus that had put those people in hospital. Within a week, she had its complete genetic sequence.

Not long before, publishing that sequence would have involved mailing it to a journal editor who, if they decided to fast-track it, might get print copies to subscribers within two or three weeks. In the first week of 2020, Shi published her sequence online, where anyone who was interested could access it.[2]

Once Shi had the virus's genome, she could test any sample for its presence, a trick she needed for her next task: tracing the outbreak to its origin. She had a pretty good idea where to start looking; of the first seven patients whose samples arrived in her laboratory, six worked at the Huanan Seafood Wholesale Market,[3] an enormous market that sold not only seafood but also live farmed and wild-caught animals of all kinds. The city authorities had already closed the market and announced that they had stopped the outbreak at its source.[4]

They had not.

It was reasonable to suppose that the outbreak started from an animal in the market, but closing the market would only end the outbreak if the microbe causing it could not transmit from one human to another. There are infections that transmit animal-to-human but not human-to-human, like anthrax and rabies, but it was dangerously optimistic to assume this new infection would behave like that without knowing what it actually was.

Nine days after closing the market, the authorities announced the first fatality: sixty-one-year-old Mr Zeng, who regularly shopped there. They did not mention that Mr Zeng's wife, who had never visited the market, fell ill five days after he did. If she had caught it from him, it would prove that the infection could indeed transmit human-to-human.

It would not have surprised the staff of Wuhan's hospitals, which were filling up with patients wheezing with pneumonia even as Wuhan's mayor delivered his annual report, spiced with promises that Wuhan would become a biomedical powerhouse with new medical schools and a biomedical industry park.[5]

Optimism was no match for a rapidly spreading virus and it wasn't long before the outbreak caught the attention of the government in Beijing.

On 18 January, the government dispatched an epidemiologist called Nanshan Zhong to Wuhan. On state television, he delivered a far less sanguine assessment. He believed the infection was transmitting between humans – and doing it enthusiastically. Zhong knew of one patient who had infected fourteen hospital staff.

The outbreak had left Huanan Market behind and was tearing its way around the city.

The authorities changed tack and announced the city would be locked down from 23 January. The warning was intended to give residents time to prepare, but instead, many opted to leave. It's impossible to blame anyone for fleeing a lockdown in a plague-ridden city, but the crowds flocking to Wuhan's railway stations and airport created the perfect environment for virus transmission; exactly what the lockdown was intended to prevent. Any infected person in those crowds would have infected many others immediately before they boarded trains or aeroplanes to every other city in China or beyond.

We all know what happened next. I'm writing this in May 2022, with the months of solitary lockdowns and the friends who died alone still very much at the front of my mind.

No doubt you bear your own scars, be they physical, psychological or both.

The COVID-19 pandemic remains far from over. Since 2020, medical science has given us many ways to treat and prevent it, but the virus Shi discovered is a moving target. Between my writing this and you reading it, the virus is likely to have pulled off a few more surprises, and medical science is likely to have added a few more weapons to our armoury. I won't try to predict them, but I dare to hope that you are reading this book in a post-pandemic world.

Enter the bat woman

Two months before Shi took that call from her director, she and her colleagues published a paper containing the statement that 'given the high diversity and recombination rate of bat coronaviruses . . . it is possible that exposure to these coronaviruses may lead to disease emergence in human populations'.[6]

Today, their dry statement reads like a screaming klaxon, but that's not how it looked in 2019. It was published in *Biosafety and Health*, a journal that is not on many people's reading lists and often publishes articles sounding such warnings, few of whom get the 'I told you so' moment that Shi has never gloated over.

Shi's entry into the world of coronaviruses was SARS, the severe acute respiratory syndrome virus that killed over 900 people in 2003.[7] By comparing the SARS coronavirus's genome to viruses circulating in animal populations, Shi showed that the SARS virus originated from a bat coronavirus that infected a human and was subsequently able to transmit between humans.[8] Fortunately, SARS was never very good at human-to-human transmission, allowing public health authorities to get a lid on it by quarantining infected people as they were treated.

If one coronavirus had crossed from a bat to a human, Shi worried, so could another. She wasn't the only one. Her Wuhan team was at the centre of a research network with close colleagues in Britain and the USA as well as in China.

She spent much of the 2000s and 2010s hiking and scrambling to the bat roosts of southern China, where she collected the coronaviruses she studied in her Wuhan laboratory. It was hard work but fruitful; she built up a picture of the coronaviruses circulating in China's bat populations[9] and earned a new nickname: the bat woman.

As they detailed in that 2019 paper, Shi and her colleagues found that among people who bought their meat in the wild animal markets of southern China, one in every 200 had at some time been infected by a bat coronavirus. They were not the first to notice. More than half the people Shi's team asked said they were worried about catching diseases from wild animal markets.

However, everyone who had been infected had fully recovered, and Shi found no evidence that any of those viruses had transmitted from one person to another.

Once, that might have been reassuring. However, the SARS outbreak showed that the occasional bat coronavirus *could* transmit between humans and cause serious disease. Now Shi had evidence that bat coronaviruses *did* infect humans fairly often. If most only caused a mild infection in one person, there had been a dangerous exception in the shape of SARS, so logically, it was only a matter of time before there was another.

That paper described a public health time bomb.

In the first days of 2020, Shi confirmed that it had gone off in the Huanan Market. Her team found the new virus smeared all over doorhandles and in the market's sewage, although they never found it in any of the market animals they tested. Shi later said the first transmission from a bat to a human might have happened somewhere else, and perhaps that person or someone infected by them brought it to Wuhan.[10]

The virus was so similar to the 2003 SARS virus that the WHO called it SARS-CoV-2, an abbreviation for severe acute respiratory syndrome coronavirus 2. The disease it caused became familiar to us all as COVID-19, an abbreviation for coronavirus disease 2019.

The WHO coined those terms in February 2020,[11] a month before they formally declared that COVID-19 was a pandemic,[12] but by the first week of January, the virus was spreading so fast that everyone paying attention knew the world had a fight on its hands.

Shi found herself cast as the Cassandra of COVID-19: her warnings were ignored until they proved correct, when, instead of being thanked, she was blamed. The blame started with posts on Chinese social media, accusing her laboratory of having allowed one of its virus samples to infect someone.[13]

Shi was well ahead of her accusers. She'd started worrying about an accidental release on the train home from Shanghai. After years of trying to warn the world about bat coronaviruses only to have her warnings come true on her doorstep, she was bound to worry that she might have inadvertently caused the disaster she was working to prevent. While her team was tracking the new virus through the Huanan Market, she was rooting through her records to make sure its genetic sequence didn't match any of the viruses in her laboratory.

It didn't.

The closest match differed from SARS-CoV-2 more than a human differs from a cat.[14] It was very similar to a bat coronavirus called RaTG13 that her team had sequenced several years before[15] – so similar that SARS-CoV-2 and RaTG13 probably shared an ancestor back in the second half of the twentieth century[16] – but the sequence was all they had. There was no sample of RaTG13 in the building.

'That really took a load off my mind,' Shi said later. 'I had not slept a wink for days.'[17]

It didn't shut up her accusers. The idea that it was all her fault spread around the world until even US President Trump was saying it. Her laboratory has been investigated several times, but no one has come up with a shred of evidence that SARS-CoV-2 was ever in her laboratory before the first hospital samples arrived.

In return for the research that gave humanity a head start against COVID-19, Shi has received far more accusation than appreciation. Then again, nobody ever thanks Batman, either.

What is COVID-19?

Thanks to Shi's sequence, the race to produce a vaccine was underway within weeks of SARS-CoV-2 first infecting a human, but in early 2020, it was a race that the vaccinologists weren't winning. Being about twice as infective as influenza,[18]

SARS-CoV-2 ripped across the globe. We all came to dread its signature symptom of losing our senses of taste and smell, which told us that SARS-CoV-2 had invaded our bodies.

When I was a researcher, coffee-break conversations occasionally fell to inventing the virus we really didn't want to have to deal with, and we often came up with something that, in retrospect, looked very similar to SARS-CoV-2: a virus that can be transmitted by breathing, infect the lining of the throat and then spread down the windpipe to the lungs.

Like influenza, measles and encapsulated bacteria like pneumococcus, SARS-CoV-2 infects the lining of the throat and nose and is transmitted by breathing. That's not unusual; there are over 200 common cold viruses that do that at any given time, and much as we might dislike them, we don't particularly fear them. As long as they stay in the upper part of the respiratory tract and away from the lungs, they're annoying but not particularly dangerous.

The SARS virus did infect the lungs, which is why it was so much more serious. However, the characteristic that made it so dangerous was also what made it so inefficient at infecting people; the airway between the upper respiratory tract and the lungs is not a friendly environment for a virus. It's coated with a conveyor belt of mucus laden with antiviral molecules, which wafts anything caught in it up to the nose and mouth to be exhaled out of the body.[19] If a virus manages to get past the mucus to the lungs, it's usually stuck down there. It can't get back out to infect someone else without running the gauntlet of virucidal mucus all over again.

Viruses that infect the upper respiratory tract tend to be highly infective but not particularly dangerous, while viruses that infect the lungs tend to be dangerous but not very infective. That's why the nightmare scenario of those coffee-break conversations was a virus that could do both: it combined features that made a virus both highly transmissible and very dangerous. Pandemic influenzas do that, which is why there has been a global early warning system in place for more than seventy years. It's also what SARS-CoV-2 does.

It does it so effectively that in 2020, fifteen out of every hundred people who caught it ended up in hospital,[20,21] and one of those fifteen did not come out alive[22] – at least, in places where there was a hospital to go to. In lower-income countries where there often isn't, figures remain hard to come by.[23]

COVID-19 is not an equal-opportunity killer. In the early stages of the pandemic, it emerged that age dramatically affected the chances of surviving SARS-CoV-2 infection. Someone in their late twenties only had a one-in-1,000 chance of dying if they were infected, which rose to one-in-100 by the early sixties, and one-in-ten at over eighty.[24]

Age wasn't the only factor. Being male made COVID-19 appreciably more dangerous,[25] as did underlying health conditions like diabetes and hypertension,[26] which, in the absence of SARS-CoV-2, can be managed relatively easily.

The receptor-binding domain: the prime target

Within months of the first human infection, SARS-CoV-2 became the most intensively researched virus in history. Much of that research focused on one small part of the virus: the receptor-binding domain of the spike protein, usually abbreviated to the RBD.

The coronaviruses are named for the spike proteins, which stud the viral capsid to make it look like the solar corona under an electron microscope.[27] The RBD sits at the tip of each spike, where it is perfectly placed to attach the viral capsid to a cell for the virus to infect. Block the RBD and you block the virus from infecting.

Coronavirus RBDs had been blocked before. That was how Sarah Gilbert's vaccine* against MERS, a close relative of both SARS viruses, had worked. She made it by inserting the MERS spike protein into a chimpanzee virus, triggering antibodies that blocked the MERS RBD.[28] If it worked against MERS, then why not against SARS-CoV-2? With no one funding her to take the MERS vaccine further, it was a relatively simple matter to slot the spike protein from Shi's sequence into the chimpanzee virus.

Gilbert's viral vector vaccine wasn't the only vaccine platform in need of a target. The other was the brainchild of Katalin Karikó at the University of Pennsylvania in the birthplace of many a vaccine: Philadelphia.

Karikó had left Hungary for the USA in 1985, which was not straightforward when it involved crossing the Iron Curtain. She and her husband had to leave behind everything they couldn't take in their luggage, and their Hungarian Forint were worthless in the USA. When they sold their possessions, they illegally exchanged the money for US dollars, which they smuggled out of the country, sewn into their two-year-old daughter's teddy bear.[29]

As Karikó was getting used to living in a new country, she was trying to develop a treatment for people who were unable to produce critical proteins. If their own DNA wasn't being transcribed into the messenger RNA (mRNA) that was then translated into those proteins, she reasoned, perhaps inserting synthetic RNA would fill the gap. It was a simple concept that ran into a complex problem: cells don't take kindly to having foreign RNA shoved into them.

It's a problem that viruses have been up against for as long as there have been viruses. Part of a capsid's role is to get past

* See Chapter 3.

the defence mechanisms on a cell's surface, and once its genetic material is inside the cell, every virus has its own bag of tricks for dodging the cell's internal defences. Gilbert's solution was to co-opt the bag of tricks that came with the virus she used as a delivery mechanism.

Karikó persisted in trying to find a way to do it from scratch, and persistence was what she needed. She often found it difficult to explain the value of a platform technology, meaning something that can be developed into multiple uses, to administrators who think in terms of one device being invented to solve one problem.

She later recalled trying to persuade one of the university's intellectual property officers to file a patent.

'What's it *good* for?' he kept asking her.

Karikó tried a different tack, noticing the property officer was going bald. She told him her mRNA platform might be useful for regrowing hair.

The patent was duly filed.[30]

In 1997, she met Drew Weissmann over the department's photocopier. He was trying to develop a vaccine against HIV, and between them, they realised that inserting RNA into a cell might be a viable approach to vaccination.[31] It would induce the vaccinee's cells to produce a virus's protein, and it wouldn't matter if the cell woke up to what was going on and reacted against it. Triggering an immune response is, after all, what a vaccine is supposed to do.

In 2012, she met Uğur Şahin of the German biotechnology company BioNTech, and she subsequently combined her university position with a vice-presidency of the firm. Their first foray into vaccine development, funded by the US government's National Institutes of Health, was in response to the 2015 Zika virus outbreak.

Zika, like rubella, usually causes a fairly mild disease, but if it infects a pregnant woman, it can seriously damage the developing foetus. The 2015 outbreak filled Brazilian maternity wards with babies born with microcephaly, meaning that their heads were unusually small because the infection slowed their brain development.[32] Karikó and Weissman adapted their mRNA delivery system to deliver a Zika protein into a vaccinee's cells, which the mRNA would then co-opt into producing the protein for their immune system to respond to.

In essence, their mRNA vaccine worked like a stripped-down virus. Like a virus, it used a cell's biochemistry to read a gene into a protein, but unlike a virus, it only carried one gene and it could not replicate itself.

Their Zika vaccine was ready for human trials within two years,[33] which is extremely fast by the standards of modern vaccine development. It wasn't fast enough. The Zika epidemic had already waned and the vaccine was no longer needed.

After three decades of indifferent administrators, reluctant funders and meticulous research, 2019 found Karikó's mRNA technology was in much the same place as Gilbert's viral vector vaccine. Both were ways to persuade a cell to produce the protein that could then trigger an immune response, both were platform technologies that could swiftly be adapted to whatever protein was needed, both had proved their worth in early-stage trials, and both were stuck at the bottom of the biotech valley of death because no one wanted to fund a phase 3 trial.

Then someone met the wrong bat.

The race for a vaccine

The last fourteen chapters have described how fourteen pathogens were countered with one type of vaccine each. For some, that one wasn't enough and a second type followed years or decades later. Normally, it's difficult enough to muster the resources for one vaccine, let alone two.

In 2020, the one-vaccine-at-a-time playbook went out of the window. With country after country going into lockdown, the world needed a vaccine and it needed it fast. Nobody knew which vaccine type would work, so vaccinologists tried everything. Some went with the pure Pasteur doctrine of killing the virus and injecting it. Others took the more refined approach of synthesising the spike protein alone and injecting that.

It soon became apparent that the frontrunners were the new technologies of viral vectors and mRNA vaccines, which were based heavily on Gilbert and Karikó's research and developed by several different firms. Karikó's mRNA vaccine was picked up by Pfizer, a large pharmaceutical firm that could put the sort of financial and manufacturing muscle behind it that BioNTech could not.

As 2020 ground on, reports of vaccine trials offered the occasional moment of hope as the unrelenting death toll headlined the news. By autumn, the vaccines were looking better than even the most optimistic vaccinologists dared hope. They worked. All of them. Some better than others and none better than Karikó's mRNA vaccine,[34] but even those made by the century-old technology of inactivating the virus dramatically reduced the danger of disease severe enough to put someone in hospital.[35]

On 8 December 2020, ninety-year-old Margaret Keenan was wheeled into Coventry's University Hospital wearing a grey cardigan and a 'Merry Christmas' T-shirt featuring a dancing penguin. The BBC filmed her sitting calmly while Matron May Parsons injected Karikó's mRNA vaccine into her left arm. It looked like a routine vaccination, but the cameras were there because it was far from routine.

May Parsons was the first person to give a COVID-19 vaccine outside a clinical trial, and Margaret Keenan was the first to receive one.

The hospital staff, who had spent the last year fighting – and often without success – to keep COVID-19 patients alive, did not share Keenan's insouciance. They lined the corridor to applaud her as she was wheeled out.[36]

Humanity's fightback against SARS-CoV-2 had begun.

Mutations in Kent

A month after the global vaccine roll-out began in Coventry, SARS-CoV-2 revealed that it had a few tricks of its own. When a virus replicates its genome, there's always a chance that the replication won't be perfect. The occasional mistake often slips in, and once in a while, that mistake proves to be an advantage over the virus it was replicated from.

At around the same time as May Parsons was vaccinating Margaret Keenan in Coventry, a variant appeared in Kent that spread much faster than the 'ancestral' variant that had driven the pandemic for the last year. The new variant's secret was a mutation that improved the attachment between its RBD and human cells.

It was different enough to the ancestral variant that Shi had sequenced in January 2020 that it was given a new name: the Alpha variant.[37] It was not very different to the ancestral variant, with the difference being confined to a tiny part of the RBD, which is itself a small part of one of SARS-CoV-2's twenty or so proteins;[38] the jury is still out on the exact number.

Alpha was the first 'variant of concern', as the WHO calls variants more transmissible or more virulent than the ancestral. It would not be the last. Within a few weeks, Beta appeared in South Africa and Gamma in Brazil. Both spread as enthusiastically as Alpha, but before they could spread as far, Delta appeared in India and spread so fast that it replaced every other variant. Its RBD was so much better at getting its genome into a cell[39] that it was two to three times more transmissible[40] than the ancestral variant. Worse, it was twice as likely to hospitalise or kill someone.[41]

The variants of concern appeared as the various vaccines were being rolled out, producing a moment of high suspense. The vaccines allowed us to hope that the end of the pandemic might be in sight, but just when we were starting to receive them, we had to worry that SARS-CoV-2 had mutated them into obsolescence.

At least part of the immunity triggered by the vaccines comes from triggering antibodies that bind to the RBD, physically blocking the virus from binding to its target cell. The problem was that the vaccines used the RBD of the ancestral variant, and by mid-2021, most infections involved the mutated Delta variant.

It wasn't immediately clear how big a problem that was. As small as the RBD is, there are many different places where an antibody can bind to it, and some antibodies triggered by the ancestral RBD bound every variant from Alpha to Delta.[42] On the other hand, many did not. The only way to tell whether the difference in antibody binding would translate into a difference in protection was to wait and see.

As data trickled in, the worst fears appeared unfounded. The vaccines proved less effective against Delta than against the ancestral variant,[43] but only marginally. Vaccinated people who did get infected were still far less likely to end up hospitalised or dead than unvaccinated people.[44] In the year after Margaret Keenan's five minutes of fame, COVID-19 vaccines prevented between 19 and 21 million deaths around the world, and that was with less than half the world's population fully vaccinated.[45]

For most of 2021, the biggest problem was producing enough vaccine and getting it to clinics – but in November, SARS-CoV-2 changed the game again.

The Omicron variant

In November 2021, a South African laboratory identified a new variant from a sample collected in Botswana.[46] The variant dubbed Omicron arrived in Johannesburg at about the same time as the sample, and spread through the population like wildfire.

There was bad news and good news. The bad news was that it was infecting a lot of people who had been either vaccinated or infected with an earlier variant, showing that it could infect people who were already immune. The good news was that once someone was infected with Omicron, they were far less likely to end up hospitalised or worse than someone infected with Delta.

As Omicron replaced Delta as the globally dominant variant, doctors and epidemiologists noticed a change in the disease it caused. Anosmia and dry cough were now rare, and most cases looked much more like the sniffles and sneezes of the common cold.[47]

On the face of it, that was good news. If COVID-19 was turning into a common cold, that meant the infection was staying in the upper respiratory tract and away from the lungs. Even if someone's immune memory failed to prevent SARS-CoV-2 from infecting them, perhaps it could confine the infection to where it did minimal damage. Alternatively, the difference may lie less with the people being infected than with the Omicron variant infecting them.[48]

It turned out that both possibilities contained some truth.

Omicron proved far better than Delta at slipping past immune memory. A single vaccine dose gave a substantial amount of protection against Delta, but none at all against Omicron infection, and even two doses didn't help much.[49] Worse, Omicron was more than twice as infectious as Delta,[50] far surpassing the cold viruses and making it almost as infectious as measles.

Omicron wasn't only better at binding its target cell. It was fundamentally different. It was less likely to infect lung cells than earlier variants, and while those earlier variants got their genome into a cell by fusing their capsid with a cell's outer membrane, Omicron did it by inducing the membrane to engulf it.[51]

As epidemiological results came in, it appeared that those differences made Omicron less dangerous than Delta. As Omicron replaced Delta as the USA's dominant variant in the early weeks of 2022, a Delta infection was four times more likely to put someone in hospital[52] or prove fatal[53] than an Omicron infection.

Omicron was evidently a milder variant than Delta. Emphasis on milder. As I write this, Omicron is filling hospitals in Hong Kong, where the authorities are reporting that it's at least as dangerous to unvaccinated people as the ancestral variant that tore around the world in 2020.[54] Omicron is nothing to be complacent about.

Omicron has been particularly devastating in Hong Kong, because many older people have not been vaccinated. In the USA, Omicron is six times more likely to hospitalise[55] or kill[56] an unvaccinated than a vaccinated person. Vaccination provides a substantial amount of protection, but it cannot prevent Omicron from infecting.

Between mid-2020 and mid-2022, the nature of the pandemic had fundamentally changed. Instead of the ancestral variant infecting people who had no immunity, most infections now involved the Omicron variant infecting people who had some immunity from a previous infection or vaccination. Someone infected with SARS-CoV-2 was far more likely to recover without needing hospitalisation, but not all the change was for the better.

Unfortunately, Omicron appeared as many countries were dropping measures like face masks and physical distancing. The combination of Omicron's high infectivity and widespread complacency allowed Omicron to infect far more people than Delta had. In the USA, the number of COVID-19 hospitalisations[57] and deaths[58] actually went up as the milder Omicron replaced the more severe Delta, simply because so many more people were being infected.

Omicron continues to take a deadly toll. In the first month of 2022, it killed around 7,000 people in Britain,[59] which is as many as influenza killed in a typical pre-pandemic year.[60]

Thousands of deaths would be bad enough if death was the only outcome we had to worry about, but not everyone who survives COVID-19 completely recovers.

Long-haul COVID

Under normal circumstances, social media is the last place to look for medical advice, but 2020 was the year in which normality was suspended.

In May that year, Amy Watson, a schoolteacher from Portland, Oregon, became so frustrated with her COVID-19 dragging on that she started a Facebook group called 'Long Haul COVID Fighters', a joking reference to the trucker's baseball cap she wore to her COVID-19 test.[61]

Watson hoped to connect with other people left debilitated by COVID-19, but by providing a forum for 'long-haulers', as the people flocking to her page called themselves, Watson revealed that long-haul COVID affected far more people than anyone had realised. When the WHO published a definition of long-haul COVID, it made Watson the first person to name a medical condition on social media, although most technical papers now call it 'long COVID' or sometimes, 'post-acute COVID-19 syndrome' or PACS.

Despite the WHO definition, long-haul COVID – or PACS, or whatever it's called – manifests inconsistently enough to leave the definition somewhat fuzzy around the edges. It usually means having any COVID-19 symptom for at least three months.[62] Difficulty in breathing is one of the most common, and sometimes the easiest to explain, because COVID-19 sometimes leaves the lungs laced with scar tissue – but only sometimes. Many long-haulers struggle to get enough oxygen into their bloodstream for no clear reason. Others suffer from chronic pain, chronic fatigue or the sort of heart problems that beset Lucy after her bout with seasonal influenza described in the previous chapter.

Lucy is living proof that long-term problems from short-term infections are not restricted to COVID-19, although they are far more common with COVID-19 than with influenza. In the early stages of the pandemic, when most COVID-19 involved the ancestral variant infecting people with no immunity, more than half of those people were left with at least one symptom after six months.[63]

By mid-2022, most cases involve Omicron infecting people who have either been vaccinated, previously infected or both, and fewer than one in ten become long-haulers.[64] By April 2022, that left around 1.3 million people in Britain – around one in every 50 – struggling with long COVID that had lasted at least three months, and with no idea of how much longer it was going to last.[65]

Even if the pandemic is over by the time you read this, it's safe to say that there are many, many people who have not recovered.

Doses and boosters

With the sole exception of the Johnson & Johnson mRNA vaccine, all of the COVID-19 vaccines were originally tested with a two-dose schedule. That was always something of a punt, because nobody could know how best to use viral vectors or mRNA vaccines until they were rolled out, and, as happened with the conjugate vaccines against Hib and pneumococcus, there's always some trial and error involved in finding the best way to deploy a new vaccine type.

Moreover, the coronaviruses are notorious for not triggering long-lasting immune memory.[66] However, that didn't automatically mean that immune memory triggered by a vaccine would wane as fast as immune memory triggered by natural infection. If coronaviruses had some biochemical trick that interfered with the development of immune memory, then separating the spike protein from the rest of SARS-CoV-2 would separate it from that trick.

It was impossible to know until there were an appreciable number of people vaccinated, but in mid-2021, when Delta was the dominant variant, there were enough 'breakthrough' infections among vaccinated people that several health authorities added a third dose to the schedule. The third dose was originally described as a 'booster', making it sound like it was intended to top up dwindling immunity, but it proved to be much more than that.

The first evaluation of the third dose came from Israel, where a team of epidemiologists found that compared to two doses, three doses improved protection against infection by ten times and protection against hospitalisation by a whopping twenty times.[67] That makes a third dose look less like a booster than something that should be a routine part of the dose regime.

The Israeli evaluation looked at the effect of Karikó's Pfizer-made mRNA vaccine at a time when Delta was the dominant variant. It would later emerge that three doses were less effective against Omicron.[68] Many countries are now rolling out a fourth dose, although what effect that will have remains to be seen.

Part of the issue may be that as I write this in mid-2022, all available vaccines are still based on the ancestral variant's spike protein, while most infections now involve Omicron, with its mutated RBD. Manufacturers are working on 'tweaking' their vaccines to use Omicron's spike, which may or may not prove more effective.

If it emerges that vaccines need to be tailored to variants, we can't assume that an Omicron-based vaccine will be the endgame, because we can't assume that Omicron will be the last variant to emerge. So far, the pattern has been that when a more infective variant emerges, it replaces its predecessors, presumably by spreading faster and leaving its surviving victims immune. Every current variant, from Alpha to Omicron, is a mutation of the ancestral variant, but that gives us little idea of where we go from here. The ancestral variant is rapidly heading for extinction, and Omicron now dominates the pandemic, so any future variant will probably be a mutation of Omicron.

It's conceivable that Omicron is as far as SARS-CoV-2's mutations can take it. It may be physically impossible for a variant to be more infective than Omicron. Very few viruses even come close. On the other hand, there's now a new nightmare scenario for coffee-break conversations: a variant of SARS-CoV-2 that combines Delta's severity with Omicron's ability to evade immunity.

If that variant ever appears, humanity will at least be starting the vaccine race with less of a handicap than we had in 2020. Because both mRNA and viral vector vaccines use synthetic sequences, it's relatively easy to switch the sequence of the spike protein to that of a new variant. A modified vaccine could be rolled out much faster because it wouldn't need to go through three phases of clinical trials. It would be the same sort of adjustment that's applied to the seasonal influenza vaccines rolled out every year, and at least for mRNA vaccines, the manufacturing process is much less laborious, so they could be rolled out quickly.

It would be a further success to crown Karikó's decades of

bringing mRNA technology to fruition, although in a 2021 interview she said she prefers to see her success in more personal terms. She described hearing from the residents of Meadowbrook Care Home in Plattsburgh, New York State, who had lived in terror of COVID-19 for a year before they were given her vaccine. A week later, COVID-19 got through the door for the first time. Many of the residents became ill, but they were spared the holocaust that had struck so many care homes in 2020. Not one Meadowbrook resident died.

The residents held a 'Kati Karikó appreciation day' with T-shirts and a banner thanking her for saving their lives. Then they started a campaign to get her nominated for the Nobel Peace Prize.[69]

She had come a long way from the expectations of her childhood. As she told one interviewer, 'My father wanted me to be a butcher.'[70]

III

The myths and mysteries of vaccination

Chapter 19

What is herd immunity and why is it important?

One of epidemiology's most often misunderstood concepts started with a few cages of mice at the University of Manchester. They were part of an experiment run by William Topley and Graham Wilson, who infected the mice with the salmonella bacterium. The mice looked identical but there was one critical difference; some had been exposed to salmonella, giving them some immunity to it, while others had not.

Topley and Wilson put the immune mice in cages with mice that had never been exposed to salmonella, and then infected them all. As they expected, the infection spread through the unexposed mice – but not equally. The higher the proportion of mice in a cage that were immune, the slower the salmonella spread and the more unexposed mice survived. Being surrounded by immune mice was protecting mice that were not themselves immune.

The title of Topley and Wilson's 1923 paper introduced the term 'herd immunity':[1] the concept that if enough individuals are immune to a pathogen, they protect any non-immune individuals among them by being unable to infect them.

Topley and Wilson moved on to found the Public Health Laboratory Service,* which has been diagnosing the British public ever since.[2] The rest of us are left to grapple with how herd immunity works in human populations and with the rather ugly term they gave the concept. Many textbooks call it community protection, because not being cattle, most of us prefer to think of ourselves as part of a community than a herd. However, the COVID-19 pandemic dragged the concept into the headlines as herd immunity, under which name it's caused a lot of epidemiologists to shout at their televisions.

The most egregious misunderstanding is that once a pathogen has infected enough people, a population has achieved herd immunity and nobody needs to worry about the pathogen anymore.

It doesn't work like that. The American rubella epidemic of 1965 and subsequent race for a vaccine, covered in Chapter 15, shows us why.

Herd immunity the natural way

While the rubella epidemic was underway, it divided the American population into three categories.

By far the largest category was the immune: people who had recovered from rubella and were now immune to it.

The next largest category was the non-immune: people who had never caught it but would if someone breathed rubella virus on them.

The third category was the infected: people with an active infection. This was by far the smallest category because rubella infection only takes around three weeks to run its course.[3] After

---

* Now part of the UK Health Security Agency.

that, the infected person had transitioned from the non-immune to the immune category.

The longer the epidemic went on, the more non-immune people were infected and became immune. A few were unlucky and died, but it made no difference to rubella. Whether through immunity or death, non-immune people were getting scarcer.

Most of the non-immune were children who had not been around for long enough to catch rubella during previous epidemics, and, being children, often ended up clustered in school classrooms. The illustration on page 313 shows how rubella could spread once it got through a classroom door, laying all but a few fortunate children low at the same time. When those infected children recovered, being surrounded by their immune classmates protected them from being infected.

The hypothetical classroom is a microcosm of what was playing out across the USA, with rubella passing from infected to non-immune people until it ran out of clusters of non-immune people to infect. There were still a few non-immune people around, but once they were sufficiently few and far between that they were surrounded by immune people, there was no opportunity for rubella to infect them.

The USA had achieved herd immunity.

If herd immunity could permanently protect a population from a pathogen, 1965 would have been the last year that the USA needed to worry about rubella.

It wasn't.

That's why Stanley Plotkin and Maurice Hilleman threw so much effort into developing rubella vaccines – and developing them fast. They weren't only competing with each other. They were racing the erosion of herd immunity.

With rubella, herd immunity is reached when 85–87 per cent of a population is immune, leaving the remaining 13–15 per cent uninfected and non-immune. Natural infection can make enough people immune to reach the threshold but no more than that. When infections ceased, herd immunity couldn't last long, because every baby born in America swelled the ranks of the non-immune, while every death of old age shrank the ranks of the immune.

When herd immunity depends on natural infection, it is always temporary.

The proponents of herd immunity to COVID-19 rarely acknowledged its ephemerality. They were not talking about enduring a single COVID-19 wave that would protect a population. They were talking about successive epidemics that would inevitably infect everyone sooner or later.

The herd immunity threshold depends on how many people need to be non-immune for an epidemic to get going. The answer depends on another concept that the COVID-19 pandemic dragged into the headlines: the basic reproductive number, usually abbreviated to R_0 or, for a TV pundit reporting it as if it's a football score, the 'R-number'.

The R_0 is the average number of people that one infected person will infect. Every pathogen has a different R_0, and the higher it is, the shorter the period between epidemics.

From rubella's 85–87 per cent herd immunity threshold and its R_0 of seven to eight, epidemiologists can calculate that it takes between three and five years for herd immunity to fall below the threshold and open the door to another outbreak.

Measles has the much higher R_0 of fifteen to seventeen, meaning that the herd immunity threshold is the much higher 92–95 per cent. The higher the herd immunity threshold, the less time herd immunity lasts. Before measles vaccines were available, measles outbreaks happened every year or two.

Those numbers also explain why diseases like measles and rubella are usually considered diseases of childhood. Both are perfectly capable of infecting adults, but outbreaks happen so often that few people get through childhood without being infected.

Preventing disease by adjusting R_0

If we know that a pathogen can't circulate when a population has achieved herd immunity and we know the factors that affect it, perhaps we can manipulate those factors to protect ourselves. We can't change the pathogen's infectiveness, but that's not the only factor influencing its R_0. It's also affected by the population in which the pathogen is circulating, to the extent that a pathogen can have different R_0 values in different populations. The R_0 values above were calculated from Western European and North American countries in the late twentieth century,[4] but measles, for example, can have an R_0 as high as thirty in some African populations.[5]

Because R_0 depends on the people a pathogen infects, we can reduce it by reducing a pathogen's opportunities to infect. The simplest action is for anyone who feels ill to minimise their contact with other people. The fewer people an infected person gets close to, the less likely they are to infect a non-immune person. Avoidance usually happens without anyone needing to be told; none of us is at our most gregarious when we're ill.

The catch is that many pathogens are infectious before we start feeling ill. Someone infected with rubella, for example, is infectious for around a week before they know it.[6] They're likely to assume they're still in the non-immune category and at risk of being infected when in fact they have *become* the risk to non-immune people.

When a pathogen can make someone infectious without their knowing it, sick people staying in bed does nothing to stop it from spreading. The only way to drive down its R_0 is to restructure society to rob the pathogen of opportunities to infect anyone. Historically, the most effective restructuring involved building closed sewers, closing off the faecal-oral infection route.

It's much harder to tackle a pathogen that floats out of an

infected person's mouth whenever they exhale. Many countries imposed sweeping restrictions in response to the three influenza pandemics of the twentieth century and the twenty-first-century COVID-19 pandemic, but most airborne pathogens are left to do their worst. The problem is that the more infective the pathogen, the stricter the restrictions needed to impact its R_0 and the greater the disruption they will cause to society and economy.

Airborne pathogens present policymakers with a question that has no good answers. They can only try to choose the least-worst answer, which is why much of the world spent the early 2020s dancing the lockdown hokey-cokey.

If only there were a way to make non-immune people into immune people without their having to be infected.

That's where vaccination comes in.

The immunological kindness of strangers

For the individual, vaccination confers immunity to the pathogen. For society, mass vaccination keeps the proportion of immune people high enough to sustain herd immunity.

Unlike natural infections, vaccinations do not stop when the herd immunity threshold is reached. Vaccination can make enough people immune to place the overall population comfortably above the threshold, which makes an outbreak far less likely than if the population's immunity is wobbling on that threshold and allows some breathing space if the vaccine supply is disrupted.

Once a vaccine is available, we may ask why we should care about herd immunity. If anyone wants to protect themselves or their children, all they have to do is ask. If someone chooses to take their chance with the pathogen, that's their business.

However, no vaccine is completely effective for every individual. The measles vaccine is one of the most effective available, but it protects only 99 per cent of vaccinees.[7] 'Only' is not a qualification usually applied to a 99 per cent success rate, but when a virus's herd immunity threshold is over 90 per cent, it doesn't allow a lot of wriggle room. If a small percentage of people shun vaccination, the non-immune category becomes large enough to allow an outbreak among both the unvaccinated and the unfortunate 1 per cent for whom the vaccine hasn't provided protection.

Another group dependent on herd immunity are babies who have yet to be vaccinated. While childhood vaccinations are timed to protect a child from as early as possible, giving a vaccine too early risks it being neutralised by maternal antibodies before the baby reacts to it. It's a delicate compromise that leaves a window of vulnerability between the waning of maternal antibodies and the first vaccination.

Another group who can't be protected individually are people with compromised immune systems, who are simultaneously unable to respond to vaccination and extremely vulnerable to the infections against which vaccines protect healthy people.

For a time, I was one of those people.

That was when I was being treated for a lymphoma caused by a mutation that made some of my B-cells – the lymphocytes that produce antibodies – divide uncontrollably.

Different cancers are treated with different chemotherapy drugs that target dividing cells. Cancer cells do a lot of dividing, but so do the lymphocytes of the immune system. Chemotherapy drugs can't tell the difference. Every dose hit my immune system like a wrecking ball. Every treatment left me wide open to infection for a week or two, but it was about to get worse.

When I felt I'd had more drugs pumped into me than some of the Tour de France winners who were then making all the wrong headlines, it became evident that they weren't doing the trick. The lymphoma cells were clinging on and the only thing that would get rid of them was a haematopoetic stem cell transplant.

Haematopoetic stem cells are where lymphocytes that patrol our bodies come from. They usually sit in the bone marrow, where they divide to produce the lymphocytes, but in my case, it looked like they were also the source of the mutated B-cells that were causing my lymphoma. They would have to go. All of them. Along with every lymphocyte I had.

In case you're wondering, yes, it hurt.

The plan was to replace them with transplanted stem cells from a donor. The transplant went as well as I'd dared hope, but it wasn't the end of my problems. I now faced the same problem as anyone else who receives a transplant: keeping the peace between the 'old' and the 'new' parts of my body. Like anyone else's, my donor's immune system was programmed to attack any cells it didn't recognise as being part of my donor. It was now surrounded by cells that weren't part of that donor – me – and didn't know it wasn't supposed to attack them.

People who receive an organ transplant, such as a heart or kidney, have the same problem but the other way round. Their own immune system attacks the donor cells without realising it's behaving suicidally. Either way, the internal squabbling has to be controlled with drugs that suppress the immune system.

Those drugs suppressed the civil war inside my body, but suppressing my immune system left me vulnerable to infections and unable to form immune memory to either infections or to vaccines.

Some transplant recipients need to suppress their immune systems for the rest of their lives. I was luckier. After a few months, my donated immune system stopped trying to attack me. I stopped taking the drugs and let it start trying to protect me.

At that point, it wasn't very good at it. Wiping out my lymphocytes had wiped out my immune memory accumulated from decades of infections and vaccinations. I was left with the immune memory of a newborn baby, without a newborn's ability to build new immune memory. I wouldn't be able to respond to vaccines for a year or so after I came off the immune suppressants, and it would be several more before I could handle any vaccine containing a live virus. Even the measles vaccine strain might be more than my fragile immunity could handle, which wasn't reassuring given what wild-type measles can do to even a healthy person.

Between the lymphoma, the chemotherapy and recovering from the transplant, I spent the best part of seven years being protected by the immunological kindness of strangers.

I share my experience because it's far from unique. Anyone being treated for cancer or learning to live with a transplant is in the same situation, as well as some unfortunate people born with immune deficiencies.

The most severe deficiency is rather literally called severe combined immunodeficiency, or SCID, a condition that leaves someone incapable of producing lymphocytes and therefore incapable of formulating a complete immune response, let alone immune memory.[8] There are many less comprehensive immune deficiencies, but they all have the same effect: an impaired ability to mount an immune response to an infection or produce immune memory to a vaccine.

Sara's story

A weak immune system can leave someone dependent on herd immunity, but so can an immune system that's too strong in the wrong place. That's what happened to Sara* from San Diego.

At seventeen years old, Sara had been offered a coveted college place that required an MMR booster to top up her immunity to measles, mumps and rubella. She'd had her MMR at fifteen months old without incident, so she was happy to comply.

---

* Pseudonym.

Ten minutes after receiving the vaccine, Sara wished she hadn't. Her skin broke out in hives, her hands and face swelled, her nose started running and, worst of all, her throat swelled up and made her feel like she was choking.

Sara was suffering from a severe allergic reaction called anaphylaxis, an overreaction of her immune system involving a massive inflammation. It's the same condition that causes some people to collapse after a bee or a wasp sting. People who know they are prone to anaphylaxis often carry a shot of adrenaline with them in case they're exposed to whatever triggers it, but Sara was caught unprepared. Nothing like this had ever happened to her before.

Sara dragged herself back to the clinic to ask, or rather to wheeze, for help. She must have seen TV depictions of anaphylaxis in which a life-saving shot of adrenaline or − if the screenwriter is really going for the ratings − someone willing to slice open the sufferer's windpipe, is all that stands between a sufferer and asphyxiation.

The reality is rarely that dramatic. Most sufferers recover without treatment,[9] but the clinic doctor wasn't taking any chances. With Sara's blood pressure dropping, they treated her with adrenaline and an antihistamine for the hives and swelling. Sara felt better immediately, but an hour and a half later, her throat swelled up again.

The doctor gave her more adrenaline and called an ambulance, deciding she needed treatment that only a hospital could provide. By the time she arrived at the Emergency Department, Sara was already much better, and she went home the same day.

A month later, Sara returned to the clinic to find out what had triggered her anaphylaxis. A doctor inserted tiny amounts of suspect substances under her skin to see what caused a reaction and, to no one's surprise, Sara proved allergic to the MMR vaccine. More surprising was that she didn't react to the measles, mumps or rubella viruses. She'd developed an allergy to gelatine,[10] a substance included in the vaccine to stabilise it. She could never again receive any vaccine containing it.

Anaphylaxis is a frightening word, but allergic reactions to vaccines are extremely rare. So rare that to find out how rare, someone has to monitor an enormous number of vaccinations.

One of the few studies to do that was led by Kari Bohlke of Seattle's Center for Health Studies. Her team monitored 7.5 million vaccinations against a range of diseases and found only five cases of anaphylaxis, two of which they were sure were caused by vaccines while three might have been.[11] Even if all five cases had been caused by vaccines, that would be only one case of anaphylaxis for every 1.5 million vaccinations. If only the two cases they were sure about were caused by the vaccines, that would be one case per 3.75 million. The true figure probably lies somewhere between the two.

Like most people who suffer from anaphylaxis, all five of Bohlke's cases recovered. However, anaphylaxis is a serious risk, and once someone is known to have an allergy to something, they can't receive any vaccine containing that something. People with allergies form yet another group dependent on herd immunity.

The limits of herd immunity

Herd immunity is the best protection available to the motley crew of unvaccinatables, formed of people whose immune systems are too apathetic or over-enthusiastic to handle vaccines. They can't choose to be vaccinated, which leaves their protection in the hands of people who can.

Ideally, we'd like a vaccine to give us immunity so strong that the pathogen can't get a foothold in our bodies and can't use us as a base for infecting someone else. The Hib, measles, hepatitis B, polio and rubella vaccines all achieve that. The HPV, pneumococcus and meningococcus conjugate vaccines prevent transmission of the types contained in the vaccines, but they haven't been in use for long enough to know whether that immunity lasts a lifetime or not.

On the other hand, some vaccines protect against serious disease but don't stop the vaccinated person from being infectious. Herd immunity cannot protect a child from rotavirus, even if everyone who comes near him is vaccinated. The vaccine is very effective against severe disease, but there are simply too many strains for the vaccine to confer complete immunity against all of them.

Nor is herd immunity any help against tetanus or diphtheria, where the immunity is to a toxin secreted by the bacterium rather than the bacterium itself. Immunity to the diphtheria toxin doesn't prevent infection, while the tetanus bacterium is not infectious in the first place.

Somewhere between the vaccines that prevent transmission and vaccines that permit it are vaccines that reduce it. The whooping cough, mumps, influenza and COVID-19 vaccines all trigger immune responses that are effective but don't provide lifelong complete immunity. They're the ones that send epidemiologists reaching for the headache pills, because it's extremely difficult to work out how much they reduce transmission by, which an epidemiologist needs to calculate a herd immunity threshold.

The rest of us can leave that to the epidemiologists. Herd immunity is only ever a secondary benefit of vaccination that should never be allowed to overshadow the primary benefit: to protect the person being vaccinated from disease. If that person protects others at the same time, so much the better. They will always have the gratitude of people like me, whose lives have depended on other people's vaccinations.

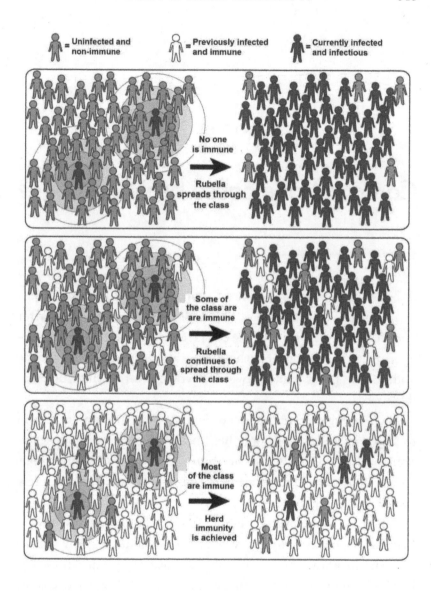

Rubella spreads through a class of previously uninfected children until too many are immune to infect those that are not, at which point the class has herd immunity.

Image produced by NIAID[12] and made available under a creative commons licence.

Chapter 20

Can a vaccine cause brain damage?

A baby's first year is a time of wonder. Her body transforms as she learns to grip things, to crawl and, one butt-plant after another, to walk. Her unfocused stare resolves to follow her parents around the room. Her babbling takes the form of language and, as she gains control over her voice, morphs into discernible words.

Each milestone gives her sleep-deprived parents another reason to celebrate, but it's not only her body that is making the developmental journey. It's also her brain, and, given the enormous complexity of the human brain, it's inevitable that there are a few things that can go wrong.

When a child's development goes awry, her parents will want to know the reason why. If it was someone's fault, it's only human to want to know whose, if only because of the question that haunts so many caring parents: what if they made a bad decision?

That search for a reason has led some parents, and indeed some doctors, to focus their attention on vaccines. Childhood vaccines are, after all, an event that happens to a baby at a time in her life that her parents strive to make uneventful. Moreover, it's an event that nearly always makes the baby cry.

Many concerns about vaccines revolve around the idea that they may somehow damage the developing brain, but is there any evidence that it's even a possibility?

To answer the question, we need to go back to where the idea first arose.

The Byers and Moll case series

In 1948, Randolph Byers and Frederic Moll, at respectively Harvard Medical School and Boston Children's Hospitals, published a report of fifteen children who developed convulsions within three days of being vaccinated against whooping cough.[1] Ten were later diagnosed with epilepsy, learning disabilities or cerebral palsy, all of which fall within the broad category of brain damage.

A few years after the whooping cough vaccine was rolled out across America, doctors like Byers and Moll would have been looking for hitherto unnoticed side effects. Unfortunately, their paper was far more influential than it was rigorous.

What they published was a case series: several patients with a similar condition or combination of conditions that Byers and Moll had seen in their clinics. Case series are important because they are often the first indication that something is awry. Chapter 15 described how Norman Gregg's case series of babies born with cataracts pointed the way to the discovery of congenital rubella syndrome, but, as Gregg understood, a case series is only a starting point. Without deeper investigation, it doesn't prove that one condition causes the other.

To show that two conditions are related, someone needs to show that they occur together *more often* than they occur independently. Even that doesn't prove that one *causes* the other; there may be a third factor that causes both.

If one of the conditions is a developmental disorder then, by definition, it will emerge during a child's development, and will probably put the child in front of specialists like Byers and Moll. The precise point in the child's development is as likely to be within three days of vaccination as at any other time. The timing doesn't prove that the vaccination *caused* the disorder.

Having noticed that some children developed disorders soon after being vaccinated, the next step should have been to look into whether those disorders were more frequent in vaccinated or unvaccinated children, and whether they were more likely to occur immediately after vaccination than at any other time.

Byers and Moll didn't do either.

Instead, they made an assumption: that if a child developed convulsions soon after vaccination and then developed a permanent disorder, the vaccine must have caused both the convulsions and the disorder.

They didn't look at how often convulsions or disorders happened at any other time, so they had no idea whether vaccination made convulsions or disorders more likely.

Their paper might have received more scrutiny if Byers and Moll had argued for the withdrawal of the whooping cough vaccine. Instead, they concluded that serious side effects were so rare that vaccination was less of a risk than catching whooping cough.[2]

Their conclusion depended on another assumption: that whooping cough was more dangerous than the vaccine. They didn't calculate that risk, but left one assumption teetering on top of another.

It was terrible science, but for decades to come, it framed a debate over whether a few brain-damaged children were a price worth paying for protection against whooping cough without addressing a more fundamental question: did the whooping cough vaccine cause brain damage at all?

It was a debate that would drag on for the next fifty years.

John Wilson's fifty(ish)

For the first twenty-five of those years, the debate was confined to the pages of scientific journals and the floors of scientific conferences. As heated as the debate sometimes became, few parents knew about the question mark that hung over the whooping cough vaccine being jabbed into their children's arms.

The man who made the debate public was a pillar of the British medical establishment. John Wilson was a consultant paediatric neurologist at London's Great Ormond Street Hospital for Sick Children and a founder of the British Paediatric Neurology Association.[3]

In 1973, Wilson detonated a bombshell in the heart of his establishment.

In a presentation to the Royal Society of Medicine, he announced that in eleven years, his hospital had seen fifty children who had suffered neurological complications – a technical term for brain damage – from the whole-cell whooping cough vaccine given at three, five and ten months, combined with the diphtheria and tetanus toxoids in the DTP.[4]

Fifty was a worrying number, but it was his next move that changed the tone of the debate. Wilson appeared on ITV's flagship documentary series, *This Week*, where his fifty children somehow became 'in the region of eighty patients'.[5]

Numerical inconsistencies were a recurring feature of Wilson's pronouncements, but on camera, what mattered was that he declared the whooping cough vaccine caused brain damage as a proven fact.

Wilson played well on the small screen. He spoke, as one journalist put it, 'in the voice of a bishop, with cultivated, drawn-out vowels',[6] which complemented his well-worn suit and unkempt hair. He was the sort of academic that Saturday afternoon drama had primed the nation to trust without wondering if he was as good an epidemiologist as he was a paediatrician.

The whooping cough vaccine debate was no longer academic.

George Dick's guess

Like Byers and Moll, Wilson showed no awareness of the limitations of a case series. Like them, he called it definitive proof without doing any further investigation. Many scientists pointed out those limitations, but epistemological critique does not make headlines that editors want to see on news-stands.

With many in Britain's medical establishment still dubious about vaccination, Wilson was not fighting his corner alone. One ally was George Dick of Queen's University, Belfast, one of Britain's leading microbiologists, whose attitude towards vaccination had been shaped by a sometimes well-placed scepticism towards America's hard-charging vaccine pioneers.[7]

In 1975, Dick announced to the Royal Society of Medicine that the whooping cough vaccine caused severe reactions in around one in every 10,000 children. Among those children, a third fully recovered, a third died and another third had permanent brain damage.[8] If Dick's claim was true, it was a lot more alarming than Wilson's, because with whooping cough now very rare in Britain, it added up to many more children being harmed by the vaccine than by whooping cough itself.

It turned out to be a big 'if' because, on being pressed, Dick admitted that his numbers were a 'guess' and then doubled down, guessing the true number might be twice his original guess.[9]

Wilson and Dick's opponents pointed out that before the whooping cough vaccine was rolled out, it had been given to 30,000 children in clinical trials.[10,11] If Dick's guesses were right, between three and six children in those trials should have developed the conditions Dick was talking about. None had, which was much harder evidence than the most fervent assumptions and guesses.

It was one thing for public health experts and epidemiologists to weigh evidence. It was another for a parent to subject their baby to any risk of brain damage, or indeed for a GP to wield the syringe that might cause it. Parents across Britain took to refusing the whooping cough vaccine, and in 1977, a survey by *The Times* found that around half of British GPs wouldn't recommend it.[12]

That was the year that whooping cough came back to Britain. Between 1977 and 1979, it hospitalised 5,000 children and killed thirty-eight.[13] It pushed anxious parents back to vaccine clinics and brought the controversy to a head. Finally, the assumptions based on the case series were tested with further investigations that asked the right question: not whether the occasional brain-damaged child was a price worth paying to keep whooping cough out of Britain, but whether the vaccine caused brain damage at all.

The National Childhood Encephalopathy Study

Foremost among those investigations was the National Childhood Encephalopathy Study (NCES), led by epidemiologist David Miller and paediatric neurologist Euan Ross, both based at Middlesex Hospital, although they headed down Marylebone Road to St Mary's Hospital before the end of the saga. The NCES was one of the largest epidemiological studies ever carried out and also one of the most controversial, which was unfortunate for a study intended to resolve a controversy.

Ideally, Miller and Ross would have compared large groups of children given either the vaccine or a placebo but that wasn't an option. It's one thing to use a placebo in a trial of an untested vaccine, which, by definition, may or may not protect the people it's given to. It's another to withhold a proven vaccine that national guidelines say should be given to every child.

Their solution was to ask hospitals across England, Scotland and Wales to report every case of 'neurological illness' in children aged between two months and three years between mid-1976 and mid-1979. Whenever a case was identified, the NCES team would randomly designate another child in the same community as a control. They would then see whether more of the children admitted with neurological illness had recently received a whooping cough vaccine than the controls.

Neurological illness encompasses everything from a single seizure or convulsion to lifelong epilepsy and intellectual disability. Like Byers and Moll, Wilson described a grab-bag of different conditions that related to the developing brain in one way or another, and so Miller and Ross needed their investigation to be as broad as his claims.

The NCES needed to search across most of Britain, because brain damage in babies is extremely rare. They were able to find only thirty-two children whose neurological conditions first appeared within a week of the whooping cough vaccine.[14] However, twenty-three fully recovered within two weeks, so whatever had been ailing them, it wasn't the permanent brain damage that Wilson was talking about. The NCES was left with nine children whose conditions had appeared within a week of the vaccine with no other obvious cause.

Unfortunately, the NCES report doesn't give much detail on what sort of brain damage those nine children suffered. Three had 'minor delays' in development while six had 'major delays'. The latter could mean lifelong intellectual disability or epilepsy. Alternatively, it could mean something they would outgrow. It's unlikely that the brain damage amounted to serious impairment in all nine.

It was such a small number that Miller and Ross could only calculate the risk at somewhere between one case in every 54,000 vaccinations and one in every 5,310,000. They added a caveat that their figures 'must be interpreted with caution owing to ... the breadth of the confidence limits'.[15]

It was a spectacular understatement. When they acknowledged that they didn't know whether they were looking at one case among tens of thousands, hundreds of thousands or millions of vaccinations, many wondered whether they had shown anything at all.

Others ignored the caution that Miller and Ross urged, arguing that whatever the uncertainties, the NCES had shown there was indeed a risk.

In short, the NCES's result left enough room for debate that everyone interpreted it as evidence for whatever position they already held.

Beneath the uncertainties about frequency lay a deeper uncertainty. The NCES nine had no obvious cause for their neurological conditions other than having been recently vaccinated, but that wasn't the same as proving the whooping cough vaccine had *caused* their neurological illness.

After three years of epidemiology on a monumental scale, the NCES produced a question rather than an answer: was it really more likely that a vaccine could leave the brains of hundreds of thousands (or tens of thousands, or millions) of children unmolested for every one it damaged, or could there, somewhere in the unfathomably complex development of the human brain, lie another explanation?

Beyond the NCES nine

The NCES wasn't the only study to look for an association between the whooping cough vaccine and brain damage. By the early 1990s, six other epidemiological studies had asked the same question. One was in Britain,[16] one in Denmark[17] and four in the USA.[18] None found any association among the hundreds of thousands of children they looked at between them, but then the NCES needed to look at over 3 million children to find nine cases.[19]

After all the guesses and assumptions, the NCES nine remained the only evidence that the whooping cough vaccine might cause brain damage and, as evidence goes, it wasn't exactly conclusive. It raised the question of how Wilson had managed to find so many children for his case series.[20]

Wilson's claim wasn't backed up by what he committed to writing.

His paper listed only thirty-six cases of neurological illness admitted within two weeks of vaccination. So much for the fifty he'd announced to the Royal Society, let alone the eighty he'd claimed on *This Week*. Nevertheless, the NCES data suggested that he couldn't have found thirty-six cases in eleven years if he'd searched the whole country, yet Wilson claimed to have found them in a single hospital.

Except, a careful read of his paper reveals, he hadn't. Wilson included six whose neurological illnesses had appeared *before* they were vaccinated, neglecting to explain how their conditions could have been caused by a vaccine they had yet to be given. Another five had recently recovered from infections or still had them when they were vaccinated. Their GPs should not have vaccinated them before they fully recovered but they did, and Wilson did not explain why he thought it was the vaccine rather than the infection that sent them to hospital.

Wilson would later admit that another two were included by mistake; they'd never received the whooping cough vaccine at all.[21]

Between the various ambiguities, that leaves between twenty

and twenty-five children who developed epilepsy, learning disabilities or both with no named explanation other than the vaccine. It's still a case series, but when a headline claim isn't supported by the rest of the paper, we have to ask how well the research was conducted.

When someone did ask, Wilson's claim fell apart completely. In his paper, he wrote that the children had been admitted to the Hospital for Sick Children 'because of neurological illness thought to be due to DPT inoculation',[22] without saying who thought it or why.

The truth emerged years later. Wilson had sent a couple of trainees to trawl the hospital's records for children admitted with neurological illness within his arbitrary two-week window.[23]

Wilson had proved that if he told trainees to find records of children admitted within two weeks of vaccination, trainees would put those records in front of him. He had not proved that children were any more likely to be admitted within those two weeks than at any other time, because he hadn't looked at children admitted at any other time.

Wilson's paper is a valuable cautionary tale. It teaches us that papers published in scientific journals should be read as critically as the media reports of them. It teaches us nothing about whether or not the whole-cell whooping cough vaccine can cause brain damage.

'Everyone lost interest'

The whooping cough vaccine controversy wasn't resolved so much as it ran out of steam. Euan Ross, co-lead of the NCES, told me, 'The whole question blew away and everyone lost interest.'[24]

The NHS didn't replace the whole-cell vaccine with the acellular vaccine until 2004 – not because anyone was still worried about its side effects, but because only the acellular vaccine was available in combination with the inactivated polio vaccine. By then, the acellular vaccine had been available for twenty years, but nobody had cared enough to push for the change.

If the furore looked like an enormous fuss about nothing by the early 2000s, we have to ask why so many doctors were convinced the vaccine was damaging brains for so long. Byers and Moll were no charlatans, and even at their most irritated, John Wilson's detractors didn't question his sincerity.

One reason is that killed-bacteria vaccines are more likely than any other vaccine type to cause side effects, and only one killed-bacteria vaccine was ever routinely given to children: the whole-cell whooping cough vaccine.

Those side effects usually amounted to swelling at the injection site, some fever, and possibly vomiting and loss of appetite. They could mean that parents got even less sleep than usual for two or three days, but the children recovered soon enough. However, one in every thousand doses caused a reaction called the 'cerebral cry',[25] a grating scream that convinced parents that the vaccine was doing something awful to their children. It invariably passed, leaving no ill effects, but it's a sound that no one ever wants to hear from a baby, especially their own.

Then there were the fevers themselves. It's a rare baby who never has a fever, but for a particularly unlucky baby, fever triggers a febrile convulsion: her limbs thrash uncontrollably while her eyeballs roll back in her head.[26] Many parents are convinced they're watching their child's death throes,[27] but in fact, the overwhelming majority of children recover completely.

Febrile convulsions are not particularly rare. Between one in twenty and one in fifty children suffer at least one, so Wilson, a paediatrician who specialised in neurological disorders, must have seen a lot of children whose convulsions had prompted their parents to call an ambulance. If those children had recently received a whooping cough vaccine, it wouldn't be unreasonable to blame the vaccine for the convulsion. Febrile convulsions are, by definition, brought on by fever and, as Euan Ross put it to me, 'If you give a whole-cell vaccine, you're bound to get some fevers.'[28]

If one of those children went on to develop a learning disability, then her parents, traumatised by witnessing the convulsions, and Wilson, who took the dangers of the vaccine as a given, might assume that the vaccine caused the convulsion and either the vaccine or the convulsion caused the learning disability.

They would have been half right: the whole-cell whooping cough vaccine could cause a fever and a fever could cause a febrile convulsion.[29] More importantly, it was also half wrong: terrifying as they are to watch, convulsions are not associated with brain damage.

We know that thanks to the Child Health and Education Study, which set out to follow the development of every child born in Britain in April 1970. They didn't quite get them all, but they did manage to recruit over 16,000.

In their early childhood years, 381 had febrile convulsions, which is squarely in the middle of the expected one in fifty to one in twenty.

When those children reached ten years old, the researchers went back to them and found they were no more likely to have learning disabilities than children who had never had a convulsion in their life.[30]

Whether or not the whooping cough vaccine caused those convulsions, they were not associated with brain damage.

Epilepsy and its causes

Another 'neurological complication' that Wilson mentioned was epilepsy, a disorder that makes someone prone to seizures that look similar to febrile convulsions. Epilepsy is a lifelong condition, although many people who have it can control it with medications.

An epileptic seizure may be triggered by many different things or none at all. One of the triggers is fever and because the whole-cell whooping cough vaccine can cause a fever, it follows that vaccination can trigger an epileptic seizure. However, triggering a seizure in a child with epilepsy is not the same as causing epilepsy in a child who didn't previously have it.

To further confuse the issue, the vaccine was given to babies young enough that it sometimes triggered an epileptic child's first seizure. To Wilson, the causal chain from vaccination to seizure to lifelong epilepsy might have looked straightforward. Where it falls flat is in the several studies that showed vaccinated babies are no more likely than unvaccinated babies to develop epilepsy.[31,32,33]

Moreover, 1970s paediatric neurologists like Wilson were labouring under the misconception that epilepsy was either genetic or was caused by a head injury. A paediatrician diagnosing epilepsy would usually ask if anyone else in the family had it, and if the answer was yes, they would attribute their epilepsy to genetics. If the answer was no, it followed that the child must have had some sort of accident.

The parents of most one-year-olds go out of their way to avoid epilepsy-inducing head injuries, but if *something* must have caused it, Wilson's thoughts might alight on the vaccine most likely to be followed by febrile convulsions.

Wilson would also have known that whooping cough can itself cause brain damage,[34] and because the whole-cell vaccine is made of the toxin-riddled bacterium that causes whooping cough, the idea that it might have similar effects wasn't too wild a speculation.

Where the logic fails is that those toxins do not directly damage a child's brain. Whooping cough causes brain damage because the coughing paroxysms stop a child from breathing and starve her brain of oxygen.[35] None of the vaccine's side effects interfere with a child's breathing.

Yet *something* was causing epilepsy in children that wasn't genetic and wasn't caused by an injury. The whole-cell whooping cough vaccine emerged as the prime suspect largely for want of any other suspects.

'The real problem,' Euan Ross, co-lead of the NCES, told me, 'is people didn't know about Dravet syndrome.'[36]

Dravet syndrome was named after its discoverer, Charlotte Dravet of Marseille's Centre Saint-Paul-Hôpital Henri Gastaut, who discovered a form of epilepsy caused by a mutation after a child is conceived.[37] That makes it genetic but not inherited, explaining those mysterious cases of epilepsy in children who had no relatives with epilepsy and hadn't had an accident.

Dravet made her discovery in 1978, when the whooping cough controversy was at its height, but no one realised that it might resolve the controversy until after it fizzled out. The first to make the connection was Samuel Berkovic of the University of Melbourne, who re-examined fourteen people with epilepsy whose first seizure had been within three days of the whole-cell vaccine. Eleven of them had the Dravet syndrome mutation.[38]

Dravet's later research revealed that the syndrome may be caused by mutations other than those that Berkovic knew to look for,[39] which probably explains the other three.

Berkovic's 2006 paper didn't attract the attention it would have done twenty years earlier. It wasn't until five years later that anyone else followed up, when five American children whose epilepsy had been blamed on the whooping cough vaccine were shown to have Dravet syndrome.[40]

By then, most high-income countries had already switched to the acellular vaccine. The whole-cell vaccine is still widely used in low-income countries as it is both cheaper and more effective, so it's reassuring to have evidence that it does no long-term damage.

The NCES nine remain the only unresolved evidence for brain damage caused by the whole-cell whooping cough vaccine, and, so far, no one has checked those individuals for Dravet syndrome.

The Pandemrix affair

The history of the idea that vaccines cause brain damage is the history of the whole-cell whooping cough vaccine controversy; a half-century-long saga of well-publicised bad science belatedly trumped by under-reported good science.

However, another vaccine was put in the frame more recently, although it attracted far less attention and revolved around a vaccine that has not been given to anyone for more than ten years.

The Pandemrix affair started on 10 August 2010, when the Swedish Medicine Product Agency reported narcolepsy in six children and adolescents who had received an influenza vaccine called Pandemrix. On the same day, Finland's National Institute for Health and Welfare reported another six cases.[41]

Pandemrix was developed by GlaxoSmithKline to counter the 'swine flu' influenza virus that appeared in 2009. It was an inactivated split vaccine like the annual seasonal influenza vaccine,* albeit with two differences. One was that while seasonal vaccines cover several different strains, Pandemrix only contained proteins from the swine flu strain. The other was that Pandemrix contained a new type of adjuvant, which is a chemical added to a vaccine to enhance the immune response. The adjuvant in question, AS03, has since been widely used without causing narcolepsy or any other serious side effect,[42] so

---

* See Chapter 17.

to examine the Pandemrix affair, we need to focus on the vaccine and not the adjuvant.

Narcolepsy is a type of brain damage often caricatured as a tendency to fall asleep at amusing moments. Cataplexy, to use the formal term, isn't falling asleep so much as sudden paralysis, often brought on by extreme emotions,[43] and is far from amusing for anyone whom it strikes. It's an extreme and mercifully treatable manifestation of narcolepsy.

Narcolepsy is far more likely to manifest as an inability to sleep properly, leaving a sufferer drowsy and unable to concentrate. It usually appears between the ages of ten and twenty, so it surprised nobody that the new Swedish and Finnish cases were reported as children and adolescents.

A case report of a dozen Nordic narcoleptics didn't prove that the vaccine caused narcolepsy any more than Byers and Moll's proved that whooping cough vaccine caused brain damage. However, sixty years had dramatically improved understanding of what a case series was and was not. Instead of leaping to conclusions for the next twenty-five years, further investigations were initiated immediately.

In the six countries where Pandemrix had been used, health authorities searched for more cases, and they found them. Cases turned up in Britain, Ireland, Norway and France, as well as Finland and Sweden, amounting to one case of narcolepsy for every 16,000 to 21,000 doses of Pandemrix given.[44]

But did that prove that Pandemrix had caused the narcolepsy?

The very low incidence raised a similar question to that raised by the NCES nine. Could such a tiny number of people have had a serious reaction to a vaccine that caused no problems in thousands of others? Or was it more likely that a search for people with narcolepsy had found people with narcolepsy caused by something other than the vaccine?

Narcolepsy is notoriously difficult to recognise. By the time someone is diagnosed, they've usually had it for between five and ten years,[45] which means that at any given time, people are walking around with undiagnosed narcolepsy. When health authorities went looking for cases, those undiagnosed cases were there to be found.

Unless someone suffers from full-blown cataplexy, narcolepsy's symptoms are vague enough to make it difficult to nail down exactly when they started. A year or more after receiving Pandemrix, someone may well answer the question of when it was when they started feeling drowsy with, 'Around then, I guess.'

To further muddy the waters, Pandemrix vaccination was not the only thing happening in the winter of 2009–2010 that might cause narcolepsy. Swine flu itself was associated with narcolepsy in countries that didn't use Pandemrix,[46] and in the countries that did, many people would have caught swine flu before they were called for vaccination.

If there was narcolepsy where there was both swine flu and Pandemrix, but there was also narcolepsy where there was only swine flu, we can't tell whether it was the swine flu or the Pandemrix that caused the narcolepsy.

If there were a third place where there was Pandemrix but no swine flu, then the presence or absence of new cases of narcolepsy in that place would tell us whether it was the Pandemrix or the swine flu that was to blame. Unfortunately, there was no such place.

The most useful comparison came from Canada, which responded to swine flu not with Pandemrix but with Arepanrix, a very similar vaccine made by the same manufacturer. Arepanrix used the same parts of the same influenza virus and the same adjuvant as Pandemrix, but it was not associated with narcolepsy. However, Arepanrix was prepared in a different way to Pandemrix and without knowing what causes narcolepsy, we can't be absolutely certain that the cause did not lie in the different preparation techniques.

Another argument against Pandemrix causing narcolepsy is that among the millions of influenza vaccines given out around Europe every year, Pandemrix is the only one to be associated with narcolepsy.[47] They're monitored by the same surveillance systems that picked up the possible association with Pandemrix, so if they haven't detected a problem with the seasonal influenza vaccines, we can be confident that it's not there to be detected. Yet Pandemrix is, in essence, just another inactivated split vaccine. It would be very strange indeed if Pandemrix alone could occasionally – very occasionally – cause narcolepsy.

By the time the Swedish and Finnish authorities sounded the alarm, Pandemrix had already been withdrawn because mutations in wild-type influenza virus had made it obsolete. It left behind a small amount of evidence that it may have caused narcolepsy and a similar amount of evidence that it did not.

The answer

We started with the question of whether a vaccine can cause brain damage.

In answer, we can be confident that no vaccine currently in use poses any danger to a child's brain.

We can go further and say there is no firm evidence that any vaccine has ever caused brain damage.

We can't say there is no evidence at all.

We can rule out the whole-cell whooping cough vaccine, which was the prime suspect for over forty years. The NCES nine remain the only unexplained cases, and not even Euan Ross, who co-led the study that found them, believes their condition was caused by vaccination.

Pandemrix is a trickier one. It's unlikely but not impossible that it caused narcolepsy in a small number of people, which is an unsatisfyingly inconclusive conclusion.

Even if we could be absolutely certain that no vaccine has ever caused brain damage, we still wouldn't be certain that no vaccine ever could. Saying something has never happened doesn't prove it cannot happen, just as flipping a coin ten thousand times and getting only heads or tails doesn't prove that the coin won't ever land on its edge: it's not impossible but vanishingly unlikely.

Chapter 21

Does the MMR vaccine cause autism?

No.

It's a much easier question to address than the one about brain damage.

You may find a simple 'no' less than satisfactory. You may be wondering why, if the answer is that simple, everyone has heard someone say that it does? That's a more complicated question, and it needs a longer answer.

The story starts in around 1990 when, at least by his own account, a young gastroenterologist working on Crohn's disease opened a textbook. 'I got to measles virus and it described how it gets into the gut, causing ulcers and inflammation,' Andrew Wakefield told a journalist twenty years later. 'You could have been reading an account of Crohn's disease ... It was very exciting.'[1]

Spend enough time in medical research and sooner or later, you'll meet *that* guy.

A young researcher who knows they're going to change the world. Who has chosen the discovery they're going to change it with and is committed to torturing every morsel of data into proof that they were right all along.

That guy hasn't grasped the critical difference between the brilliant intuitive leap and the crackpot pseudotheory: it's not how clever the idea is but whether it survives trial by evidence. This book is full of scientists who had ideas by the dozen and ruthlessly winnowed them by evidence, logic and experiment until only the good ones were left standing.

In short, they were good scientists.

A particular type of bad scientist has one idea and, in the absence of any others, convinces themselves that it's the only one that matters.

A good mentor might coax open a one-track mind, perhaps converting a bad scientist into at least a mediocre scientist. A bad scientist who isn't blessed with such a mentor – or who chooses to ignore good mentorship – is blind to the flaws in their idea, however many times their colleagues point them out. They wave away anyone who points out the lack of evidence as airily as they wave away anyone who suggests the experiments that might test their claim.

If they can't learn a less rigid mindset, they usually decide that science isn't for them. Wakefield did that in 2015 when he announced: 'I am now a filmmaker.'[2]

This chapter is about what he set in motion before his career change.

The Wakefield hypothesis

If Wakefield had stuck with his textbook epiphany, that wild-type measles causes Crohn's disease, he would have been wrong, but he would not be famous. Crohn's disease is an inflammatory disorder of the lower intestine that, while very debilitating for its sufferers, does not command headlines.

Instead, he asserted that the measles vaccine makes children autistic as part of a condition he gave various polysyllabic names. In 1998, it was ileal-lymphoid-nodular hyperplasia;[3] in 2000, it was autistic enterocolitis;[4] and by 2002, it had become ileocolonic lymphonodular hyperplasia.[5]

One gets the impression that he was trying different jaw-breakers to see which made him sound cleverest. His description of children with autistic enterocolitis – to pick the shortest and most literal of his terms – combined three different features. First, they had inflammation of the largest part of their lower intestine, called the colon. Second, they had a regressive form of autism, in which cognitive and emotional development appeared normal until either it 'failed to progress beyond a certain point'[6] or they lost their verbal skills and regressed to that point. Third, and most problematically, Wakefield claimed that the first two conditions were triggered by the MMR vaccination, containing the live measles, mumps and rubella vaccine strains.

Britain introduced the MMR in 1988, and over 90 per cent of all children received it,[7,8] mostly as scheduled at around one year of age. That's also the age when the first signs of the sort of severe autism that Wakefield was talking about are likely to appear.[9] It would have been stranger if Wakefield had found a cluster of autistic children who *hadn't* received the MMR. Blaming the MMR for autism that appeared soon after a child's first birthday made as much sense as blaming their first birthday cake.

Severe autism is often linked to digestive disorders,[10] which is how a gastroenterologist ended up associating his name with a disorder of the brain – and make no mistake, regressive autism is a serious disorder. Children with regressive autism do not mature into eccentric but essentially capable adults who might be played by Dustin Hoffman or Benedict Cumberbatch. They cannot communicate verbally and many cannot feed themselves or use the toilet independently. They need twenty-four-hour care throughout their lives.

Wakefield's first paper on autistic enterocolitis[11] was published in the *Lancet*, one of Britain's foremost medical journals. It presented a case series of twelve children with inflammatory bowel disease and autism, from which he concluded that the two conditions were linked.

An earth-shattering discovery it was not. Severe autism and digestive problems were already known to occur together.[12]

Wakefield and his colleagues speculated that measles might be behind the condition, and by the 1990s, the wild-type was so rare in Britain that those children could only have encountered measles as the vaccine strain in the MMR.

The paper contained no evidence of measles infection, either vaccine strain or wild-type, in any of the twelve children. Nor did Wakefield ever explain why he assumed autistic enterocolitis was caused by measles instead of the mumps or rubella vaccine strains.

A *Lancet* paper looks good on an academic CV, and if he'd left it there, it would have been a solid step towards a professorship and perhaps a civil honour before he retired. With a readership – one up from a lectureship – in his early forties and plenty of research funding, his career path was looking solid if not spectacular.

He didn't leave it at a paper.

Like John Wilson a quarter-century earlier, Wakefield went public. In February 1998, he called a press conference at his department in London's Royal Free Hospital and, freed of the constraints imposed by the *Lancet*'s editors, announced that the MMR's measles strain[13] caused the condition he'd discovered. He didn't mention that his paper explicitly acknowledged that 'we did not prove an association between measles, mumps, and rubella vaccine and the syndrome described'.[14] He probably trusted that very few of the journalists excitedly scribbling notes would bother to read it.

The few who did noticed that the same issue of the *Lancet* contained a paper disproving Wakefield's earlier claim that measles causes Crohn's disease.[15] It also contained a commentary by two experts who pointed out that by selecting children who developed a disorder immediately after being vaccinated, Wakefield's paper made the same mistake as John Wilson's paper on the whooping cough vaccine. Like Wilson, Wakefield assumed that if a child developed a condition after being vaccinated, the vaccine must have caused the condition. He didn't confirm that vaccination made the condition more likely, which, with a condition often diagnosed at around the age at which children were given the MMR, was a critical flaw.

None of that mattered when Wakefield told the assembled journalists that, 'in all conscience, I cannot support the idea of using all three vaccines together'.[16]

Interesting choice of words.

Not 'the evidence supports' withdrawing the MMR, which is what we'd expect from the scientist he claimed to be – although, as we'll see, the evidence certainly did not. Instead, he packaged his conscience into a soundbite that was quoted in most of the following day's newspapers.

Wakefield has always known what plays well with the press.

It played less well with the dean of the Royal Free Medical School, Arie Zuckerman, who was sitting next to Wakefield. Zuckerman's more prosaic warning that 'If this were to precipitate a scare that reduced the rate of immunisation, children will start dying from measles,'[17] was far less widely reported. Wakefield steamrollered his superior's arguments, reducing Zuckerman to banging his lectern in frustration.[18] Wakefield cast himself as the plucky challenger to Zuckerman's establishment and his audience lapped it up.

'Ban three-in-one jab urge doctors after new fears,'[19] screeched the *Daily Mail*. 'Undetected bowel illness led to baby's misery,'[20] wailed the *Guardian*. Exactly the sort of headlines that Zuckerman had feared when he banged that lectern.

Zuckerman thought Wakefield was reaching beyond the evidence, but at the time, he didn't know the half of it. He couldn't know that Wakefield had fabricated the evidence himself.

What Wakefield didn't say

We know this thanks mostly to Brian Deer, a *Sunday Times* reporter who specialises in uncovering pharmaceutical and medical malpractice. In the twenty years following Wakefield's press conference, Deer became Wakefield's nemesis. He uncovered one inconvenient fact after another that Wakefield had concealed from the *Lancet*'s editors and his colleagues at the Royal Free.

Deer discovered that, like Wilson, Wakefield hadn't *looked* for the association between MMR and autistic enterocolitis that he claimed to have found. He started by *assuming* the association and then sought case histories that fitted his assumption.

While Wilson had looked in his own hospital's records, Wakefield found his twelve by soliciting patient support groups around Britain, which raises the question of why he needed to cast such a wide net. Deer's investigation found that Wakefield was not the conscience-driven academic he claimed to be. The search that led him to those twelve children was funded by a legal firm that 'hoped to bring a lawsuit against vaccine manufacturers'.[21]

It raised an obvious conflict of interest; the lawyer wanted evidence to support his case, not an investigation into whether he had a case at all. However, it's a mistake to assume that a funder's vested interest automatically leads to dishonest research. Much academic research is funded by pharmaceutical firms, which are rarely disinterested but there is usually a written agreement allowing the scientists to publish whatever they find, whether it's what the funder wants them to find or not. There are exceptions, which occasionally blow up in someone's face, but publishing all results – including the inconvenient ones – remains the norm in academic research.

Wakefield's study was an exception and it blew up in his face. When Deer got hold of the twelve children's medical records, five of them had been diagnosed with developmental disorders *before* they were given the MMR.[22] Another three didn't have autism at all.

For all his canvassing, Wakefield hadn't been able to find twelve children who developed autism immediately after receiving the MMR, let alone show that the MMR caused the autism.

Deer chronicles the whole sorry story in his book, *The Doctor Who Fooled the World*,[23] from Wakefield's textbook epiphany to that fateful press conference, via falsified evidence and research methods so unethical that they belong to the American mid-twentieth-century vaccine boom rather than 1990s Britain.

Wakefield used procedures like colonoscopy and lumbar puncture, which, even under general anaesthetic, are invasive and extremely distressing to children whose condition made them unable to understand what was being done to them. It's one thing to piggyback research on invasive procedures needed for a child's clinical care. It's quite another to inflict them on a child purely for research, which is why Wakefield didn't tell the Royal Free's ethics committee what he was doing. Nor did he mention that he'd collected blood samples from children at his son's birthday party and slipped them a fiver for doing it.

The latter was the sort of behaviour that Albert Sabin, developer of the live polio vaccine, had boasted about when he said he couldn't do anything to other people's children that he hadn't done to his own children and their friends first.* It's also the sort

---

* See Chapter 11.

of thing that Sabin's daughter found deeply distressing,[24] which is why such things were no longer allowed by the 1990s.

The General Medical Council decided Wakefield's cavalier approach amounted to medical malpractice. He was struck off the medical register[25] in 2010, barring him from practising as a doctor.

Deer's narrative follows Wakefield across the Atlantic and down a convoluted rabbit hole of conspiracist beliefs until 2016, when, in a twist of rehabilitation worthy of a Hollywood screenwriter, he emerged from obscurity at one of President Trump's inauguration balls and started dating ex-supermodel Elle Macpherson. At the time of writing, he is an elder statesman of the American conspiracist community, who lap up his rants about how COVID-19 vaccination is an excuse to inject everyone with cryptocurrencies.[26] His gift for moulding sciencey terms into terrifying, if not entirely coherent, pronouncements has not faded with age.

While ghoulishly fascinating to follow, Wakefield's story does not answer the question we started with. Wakefield's assertion that the MMR vaccine causes autism was disproved not by examination of his lifestyle but by scientists who took his assertion at face value and subjected it to the trial by evidence that Wakefield skipped over.

Was it ever plausible that measles could cause autism?

Wakefield's assertions were premised on measles causing a long-term infection.

It was, to say the least, a weird premise.

That textbook would have told him that a measles infection only lasts for two or three weeks before the lymphocytes see it off.[27] Such time-limited virus infections are called 'acute' and, as Chapter 13 described, acute infections like measles often leave some damage behind them. Wakefield, however, claimed that both Crohn's disease and autistic enterocolitis were caused not by unrepaired damage but by measles clinging on in the colon.

There have been occasional cases of measles clinging on, but in the brain rather than in the colon. Such cases are extremely rare and have all been in children whose immune system is not functioning properly.[28]

Wakefield was claiming that the vaccine strain of measles clinging on in the colon happened far more often than that. If it were true, it should not have been impossible to prove. It's a lot easier to look for a virus in the colon, which has a ready-made point of entry, than to poke around in someone's brain.

There are two different ways to find a virus in a tissue sample, and when Wakefield was working on Crohn's disease, he claimed to have succeeded with both.

One way is to look for the virus's proteins by using a trick the immune system uses to clear it. An antibody recognises one particular protein, so if you purify a solution of identical antibodies, you can use those antibodies to probe for a given viral protein.

Alternatively, you can go straight for the virus's genetic material. If you know the genetic sequence you're looking for, you can tag it with a probe that carries a marker that you can see. The catch is that even the most virus-infested samples don't contain enough genetic material to see directly.

The solution is the polymerase chain reaction or PCR, the same technique that would later be used to test for the COVID-19 virus in the throat swabs that most of us had to use at one time or another. It works by repeatedly doubling the sequence you're looking for, turning one copy of the virus sequence into two, then four, then eight, and so on until there are enough copies to detect. The key to PCR is that it *only* doubles the sequence you're looking for and leaves any other genetic material in the sample alone. If you detect a sequence in the sample when you've done the PCR, it must have been there in the first place. If you can't, you know it wasn't there to be doubled.

If you do it right.

Whether you're looking for proteins or genetic code, there are a lot of ways to do it wrong. If you think you're seeing what you're looking for, you need to be very sure it *is* what you're looking for. A section of colon tissue contains more different chemicals than anyone can ever list, and if one of those chemicals can stick to your antibody or your genetic probe, it will fool you into thinking you've found what you're looking for.

To be certain that what looked like measles really was measles, Wakefield would have needed to run a tissue sample that he was sure contained no measles alongside his test samples, confirming that his test found no measles when there was none to be found.

When Wakefield presented a paper that he claimed showed both viral proteins and genetic material in tissue from someone with Crohn's disease,[29] he claimed to have included such negative controls but showed no data from them. However, when other research groups tried it, none were able to find measles virus in the intestines of Crohn's disease patients.

Wakefield responded with a series of rather desultory letters of rebuttal, each coming up with a reason why his detractors must have done it wrong. Instead of presenting more data to back up his point, he left Crohn's disease behind and moved on to autistic enterocolitis.

What he didn't do raises as many questions as what he did.

If he'd believed his techniques worked, he could have used them to show the colons of the twelve children in the *Lancet* paper were infected with measles. He had the samples. He claimed to have the techniques. All he had to do was put them together.

He didn't.

He never published any data derived from those techniques again. Instead, he partnered up with John O'Leary at Coombe

Women's Hospital, Dublin, who developed an entirely new PCR from scratch. O'Leary reinvented Wakefield's wheel for him, which is hardly a statement of confidence in the wheel Wakefield insisted was spinning merrily at the Royal Free.

In fairness, Wakefield and O'Leary were trying to do what John Wilson didn't: they were building on a case series with further investigation. That was good science, although there's reason to question how they went about it. One five-year-old ended up in intensive care after a colonoscopy perforated his bowel in twelve places.[30]

If Wakefield believed there was measles in their colons, he could have at least tried looking for it in stool samples before trying colonoscopies.[*]

When Wakefield was orchestrating the Royal Free's colonoscopies, O'Leary found measles in seventy-five of ninety-one children with autistic enterocolitis and in only five of seventy healthy children. He and Wakefield claimed they could 'confirm an association between the presence of measles virus and gut pathology in children with developmental disorder'.[31]

They gave a lot of weight to having found measles in more children with the disorder than without, but, as with many of Wakefield's papers, what he didn't mention jumps out as prominently as what he did. He didn't talk about what measles was doing in the colons of five healthy children *at all*.

If he and O'Leary had found measles hanging around in healthy children, they had made a fundamental discovery. So

---

[*] The Royal Free has come a long way since then. I was referred there for a colonoscopy in 2021, which would have been anxiety-inducing enough without the Wakefield story at the front of my mind. I needn't have worried. The team's blend of competence and compassion quickly calmed me down. One nurse launched into an anecdote about not being allowed to ride a camel in Dubai until she'd drunk its milk, and how she couldn't get the taste out of her mouth for a week. She'd polished her delivery into the perfect distraction for someone enduring a light being shone where no light is supposed to shine.

fundamental that researchers around the world would have tried to repeat it, which may be why their paper breezes past the point without sparing it a single word.

If they were trying to duck the issue, it didn't work. The paper attracted enough attention that several PCR experts visited O'Leary's laboratory. They were not impressed.

Foremost among them was Stephen Bustin, one of the world's leading experts on PCR and author of the textbook feted as the 'PCR bible'.[32] In 2008, Bustin tore into O'Leary in an article detailing how O'Leary was doing PCR wrong.[33]

Bustin listed six ways in which O'Leary's PCR technique was likely to show measles was there when it wasn't, but more importantly, O'Leary had made it impossible to know if he was getting misleading results or not. Every time a PCR – any PCR for anything – is run, it needs to be run alongside a negative control sample that contains everything in the test sample except the genetic sequence being looked for. If that negative control shows a positive result, it shows that something has gone wrong and that run's results are invalid.

O'Leary was not running negative controls.

It was impossible to know whether a positive result from a colon sample meant he'd found measles virus or that something had gone wrong with his PCR.

By omitting the negative control, O'Leary had rendered his results meaningless.

A few months after Bustin's takedown, another paper described how research groups in three different laboratories had been unable to repeat O'Leary's results. When PCR was done properly, there was no sign of measles.[34]

Among the authors was John O'Leary himself. Even he hadn't been able to find measles in his samples when he improved his technique.

Bustin described O'Leary's co-authorship of a paper disproving his own results as 'wonderfully ironic' and added that 'the expectation now is that [O'Leary] will publicly retract'.[35] More than ten years later, O'Leary has not retracted.

That was Wakefield's last attempt to back up his hypothesis with experimental data, but we don't need to depend on Wakefield's less-than-rigorous attempts to prove his point. His hypothesis was worrying enough that several other research groups tested it.

Did introducing the MMR increase the autism rate?

To be scrupulously fair, Wakefield's argument did not depend on finding measles virus in the colons of children with autistic enterocolitis. It was based on twelve children who were completely healthy until they were given the MMR vaccine. As we've seen, several weren't, but in the spirit of taking his claims at face value, let's put that to one side for now.

Autistic enterocolitis was defined by autism, and if the MMR did indeed cause autism, we would expect the MMR's introduction to lead to more children developing autism.

The largest available dataset of autism rates was published by the Autism Society of the San Francisco Bay Area. In 2015, the Society put together a report of every male Californian that the California Department of Developmental Services had registered with autism.[36]

As the plot on page 351 shows, the oldest was born in 1931, while the youngest they considered were born in 2010. It's important to look at the year of birth rather than the year of diagnosis, because as the twentieth century progressed, doctors became better at recognising autism. Some people were well into middle age by the time they were diagnosed.

The plot shows that autism was extremely rare among Californians born in the 1930s, but became steadily more frequent among boys born from the 1940s through to the 1970s. That matters because when the USA began mass measles vaccination in 1967,[37] it changed how children experienced measles.

Before vaccination, nearly all children were infected with the virulent wild-type measles, usually when they were a few years old.

We might hypothesise that the mild vaccine strain would be *less* likely to damage a developing brain than the much more virulent wild-type, in which case we'd expect fewer boys with autism born after 1967. On the other hand, a child vaccinated at one year was encountering measles at a much younger age than most natural infections, so we might hypothesise it posed *more* danger because brain development was at an earlier stage.

In fact, we see neither. The steady increase breezes past 1967 as if nothing changed.

That's what we'd expect to see if measles has nothing to do with autism.

However, it wasn't the single-dose vaccine that Wakefield blamed for autistic enterocolitis, but the MMR.

In the USA, the MMR replaced the single-dose measles vaccination in 1971. If Wakefield was correct, we'd expect to see a marked step-up in California's autism rate among boys born in the early 1970s.

There is no such step.

The gradual increase continues until the late 1980s, when the rate of increase suddenly speeds up, rising from around one boy in 500 in 1988 to one in 200 in 1995, topping out at around one in eighty in 2003. After that, the autism rate levelled off until 2010.

The increase is certainly disturbing, but it's not the pattern we'd expect if it was caused by the MMR.

In Britain, we don't have data that goes back that far, but we do have the results of a collaboration between Public Health England* and scientists at the Royal Free, who probably shared a coffee room with Wakefield. They looked at the North Thames Region, covering much of north and north-west London as well as Hertfordshire and Bedfordshire.[38] They were only able to go back as far as 1979, by which time the single-dose vaccine had already been in use for more than ten years. However, Britain didn't introduce the MMR until 1988, so they were able to look for a telltale step-up that would confirm Wakefield's claim.

It wasn't there.

They saw the same trend as in the Californian data, with a steady rise in cases throughout the 1980s that levelled off in the mid-2000s.[39] Between 1988 and 1989, the MMR replaced the single-dose measles vaccine without affecting the trend in autism rates.

The British and American data concur: introducing measles vaccination does not affect autism rates.

Should we switch from the MMR to single-dose vaccines to be on the safe side?

If a reasonable man genuinely believed that the measles vaccine causes autism, he might call for the withdrawal of the measles vaccine.

Wakefield didn't. He argued that children should still be vaccinated against measles, but not in combination with the rubella and mumps vaccine strains. He did not present one iota of evidence that receiving the measles vaccine as part of the MMR is any different to receiving it on its own.

Not then, not in the two decades since.

---

* Now the UK Health Security Agency.

But once again, let's give him the benefit of the doubt. We've seen that introducing the MMR didn't increase autism rates. Let's look at what happens if Wakefield's advice is followed and the MMR is withdrawn.

The first place we might look is in Britain, where Wakefield's 1998 press conference got the most airtime. However, dire predictions of Wakefield-inspired headlines emptying vaccine clinics never came to pass. As we saw in Chapter 13, uptake fell after the 1998 press conference, but it remained above 80 per cent.[40] Wakefield had never claimed that the MMR caused autism in any but a tiny number of children. A 10 per cent fall in uptake may not have been enough to make a discernible difference.

We need to see what happens if the MMR is withdrawn completely, which happened in Japan after the Urabe mumps vaccine, which, as described in Chapter 14, turned out not to be as attenuated as had been thought. In most countries, the Urabe strain was replaced with very little media attention, but in Japan, it caused enough of a scare that parents declined the MMR vaccine for their children.

That was in the late 1980s, while Wakefield was still working on Crohn's disease. It was only after several years of wrangling that anyone realised that his suggestion of giving the measles vaccine separately had already been tested. First to notice was a team led by Hideo Honda of the Yokohama Rehabilitation Centre, who documented Yokohama's MMR coverage falling from 70 per cent in 1988 to below 30 per cent in 1991. In 1993, the government replaced the MMR with separate measles, mumps and rubella vaccines.[41]

None of this had any effect on the incidence of autism, which followed a similar trajectory to those seen in the USA and Britain. As fewer children received the MMR, more developed autism.

Wakefield's solution had been tried before he even suggested it. It made no difference at all.

If the MMR doesn't cause autism then why the rise in autism rates?

One effect of Wakefield publicising his hypothesis is that it's been tested far beyond the point where most hypotheses are discarded. Not one shred of evidence has been found, which makes it one of the most comprehensively disproven hypotheses in scientific history.

The MMR vaccine *does not* cause autism.

A more disturbing question lies beyond the brouhaha that Wakefield stirred up. What *does* cause autism, and why did the autism rate rise between the 1970s and the 2000s in the USA, Britain and Japan alike?

Unfortunately, those are questions with no clear answers. Autism is a syndrome: a cluster of features that often occur together but for which no one has found a single cause.

We know that part of its cause lies in genetics, but if genetics were all that mattered, then in every pair of identical twins, who share the same genome, either both would be autistic or neither would. In fact, being genetically identical increases the probability of equivalent autism status – an autistic identical twin makes a child seven times more likely to be autistic than if they had an autistic non-identical twin[42] – but many identical twins do not have the same autism status.

Something else must be involved. That something may operate by causing mutations after conception, similarly to the cause of Dravet syndrome – and, indeed, autistic children do tend to have more mutations than non-autistic children.[43] Alternatively, it could be something that directly impacts brain development, like rubella infection during pregnancy, which remains the external factor most clearly associated with autism. However, in the USA, vaccination made rubella a rare disease well before the 1980s rise in autism rates. There is a certain irony that the MMR, while being erroneously blamed for autism, contains the only known preventative against it.

Another possible culprit is air pollution, although not every study to look for an association has found it.[44] Many that did were looking at the notoriously smoggy downtown district of Los Angeles, but the rise in autism rates has not been restricted to areas with such high pollution. Moreover, tightening regulation has seen air quality improve in most high-income urban centres while autism rates continued to rise. The evidence for an association with air pollution is stronger than with the MMR, but that's not a high bar to clear.

Another association is that older parents are more likely to have autistic children.[45] The association holds for both mothers and fathers, but then most couples are only a few years apart. If only the mother's age or only the father's age mattered, it wouldn't be possible to see the difference.

The associations with air pollution and parental age are both tenuous, but research into the causes of autism continues. We can only hope for better answers soon.

The scientists conducting that research have refrained from Wakefield's approach of backing up overblown claims by hiding inconvenient data. Being good scientists, they recognise that if you have to hide evidence to make your point, then you don't have a point.

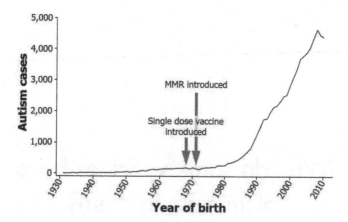

The birth years of males diagnosed with autism in the caseload of the California Department of Developmental Services, recorded in 2015.[46]

Chapter 22

Why do some vaccines have aluminium in them?

In 2013, a team from the Dutch Centre for Infectious Disease Control asked parents what made them nervous about vaccines.

One parent* said their child would never be vaccinated because 'there are adjuvants in vaccines that are poisonous, such as mercury and aluminium ... and you really do not want that in your body, even in small quantities'.[1]

Mercury compounds are not adjuvants but preservatives, and we'll deal with them in the next chapter. Aluminium compounds are indeed used as adjuvants, meaning they enhance the immune memory triggered by the vaccine. They're not biologically inert – there would be no point in putting them in vaccines if they were – but was that Dutch parent right to call them poisonous?

If they didn't want even small quantities of aluminium in their child's body, they were in for a disappointment. It's the third most abundant element in the earth's crust, and it finds its way into everything we eat or drink. Take a sample of tissue, hair, blood

---

* Name and gender not given.

or breast milk, and you'll find trace amounts of aluminium in it. That's nothing to be afraid of because the human body is perfectly capable of handling trace amounts. If aluminium was as terrifyingly toxic to us as that Dutch parent believed, we wouldn't be around to worry about it.

Pointing that out may not have assuaged their anxieties. Eating or drinking a trace amount of aluminium isn't the same as injecting the stuff. They probably wanted to know whether the aluminium in a vaccine is a harmless trace amount or whether there's enough of it to be toxic.

However, asking whether a vaccine component is toxic is only the second question to ask about it. The first, as with anything injected into anyone, is whether there's a good reason to inject it at all.

With aluminium adjuvants, that reason lay behind the decision to add it to vaccines in the first place.

The accidental discovery of aluminium adjuvants

Alexander Glenny at the Wellcome Laboratories in Beckenham, Kent, discovered the adjuvant properties of aluminium salts by accident in the early 1920s. He was trying to come up with a better way to produce diphtheria antiserum,* for which he needed to purify diphtheria toxin out of liquid culture medium. He knew the bacteria were producing far more toxin than he was able to extract, so he tried various chemicals until he got to potassium aluminium sulphate, or simply alum, which bound the toxin and improved his yield. So far, so good, but now he needed to know if the alum affected the immune response to the toxin.

---

* See Chapter 4.

When Glenny injected guinea pigs with the alum-bound toxin, they responded with a stronger antibody response than if he injected the same amount of toxin on its own.[2] In technical terms, alum was acting as an adjuvant.

Meanwhile, in Paris, Gaston Ramon was developing the diphtheria and tetanus toxoid vaccines. If alum could enhance the antibody response in a guinea pig injected with a toxin, it was reasonable to expect it to enhance the antibody response in a human injected with toxoid. So it proved, and in 1932, alum was added to both diphtheria and tetanus vaccines.[3]

Alum is a salt of aluminium. The most familiar salt is table salt, in which the elements held together are sodium and chlorine, but to a chemist, a salt is any chemical compound held together by the charges of its elements.

Alum is one of four different aluminium-based salts that make effective adjuvants. The other three are aluminium hydroxide, aluminium oxyhydroxide and aluminium phosphate.[4] Their names might interest a chemist, but for that Dutch parent, the salient point is that they all contain aluminium.

Glenny was more interested in application than theory and, having discovered that alum functioned as an adjuvant, he wasn't particularly interested in how it worked. He performed some rather perfunctory experiments and concluded that it enhanced the immune response by releasing the toxin slowly rather than allowing the immune system to gobble it all up at once.

More recent experiments have focused on the dendritic cells, which process and present protein fragments to the lymphocytes, including the antibody-secreting B-cells. They showed that dendritic cells take up alum-bound proteins not slower but faster than unbound protein.[5] If alum is indeed delaying the release of the protein, it's doing it from inside a cell.

It's a long way from a complete explanation, but if we still don't know *how* aluminium salt adjuvants vaccines, we have nearly a century's worth of data to show that it *does*. That Dutch parent is likely to be more interested in the other question we can answer with all that data.

Is it safe?

How toxic are aluminium salts?

The toxicologist's mantra is that the poison is in the dose. Substances we usually regard as harmless and wholesome, like the vitamin C sold as a health supplement or the chlorophyll that makes a salad green, are toxic in large enough quantities. Alternatively, take the most potent toxin known to science, rebrand it from botulin to Botox, and watch people queue up to have it injected into their faces. It's safe as long as the quantities are minuscule.

The human body is very good at clearing out chemicals before they build up to toxic doses, and that includes aluminium compounds, which are packed off to our kidneys and expelled in our urine[6] long before they build up to toxic levels.

To ask whether the aluminium salts in vaccines are toxic, we need to know if those vaccines contain a toxically high dose – and to know that, we need to know how high a dose is toxic.

The standard approach to assessing a chemical's toxicity is to calculate what's called the LD50: how much of it do you have to inject into a group of unfortunate rats to kill half of them? With aluminium salts, it's between 25 and 133 milligrams,* depending on which salt, for every kilo of rat.[7] That makes aluminium salts about as toxic as the vitamin D3[8] that's recommended to stave off the winter blues or the capsaicin[9] that gives chilli its kick.

Put like that, aluminium salts don't sound particularly nasty,

---

* A milligram is a thousandth of a gram.

but there's more to toxicity than dying or not dying. We need to look deeper into how the human body interacts with aluminium before we can feel comfortable with it.

When a rat, or indeed a human, takes in a toxically high dose of aluminium salts, that toxicity manifests by the aluminium accumulating in the brain. It can cause some nasty effects at well below the lethal dose. That happened in 1988, when 20 tonnes of aluminium was accidentally emptied into a drinking water reservoir near the Cornish town of Camelford. Residents suffered from aching joints and loss of concentration and memory.[10] Most recovered quickly, but the incident serves as a warning not to be complacent about aluminium.

It also shows us what happens when someone takes in too much aluminium at once. The next question is whether the childhood vaccination schedule comes anywhere near delivering too much aluminium.

Twelve years of vaccines or two kilos of bread

Not all childhood vaccines contain aluminium adjuvants. Because they work by binding proteins, they only work with vaccines based on single proteins. They won't do anything with live-virus vaccines like the MMR, rotavirus or childhood influenza vaccines.

That still leaves a lot of the childhood vaccines, including the first that a child gets in most national vaccine schedules. The British schedule starts at eight weeks, when children get both the meningococcus B vaccine and the '6-in-1' containing diphtheria, tetanus, whooping cough, Hib, polio and tetanus. Over the next decade, twelve aluminium-adjuvanted vaccines are scheduled, concluding with the last dose of the HPV vaccine given at twelve or thirteen years old.

Between them, those vaccines contain less than 4.5 milligrams of aluminium. Over twelve years, a child gets between a fifth and a thirtieth of a dose with a fifty-fifty chance of killing a one-kilo rat – depending on which LD50 figure you use – if it were all injected at once.

More pertinently than how it might affect a hypothetical rat, 4.5 milligrams is less than the 5 milligrams that passes through an adult every week. It's about as much as is found in a couple of kilos of bread,[11] which is a lot less bread than most children get through by the time they're twelve. Over more than a decade, 4.5 milligrams isn't even a blip.

A concerned parent could argue that what an adult can cope with may not be the same as what a baby can cope with. Babies, after all, do not eat bread by the kilo. They do, however, ingest aluminium through breast milk, and a litre of breast milk contains around a tenth of a milligram of aluminium.[12] The most that a baby gets at any vaccination is in that eight-week combination, when the meningococcus B vaccine contains half a milligram and the '6-in-1' another half.

In other words, the largest dose of aluminium that a baby will get from a vaccination is about the same as they might get from ten litres of breast milk, which they are well equipped to process.

Allergic Danes and baby Bostonians

Saying it doesn't look like there's anything to worry about is well and good, but not as well and good as direct proof that aluminium in vaccines does no harm.

The best safety data on aluminium salts comes not from vaccinology but from allergy treatment. One way to treat an allergy is to give the sufferer regular doses of the substance to which they are allergic, which builds up a tolerance to it. Like vaccines, those substances are usually adjuvanted with aluminium salts. Regular doses can add up to as much as 350 milligrams of aluminium over five years,[13] which is a lot more than the 4.5 milligrams over twelve years given in vaccines. Even allowing for the fact that the allergy treatments are usually given to older children or adults, the dose per body weight is still many times what anyone gets from vaccines.

Some epidemiologists worried that allergy patients might be getting enough aluminium to push the limits of what they can safely handle. No allergy patients were being rushed to hospital with aluminium poisoning, but low-level toxicity might manifest in ways that doctors wouldn't immediately connect to aluminium.

Those epidemiologists needed a large database of patient records that they could scour for any health problem that appeared more often in people treated with aluminium-adjuvanted allergens. When you need a lot of medical records, the place to look is usually Denmark. The Danish Civil Registration System has been compiling records of every medical procedure on every Danish resident since 1968, and researchers can access the records without being able to see whose records they're looking at. Thanks to the huge amounts of anonymised data, Danes have answered many pressing questions about health and disease simply by going about their daily lives.

The epidemiologists looked at records from nearly 19,000 people who had been prescribed aluminium-adjuvanted allergen treatments between 1997 and 2006, and compared them to 430,000 people who had received the aluminium-free allergy treatments of antihistamines or glucocorticoids.

If some aluminium-related health problem was manifesting in even a small percentage of allergic Danes, 19,000 of them would have been enough to show it up.

The epidemiologists detected no such thing.[14] The only difference was that the people receiving aluminium-adjuvanted allergens were slightly *less* likely to die or to develop autoimmune diseases. Quite why was never resolved, but it was clear that the aluminium salts were doing no harm at much higher doses than are used in vaccines.

The Danish study looked at adults aged eighteen and above, so if we want to be absolutely sure that 4.5 milligrams of aluminium over twelve years doesn't poison children, there's further reassurance in a study led by Mateusz Karwowski at the Boston Children's Hospital. He looked into whether aluminium in vaccines had any appreciable effect on the aluminium level in a baby's body. Karwowski's team compared babies who had all their scheduled vaccines with babies whose parents declined, and found that vaccines did not affect the trace aluminium in their blood or hair.[15] The aluminium in vaccines didn't even register against the aluminium they processed every day.

Aluminium is so pervasive that Karwowski had to go to some lengths to make sure the aluminium he was measuring was from what the babies had ingested. His team had to pre-screen every container they used to store hair and blood in to make sure it didn't already contain more aluminium than the samples. They also had to ask the babies' parents not to wash their hair before sample collection, in case the shampoo left an aluminium residue in their hair.

Karwowski's struggles to eliminate contamination must have been frustrating, but they're also reassuring. They show that aluminium in vaccines is a drop in the ocean of aluminium in our environment.

The downside of enhancing an immune response

Thanks to allergic Danes and Karwowski's Bostonians, we can be confident that the Dutch parent's fears about aluminium toxicity were groundless. However, if adding aluminium to a vaccine increases the immune response, it follows that it may also increase the inflammation that causes sore arms and fevers after a vaccination.

One of the first studies on the subject was done in a Hertfordshire school in 1979, when the schedule included a booster dose of tetanus vaccine at fifteen or sixteen years old. When adjuvanted vaccine was compared to unadjuvanted vaccine, teenagers who got the adjuvant ended up with sorer arms and were more likely to have an elevated temperature,[16] albeit not elevated by very much. Few of them felt feverish, and most wouldn't have known their temperatures were elevated if the researchers hadn't measured them. It wasn't serious enough to affect how many teenagers took time off school.

Similar results were reported from a study on babies in Australia's radiantly named Municipality of Sunshine. When they were due for their diphtheria, tetanus and whooping cough vaccines (DTP), some received aluminium-adjuvanted vaccines and some received identical vaccines without the adjuvant. The adjuvanted vaccines left arms redder than unadjuvanted vaccines but didn't make any difference to whether the babies developed fever or cried.[17]

Swellings and fevers often happen when the immune response is swinging into action. We see that when we get a splinter and the skin around it swells up. If the aluminium adjuvants enhance the swelling, that's a side effect of an enhanced immune response.

It is not evidence of toxicity, which, as the Camelford incident showed, manifests in a very different way. There is ample evidence that the aluminium in vaccines amounts to nowhere near enough to be toxic, and the anonymous Dutch parent need not have worried.

Chapter 23

Can mercury in vaccines be harmful?

Another parent was in another dilemma about another metallic element.

'Talk about being between a rock and a hard place! As a parent, I am loath to having anything that contains mercury injected into my son.'[1]

That was Jas Singh, a Canadian engineer writing to the *British Medical Journal* in 2009. Their son had been offered a vaccine against the swine flu influenza that appeared that year. Being an engineer, Singh knew that mercury is toxic and didn't want it injected into his son.

He wasn't alone. Mercury in vaccines worries a lot of parents, and it's worried enough vaccinologists that some have looked into it. They found there's nothing to worry about.

The first reason to be reassured is straightforward: very few vaccines still contain any mercury compounds. In Britain, the last mercury-containing vaccines were withdrawn from the childhood vaccination schedule by 2005. With the brief exception of some of the vaccines issued in response to the 2009 swine flu, British vaccines have been mercury-free ever since.

It may be used in vaccines licensed in the future for a simple reason: there's no evidence that mercury used in vaccines ever harmed anyone.

That might sound strange to an engineer like Singh, who wouldn't have been allowed near it without sating some health and safety officer's voracious appetite for meticulously filled forms. However, Singh probably used a different mercury compound from that used in vaccines.

When we think of mercury, we usually think of the stuff that spilled out of old-fashioned thermometers when they were broken, forming a silver blob that skittered across a surface if we poked it. Not that it was a good idea to poke it. Pure mercury is toxic, which is why we no longer see mercury thermometers on pharmacy shelves.

The mercury used in vaccines was not in that pure form, but in a compound called ethyl mercury or thimerosal, or sometimes thiomersal, which was used precisely because it's not very toxic.

As with aluminium adjuvants, whether something is toxic or not depends on how much of it we take in at once. Thimerosal's LD50 is similar to aluminium salts,[2] making it similar to vitamin D3 and capsaicin. It's hardly the sort of thing that Hercule Poirot would explain a mysterious murder with, but that wouldn't necessarily reassure a worried parent like Singh who, if they had been trained on mercury toxicity, would have known that mercury can cause brain damage at far lower doses than would be needed to murder someone.

Fortunately, there is ample evidence to show that thimerosal doesn't do that, either.

Why was thimerosal used in vaccines?

As with aluminium adjuvants, the question of whether thimerosal is safe is only the second question to ask. The first is whether there was a good reason for injecting it into small children at all. Unlike with aluminium adjuvants, regulators decided there was not, raising the question of how it ended up in vaccines in the first place.

The answer lies back in the 1920s, when killed-bacteria vaccines were improvised in hospital laboratories and hypodermic needles were reused. Ethyl mercury was first synthesised by Eli Lilly, a US pharmaceutical company, and marketed under the brand name Merthiolate. It proved highly effective at killing bacteria at levels that weren't toxic to humans, solving several problems at once.

Scientists in hospital or state laboratories often reacted to outbreaks by applying the modified Pasteur doctrine of isolate, inactivate, inject to improvise a vaccine. It was a hit-and-miss approach that sometimes got a lid on an outbreak and sometimes did nothing but make a lot of arms sore.

They usually did the inactivation with chemicals that reliably killed bacteria but were too toxic to be left in the vaccine. The process of removing them often removed most of the killed bacteria as well, so that by the time the vaccine was injected, it didn't contain anything for the immune system to react to.

Another problem was keeping the vaccines sterile. One vial might contain fifty doses, so it would be left open while one syringe after another sucked up one dose at a time. It was asking for contamination, and even a usually harmless bacterium can be dangerous if it's injected under the skin.

Ethyl mercury solved both problems. It reliably killed bacteria and viruses at concentrations harmless to humans, allowing vaccinologists to eliminate complex purification procedures and ensuring the vaccine stayed sterile if a contaminating bacterium got into it.[3] It became the go-to chemical for killed-bacteria vaccines and was central to Pearl Kendrick's whole-cell whooping cough vaccine.

The second half of the twentieth century saw pharmaceutical firms take over vaccine production, replacing improvised vaccines with mass-produced products. The problems solved by thimerosal, as ethyl mercury was now called, were smoothed out of the process. Reusable needles were replaced with cheap single-use models, while multidose vials were replaced with single-use preparations sealed under conditions of strict sterility.

There's still a role for thimerosal because multidose vials are still used in low-income countries, but by the 1990s, single-dose vials were the norm in high-income countries. Thimerosal was on its way out, but not because of safety concerns. It simply wasn't needed anymore.

Is there any evidence that thimerosal causes autism?

Thimerosal's quiet departure was interrupted in 1999 when, as part of the USA's Food and Drug Administration's modernisation act, the FDA was required to calculate how much mercury was in every product they approved. They realised that American children were receiving 187.5 micrograms* of mercury in their first six months. That was well within the FDA's safe limit, but it exceeded the more stringent limits set by the Environmental Protection Agency.[4]

No one who has dealt with the arcana of government regulation will be surprised that two departments of the same government had come up with two different safe limits. For once, it wasn't only the age-old failure of the right hand to tell the left hand what it was doing: the EPA had based their figures

---

* A microgram is a thousandth of a milligram; a milligram is a thousandth of a gram.

not on ethyl mercury, or thimerosal, but on its evil twin. Methyl mercury is used in industrial processes and as a pesticide, so it's a lot more toxic.[5] It may well have been methyl mercury that Jas Singh had in mind when he worried about it being injected into his son.

As their similar names suggest, ethyl and methyl mercury are chemically very similar, differing only by one carbon and two hydrogen atoms. However, three atoms can make a big difference to how a chemical interacts with the human body. One carbon and two hydrogen atoms are the difference between ethanol, the alcohol that makes wine or beer pleasant to drink, and methanol, the 'meths' that renders habitual drinkers blind.

Those three atoms are equally important when they're attached to mercury. Ethyl mercury passes through the body so quickly that half the thimerosal in a vaccine is flushed out of a child's body within a week,[6] clearing it before it has time to build up to toxic levels.

Methyl mercury, on the other hand, stays in the body for much longer, so with repeated exposure, far lower doses can build up to toxic levels.

The EPA's safe limit for methyl mercury allowed a generous margin of error that the much faster-clearing thimerosal in childhood vaccines only just breached. Nevertheless, the EPA's limits made no distinction between ethyl and methyl compounds. The vaccine schedule breached the EPA's stated limit, which led to a flurry of meetings between an alphabet soup of federal agencies, government departments and medical associations. It culminated in a policy statement by the Public Health Service and the American Academy of Pediatricians issued in July 1999,[7] announcing a move away from thimerosal-containing vaccines and recommending that until the move was completed, the hepatitis B vaccination should be delayed to lower the total mercury exposure at any one time.

Where America led, the world followed. The European Medicines Evaluation Agency (EMEA)* issued a similar statement, acknowledging that there was no evidence that mercury in vaccines had ever harmed anyone, but stating it was 'prudent to promote the general use of vaccines without thimerosal'.[8]

Like their US counterparts, the EMEA was applying the precautionary principle: a safety concern had arisen and there was no good reason to go on using thimerosal, so it made sense to stop using it.

The whole process of identifying, discussing and rectifying the problem was completed in a few weeks, which led to differing opinions among the doctors and policymakers involved. Some thought it exemplified the efficiency with which government bureaucracy should respond to even a minor safety concern. Others, mostly those who were engaged in countering rumours being put about by antivaccine lobbyists, took a different view.

Stanley Plotkin, inventor of the rubella vaccine, called it 'nothing less than a public health disaster'.[9] He didn't object to withdrawing thimerosal, but he was worried that the precipitate rescheduling of hepatitis B vaccination looked more like an emergency response to a crisis than a response to a box-ticking exercise.

In the year after Andrew Wakefield's false claim that the MMR vaccine caused autism, and two years after the RotaShield rotavirus vaccines were withdrawn, a lot of parents were already nervous about vaccines. The last thing Plotkin wanted was an evidence-free issue that would make them even more nervous.

His fears were realised.

In 2001, while autism cases were rising rapidly around the

---

* Now the European Medicines Agency.

world, a marketing consultant called Sallie Bernard and a nurse called Lyn Redwood founded a US-based charity called SafeMinds and published a paper arguing that the rise in autism cases was down to thimerosal.[10]

It appeared in a journal called *Medical Hypotheses*, which, as its title suggests, publishes suggestions for things that might be worth looking into rather than completed research. Unfortunately, the distinction between hypothesis and evidence was lost on reporters looking for a headline story, who enthusiastically added fears about thimerosal to whatever other worries parents like Singh may have had about vaccines.

Unlike many who jumped on the vaccine-blaming bandwagon, SafeMinds put its money where its mouth was and funded a study in which infant monkeys were dosed with childhood vaccines with or without thimerosal. They found thimerosal made no difference to the monkeys' brain development.[11] SafeMinds moved on from vaccines and continues to fund research into the environmental causes of autism.

It wasn't a particularly rigorous test of the SafeMinds hypothesis. There's no reason to assume that thimerosal or anything else would affect a monkey's brain development in the same way as a child's. However, SafeMinds did something that remains almost unheard of in the history of the antivaccine movement: they put their ideas to the test, and when the evidence didn't support their ideas, they accepted the evidence and refocused their efforts in more productive directions.

Unfortunately, if not unpredictably, their results received less coverage than their hypothesis. The fears of parents like Singh were not assuaged.

Something else that received little coverage was the evidence that might have assuaged them, which was far more rigorous than the SafeMinds-funded experiments on monkeys.

The epidemiology of thimerosal and autism

If thimerosal was indeed a major cause of autism, we would expect to see the proportion of children developing autism rise whenever a thimerosal-containing vaccine was added to a national vaccine schedule and fall whenever one was removed.

As with aluminium adjuvants, the best place to find a large enough database to see such steps is the Danish Civil Registration System. The Danish data was particularly useful here because Denmark's last thimerosal-containing vaccine had been replaced in 1992, years before the American policy change was followed around the world.[12]

Between 1971 and 1990, diagnoses of autism in Danish two- to four-year-olds were consistently below 0.004 per cent. From 1990, Denmark saw the same rise in autism that affected Britain, the USA and Japan, even though the amount of thimerosal in childhood vaccines hadn't changed in more than twenty years. When the last thimerosal-containing vaccine was withdrawn in 1992, the autism rate had reached 0.012 per cent and continued to rise rapidly. By 1994, 0.02 per cent of two- to four-year-olds were diagnosed with autism, and by 2000, eight years after the last Danish child had been injected with a thimerosal-containing vaccine, the autism rate hit 0.045 per cent,[13] nearly four times where it was when vaccines contained mercury.

Researchers in Britain,[14,15] the USA[16,17] and Canada[18] also looked for an association between thimerosal dose and autism diagnosis, albeit with smaller datasets than the Danish Civil Registry. They all found the same pattern – or rather, the same lack of a pattern. Autism continued to rise long after thimerosal-containing vaccines were withdrawn.

Nor did those epidemiologists confine themselves to looking at autism. They covered a whole range of outcomes ranging from developmental progress, measured by the rate at which speech and language developed, to developmental disorders such as attention deficit and stammering. Between them, the various studies collected data from over three quarters of a million children. No aspect of child development was related to how much thimerosal they received with their vaccines.

Is there any possibility that mercury might cause autism?

An engineer like Singh, who would be trained in risk assessment, might point out that a small risk factor can be obscured by a change in a large risk factor. If thimerosal were that small risk factor, its effect might have been buried if a much larger risk factor came into play in the 1990s. After all, *something* caused a worldwide rise in autism diagnoses in the late twentieth century, even if we still don't know what that something was. Before we dismiss the possibility that thimerosal might have caused autism, we need to consider whether mercury compounds can cause autism at all, which means looking into what happens when mercury doses reach toxic levels in children.

We know a lot about that because of the widespread – and deeply unwise – use of mercury chloride in a children's medicine called calomel in the late nineteenth and early twentieth centuries. Calomel-laced chocolate was used to treat intestinal worms, and mothers bought powdered calomel to rub into their children's gums to relieve teething pain. In that, it was probably effective, because one symptom of mercury poisoning is numbing.

Unfortunately, easing pain was not all it did. When it caused bleeding sores in children's gums, many mothers thought the sores were caused by teething and responded by rubbing in more calomel.

As calomel became widely used, doctors started noticing 'pink disease',[19] so-called because children's skin turned pink and peeled like sunburn, sometimes badly enough to turn fingers and toes gangrenous. Nobody connected pink disease with calomel until the late 1940s, when it was finally recognised as mercury poisoning.

This is why clinical trials matter. If calomel had undergone even the most basic safety trial, it would never have made it to pharmacy shelves, and there would never have been such a thing as pink disease.

More relevant to mercury and autism is that calomel powders were widely used until 1954,[20] when most pharmaceutical firms in Europe and the USA stopped manufacturing them. The figure on page 000 takes another look at the records compiled by the Autism Society of the San Francisco Bay Area,[21] and shows that autism rates rose among male Californians born *after* calomel was withdrawn, even though far more children born in the 1930s and 1940s had mercury rubbed directly into their gums. That's not to say that rubbing mercury into a baby's gums is a good idea, but whatever damage it was doing, it did not cause autism. The same plot shows that the rise in autism rates continues after the last vaccine containing thimerosal was issued in 2003.[22]

The misuse of mercury in medicine caused an enormous amount of misery, but at the same time, gave us an enormous amount of information on mercury poisoning. Enough that we can confidently state that autism is not among the many effects of that poisoning. When children were exposed to far more mercury than they ever get from a vaccine, they were far less likely to develop autism than today's children are.

Other researchers asked the question the other way round: if mercury caused autism, we would expect autistic children to have higher levels of mercury exposure than non-autistic children.

Lynn Wecker of the Louisiana State University Medical Centre led a study to see whether there was any evidence that autistic children were more exposed to a range of different elements, including mercury, than their fellow New Orleanians. She and her team took hair samples from children aged between two and eleven years old, and they found differences, albeit not in the concentration of mercury.[23] The autistic children's hair had lower concentrations of calcium, magnesium, copper, manganese and chromium, and higher concentrations of lithium.

The reasons behind the differences remain a mystery. Autistic children often have digestive problems[24] that might affect the way they metabolise minerals, but as Wecker didn't collect data on digestive problems, that is no more than speculation.

Wecker's results concur with twenty years of epidemiological research: the levels of ethyl mercury in vaccines have always been comfortably non-toxic. Jas Singh could have watched his son have his flu jab without the slightest concern.

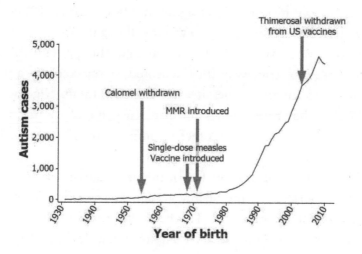

The birth years of males diagnosed with autism in the caseload of the California Department of Developmental Services, recorded in 2015.[25]

Chapter 24

Can the influenza vaccine cause the flu?

Nigel* resolved never to have another influenza vaccine.

'I had a flu jab once and I got the flu and that lasted over a week,' he told his GP. 'Never again, no more jabs ... it's no use having this stuff if it's going to give me flu again.'[1]

That GP, Rosie Telford, was asking the patients of her Manchester practice why they accepted or rejected the annual influenza vaccination when it was offered to them. Nigel raised a concern that often comes up in discussions of the influenza vaccine: that instead of protecting him from influenza, it had given it to him.

'Flu' is an abbreviation for 'influenza', but most of us use it as a generic term for feeling under the weather, especially with a sniffle of some sort. I've been working on viral disease for twenty years, and I still use 'flu' to mean 'feeling like death warmed up' instead of 'confirmed diagnosis of influenza virus infection'.

---

* Pseudonym.

Several viruses can cause a cold that we might call the flu, but we can't get it from the adult influenza vaccine. It's not only completely inactivated but also 'split', meaning that it only contains the two proteins most important to immunity. There's nothing in there that could infect Nigel.

However, Nigel is not the only person to believe he has caught flu from the influenza vaccine. His concern comes up so often that there must be something behind it.

Could the adult influenza vaccine side effects amount to flu?

In the last days of 2019, my friend Rani* asked me about influenza vaccines.

We'd met for a coffee on a winter evening, while London coughed and sneezed its way into five o'clock darkness. The latest winter bug gave a percussive background to unsettling reports of a new coronavirus in Wuhan, which, while it didn't seem particularly alarming – it was on the other side of the world, after all, and it wasn't an influenza virus that might be a pandemic strain – had got us talking about respiratory viruses.

She'd never had an influenza vaccine, and hadn't realised that she could get it by simply walking into a pharmacy and asking for it. I assured her that the worst it had ever given me was a sore arm and a couple of days of feeling tired. We finished our coffees, dropped into a nearby pharmacy and ten minutes later, she was vaccinated.

The next day, Rani phoned me to tell me she was dying.

I had a moment of panic before she assured me she didn't mean it literally. She was running a slight fever, her muscles

---

* Pseudonym.

ached and she didn't feel like getting out of bed. She was in no danger of death, but in colloquial terms, if not medical, Rani had the flu.

Her immune system had mounted an overzealous response to the vaccine. It was the same inflammation that gave me a sore arm but, in her case, it hadn't stopped at her arm. It had turned into an inflammatory response that spread through her whole body.

She told me she had plenty of ibuprofen, and I mumbled a few platitudes that made me feel I was somehow helping.

The day after that, she called me again to say she now felt fine.

I apologised for my misleading reassurance, but she said she was happy she'd been vaccinated. Rani is a freelancer whose life alternates between weeks of intense work with long gaps in between. She'd rather be flattened for a day while she wasn't working than have the flu while she was.

Nevertheless, Rani was very unlucky. Across many different trials, the number of people who complain of muscle pain or noticeable fatigue after an influenza vaccine is very low: less than twice as many who complain of the same effect after getting a placebo.[2] Rani's bad day is about as bad as it gets. With the possible exception of the long-withdrawn Pandemrix vaccine, which possibly caused narcolepsy in a tiny number of people – but probably didn't – serious adverse events following influenza vaccination are vanishingly rare.

Being a healthy woman in her forties, Rani regarded influenza as an inconvenience rather than a danger. Nigel, on the other hand, was being offered the influenza vaccine because he was over sixty-five years old and becoming more vulnerable to influenza with every passing year. In a typical year, influenza hospitalises 30,000 people and kills 7,000 in Britain.[3] That's not a lot in a country of over 65 million, but most of those 30,000 look a lot more like Nigel than like Rani.

It's possible that Nigel, like Rani, had experienced a

particularly unpleasant reaction to the vaccine, in which case he wouldn't have been entirely wrong to say the vaccine gave him the flu.

We all need to balance the side effects of the vaccine against the protection it gives us. It's easy for me, because it doesn't do anything to me that I can't handle with a couple of paracetamol. It's more difficult for the people like Rani, and possibly Nigel, who get hit harder.

That's assuming that their 'flu' was caused by the vaccine in the first place.

Is flu after an influenza vaccine always caused by the vaccine?

Rani and I assumed her achy day was caused by the vaccine because her symptoms were typical vaccine side effects that kicked in within a few hours after she was vaccinated and were gone in twenty-four hours. If her symptoms had taken another day or two to appear, or lasted a day or two longer, we'd have been less certain that the vaccine caused them.

One parent, asked why they refused routine influenza vaccine for their daughter, answered, 'Several children at my daughter's school, after four weeks of having the vaccination, were off school with flu.'[4]

That was 'Parent 14', who was interviewed as part of a study done in West Yorkshire and Greater Manchester, a region where a lot of parents refuse influenza vaccination for their children. Parent 14 didn't want their daughter to have a day like Rani's, but unlike Rani, the children Parent 14 was talking about were not feeling ill the day after being vaccinated. They were talking about children falling ill up to a month later.

The connection sounds unlikely, especially as the childhood

vaccine is even less likely to cause side effects than the adult vaccine.[5] That may seem strange given that the childhood vaccine is not inactivated, like the adult vaccine, but is a weakened form of the influenza virus. Giving children the 'flu', in the sense of an influenza virus infection, is literally what it does, but usually without causing 'flu' in the colloquial sense of being ill.

Parent 14 was saying the vaccine gave children 'flu' in the colloquial sense, but if it took up to a month to do it, it was taking its sweet time about it. Whether it's a vaccine strain or a wild-type, the influenza virus starts replicating as soon as it finds cells to infect, and at the same time, it triggers an immune response. It might take a few days for the squabble between virus and immune system to make itself felt, but not as long as the weeks that Parent 14 was talking about.

Before assuming that every absence in a classful of children between September and December was caused by the vaccine, we might ask if there was anything else that could be causing children to stay home with the flu.

The annual influenza vaccine roll-out is timed to pre-empt the winter 'flu season' when the influenza virus is at its most common in Britain and across the Northern Hemisphere's mid and high latitudes. When influenza comes north, it doesn't come alone. The Northern Hemisphere winter and spring see common cold viruses of many different types at their most prevalent.[6]

We don't have a complete explanation for why. One likely reason is that our respiratory tracts are much better at expelling viruses before they attach to cells at moderate humidity levels, but not so good in the low-humidity environment created by indoor heating.[7]

Another possibility is that the schools themselves function as outbreak incubators.[8] Classrooms place children close together in rooms that are often poorly ventilated. A child bringing a cold virus to school can spread it to half their class by the end of the day. The infected children then take the virus home to their families, who then take it to work and infect their colleagues, some of whom will give it to their own children, who infect another school. The summer holidays break the cycle by taking away the cold viruses' fastest means of spreading.

If the influenza virus magically ceased to exist and the vaccine was withdrawn, there would still be plenty of cold viruses left that cause the 'flu'. It would be a strange four weeks of the winter term that saw no children coming down with it.

At least some of the flu that Parent 14 was talking about would not have been caused by influenza but by rhinoviruses, adenoviruses or COVID-19's less severe but still mischievous relatives, the endemic coronaviruses.[9]

Some of it may indeed have been influenza. In the annual race between influenza virus mutations and vaccine roll-out, the roll-out sometimes loses – and even when it wins, vaccine protection is never complete.

Without their clinical records, it's impossible to know what was behind the 'flu' suffered by Nigel and the class that Parent 14 was talking about. It might have been side effects from the vaccine, or it might have been an unfortunately timed cold. What we do know is that for adults and children, influenza vaccination cuts the chances of having an influenza infection in the subsequent flu season by 40–50 per cent[10,11,12,13] and it cuts the number of children who die of respiratory disease by a third.[14]

That's why I get my influenza vaccine every year.

Chapter 25

Can too many vaccines overload a baby's immune system?

Joanne* had a question.

'By over-immunising children, are we in the West modifying our children's immune systems, making them more vulnerable to contracting diseases in the future and damaging them in some way?'[1]

She was speaking in a Glasgow focus group in 2003, when fears that the MMR vaccine might cause autism were at their height. Joanne had chosen to have her five-month-old son vaccinated, but like many first-time mothers, she worried about whether she'd made the right decision.

She asked a fair question.

---

* Pseudonym.

Is a baby's immune system in danger of being overwhelmed?

A baby is helpless.

It's the first thing we learn about babies, and as soon as we've learned it, simply seeing a baby is enough to make us feel protective. A baby is born unable to feed himself, to see what's in front of him or even to control his own body temperature. All he can do is wail for attention.

At five months, Joanne's son would have been able to grasp his toys and might have been starting to crawl, but her protective instincts would still have been dialled up to full capacity – and with good reason.

By contrast, let's consider another sort of baby: a giraffe. The giraffe's mother hardly pauses when she drops the calf two metres to the ground. The young giraffe needs to be on his feet within the hour, because he may need to outrun a pride of lions or a pack of hyenas at any time. That giraffe looks like he's starting life in a very different way from a human.

Except, from an immunological or microbiological viewpoint, the human baby and the giraffe calf aren't very different at all.

For both the human baby and the giraffe calf, birth means passing from an almost sterile womb into a world teeming with microbes. From the baby and the calf's first breaths, those microbes colonise their windpipes and digestive systems, while their immune systems start the lifelong process of sorting friend from foe. A newborn human's brain, bones and muscles are nowhere near as developed as the giraffe calf's, but he needs to be ready for the same microbial challenge.

While Joanne was holding her newborn son close and keeping him safe, she was also giving him the bacteria he would need to digest solid food. In his first few days, he experienced the most intense exposure to new microbes of his life, and his immune system was ready to meet them. A drop of his blood would have contained twice as many lymphocytes as it would when he reached twenty years old,[2] each lymphocyte carrying the potential to respond to one tiny part of a microbe.

From his first mouthful of colostrum, his immune system was engaged in an intricate dance with the onslaught of microbes that science is only beginning to understand. He would be primed to recognise those first microbes as welcome tenants rather than to mount a full-blown response to them, while some parts of the immune system need contact with those first bacteria before they can respond at all.[3]

The human baby may be physically helpless, but his immune system is as fully formed as that of the young giraffe staggering to his feet for the first time.

How much pressure does the vaccination schedule place on the child's immune system?

That's all very well, a worried mother like Joanne might ask, but doesn't that give her son's immune system enough to worry about without injecting him with vaccines as well?

When considering how much an immune system is having to cope with, what matters is the number of antigens. One antigen is one molecule that the immune system must process and react to. For a baby, that means deciding whether it belongs to one of the bacteria he needs to tolerate or if it's something dangerous that he'll need to deal with. Either way, the immune system will need to remember that antigen.

A typical bacterium has several thousand different proteins and carbohydrates, each of which is an antigen that the baby's immune system must sort through. All those early bacterial encounters throw tens of thousands of antigens at his immune system in his first few weeks. Against that background, the few vaccine antigens hardly count at all. The current British vaccination schedule involves fewer than 100 antigens before a baby's first birthday, which is less than a twentieth of the number carried by any of the many species of bacteria that his immune system is coming to terms with.

The reason the vaccination schedule is so sparing is that for most pathogens, an effective immune response doesn't need to target all of its antigens. Some vaccines, like those against diphtheria, tetanus and hepatitis B, only contain a single protein antigen. The vaccinations against some viruses do use the whole virus, but viruses are much smaller than bacteria. The combined measles, mumps and rubella vaccine has fewer than thirty antigens that cover all three viruses in their entirety. No vaccine on the British schedule contains anything close to the thousands of antigens that make up a single complete bacterium.

It would be even more reassuring to have an idea of what the limits of a healthy baby's immune system are, but we don't know, for the simple reason that there's never been any sign of any baby coming close to them. A team led by Paul Offit at the University of Pennsylvania, inventor of the RotaTeq rotavirus vaccine, tried to calculate it from first principles and concluded that a baby can cope with at least a million antigens without difficulty.[4] That's more than 10,000 times as many as are on the British childhood schedule.

Should we worry about the vaccination schedule becoming more intense?

For a mother like Joanne, worried about overloading a baby's immune system, theoretical calculations like Offit's may be reassuring but only up to a point. Today's parents may well be concerned that their children get a lot more vaccines than they themselves received as children.

It's probably more reassuring to know that while the British schedule covers more pathogens than it did in 2003, it contains far fewer antigens. That's because in 2004, the NHS replaced the whole-cell whooping cough vaccine with the acellular vaccine. While the whole-cell vaccine contains all of the bacterium's 3,000 antigens, the acellular vaccine contains only three.

The reason for changing the vaccine had nothing to do with the number of antigens. It was a by-product of the decision to switch from a live-virus polio vaccine to a safer killed vaccine.[5]

Being the only vaccine on the schedule to contain whole bacteria, the whole-cell whooping cough vaccine accounted for the vast majority of the antigens in the vaccines given to Joanne's son. By his first birthday, he would have received more than fifty times more antigens than a baby born in 2023 will.

The most intense vaccination on today's schedule is at eight weeks, when a baby receives seventy-four antigens that protect him from nine different pathogens. It's a small fraction of what his parents received if they were vaccinated before 2004, and an even smaller fraction of the number of antigens he's receiving from the bacteria arriving from his mother.

The vaccination schedule gives a baby a tiny fraction of what he can – and does – handle.

Would a more intense vaccination schedule impair the immune system?

Being an experimentalist by both training and inclination, I tend to treat projections like Offit's million antigens as hypotheses to be tested rather than proven facts. Unfortunately, the only way to find the limit to the number of vaccines a baby can handle would be to inject him with enough to push him past that limit. Any medical researcher who thinks that experiment is a good idea needs to find a new job.

However, Joanne's concern was not about what a million vaccines might or might not do. It was about whether the vaccine schedule as it stands might make a baby more vulnerable to disease in the future. That's a question we can ask. If we know which babies received which vaccines, we can see if the babies who were given more vaccine antigens were more likely to get sick later. All we need is their medical records, and, like the epidemiologists who looked into aluminium adjuvants and thimerosal, epidemiologists concerned about vaccine overload turned to the Danish Civil Registration System.

They reviewed records from over 800,000 children born between 1990 and 2001. Several changes were made to the Danish vaccine schedule during that time, and some of the children missed some or all of their vaccinations for one reason or another, making it possible to compare children who received different numbers of antigens.

It gave the epidemiologists plenty of data with which to test the hypothesis that children who received more vaccine antigens were, as Joanne put it, more vulnerable to contracting diseases in the future. They knew that vaccinated children would be protected against the pathogens in the vaccines, but not every pathogen that can infect a child is covered by the vaccine schedule.

Between 1990 and 2001, the epidemiologists found 84,000 children hospitalised for at least one night by an infection that no vaccine was available for.[6] If vaccines were overloading Danish children's immune systems, then children who received more vaccine antigens would have been more likely to end up in hospital.

The opposite turned out to be true. Children who had received more vaccine antigens turned out to be *less* likely to be hospitalised by an infection that was not on the vaccine schedule.

A few years later, the US government's Centers for Disease Control and Prevention (CDC) funded a similar study using data collected from 495,000 children across the USA born between 2003 and 2013.[7]

Once again, more vaccine antigens did not lead to more illness.

They ran a second analysis, this time looking not at the total number of vaccine antigens but at how many the children received on any single day. They still found no difference. Children given more antigens fared no better or worse than those who had received less.

The American study was published fifteen years after Joanne asked the question. Combined with the Danish study, it addresses a concern that Joanne shared with countless other parents: more vaccines do not make a child more vulnerable to infections.

Would a more intense vaccination schedule affect the developing brain?

If the current vaccine schedule is in no danger of overloading a child's immune system, we're left with the concern that dogs any discussion of childhood vaccinations: could it affect a developing brain? We've established the lack of evidence that whooping cough or MMR vaccines interfere with brain development in previous chapters, but as we're discussing the cumulative effects of vaccines, we may ask whether vaccines that are harmless in themselves might have an effect when they're given in combination. It doesn't sound very likely, but children's brains are not a subject to make assumptions about.

The answer comes from a group of 1,047 American children that were originally recruited to look into the effects of thimerosal. Some of those children had received all their vaccines and some had not, and they were all assessed by a paediatric psychologist between their seventh and tenth birthdays. If their brain development had been affected by how many vaccines they received, it would have shown up in their language ability, coordination or memory.

Once again, it didn't.[8,9] Children who had received more vaccines showed *better* cognitive performance, which, once again, raises the question of why. Just as there's nothing in a vaccine that should slow down the development of a brain, there's nothing that should enhance it either. Vaccines are supposed to leave brains well alone.

Combined with the Danish results, we might hypothesise that vaccines help a child's brain to develop simply by allowing him to spend less of his childhood being ill. A sick child's body is more concerned with fighting the infection than with developing, and if he's confined to bed, he isn't stimulating his developing brain through learning and playing.

The researchers themselves were more cautious in their interpretation, stating that it could have been simply due to chance.

With regard to Joanne's question, it doesn't matter. The salient point is that vaccine antigens account for a tiny fraction of all the antigens that a baby handles with the same aplomb with which a giraffe calf handles being dropped on to the savannah. Joanne could rest assured that her son could cope with far more vaccine antigens than he was being given – and so can today's parents.

Epilogue

The lessons of Ali Maow Maalin

In October 1977, a hospital cook called Ali Maow Maalin caught smallpox. In itself, that was unremarkable. Countless millions had caught smallpox, sufferered from smallpox and many of them had died of smallpox.

Maalin's case was remarkable for several reasons. One is that he could easily have avoided it. In the past, he had worked as a smallpox vaccinator himself but, as he later said, 'I was scared of being vaccinated then. It looked like the shot hurt.'[1]

Another reason is what happened next. Maalin lived in Merca, a small city in southern Somalia. A few years earlier, a case of smallpox there might only have been noticed by the sufferer's friends and family. By 1977 a case like Maalin's immediately appeared on the radar of the smallpox eradication programme. They were never able to vaccinate everyone at risk of smallpox, so their approach depended on identifying any new case and vaccinating everyone in the area. If they were quick enough, the 'ring vaccination' strategy snuffed out an outbreak before it got started.

In Maalin's case, the response was quick enough. Around 50,000 people were vaccinated, and not one more person caught smallpox.

Ever.

That's the final reason why his case was remarkable. Ali Maow Maalin was the last person to be naturally infected with smallpox.

He survived the experience and returned to work as a vaccinator. His sister had died of measles, which became one of the main targets of the Somali vaccination programme, and he later became involved in the polio eradication campaign.

Like vaccinators anywhere, Maalin often encountered parents who had misgivings about vaccination, but he was uniquely placed to discuss it with them. He later described his approach:[2] 'When I meet parents who refuse to give their children the polio vaccine, I tell them my story. I tell them how important these vaccines are. I tell them not to do something foolish like me.'

He couldn't know how many lives and limbs his gentle persuasion saved, but through the 1990s and 2000s, vaccination slowly pushed polio out of Somalia.

By then, running vaccination campaigns in Somalia was not for the faint-hearted. The state was collapsing and heavily armed militias were stepping into the gap. It was the time of the events luridly depicted in the film *Black Hawk Down*, which envisaged 1990s Somalia through the sniperscope of an army with little understanding of the country in which they were operating. Meanwhile, Maalin and his fellow vaccinators were quietly defeating polio.

In May 2013, polio returned. A two-year-old girl in the capital Mogadishu developed poliomyelitis, sending Maalin and his fellow vaccinators into action to shore up the gaps in vaccine coverage.

They succeeded. Somalia's last case of wild-type polio was in August 2014. Two years later, a case in Nigeria was the last in Africa for the next eight years. It recently returned to the continent with cases in Malawi[3] and Mozambique,[4] but at the time of writing, those appear to have been isolated cases rather than heralding new outbreaks.

Maalin didn't live to see the victory that was his as much as anyone's. During his fieldwork containing the Somali outbreak, he caught malaria and died.

Ali Maow Maalin's opinion on vaccination was formed the hard way. He understood why some people are afraid of vaccination because he was one of them, and he understood that whatever a parent fears for themselves, they fear even more for their children. He'd also learned that there's something more frightening than vaccination: facing a serious disease without it.

He helped a lot of people to overcome that fear by sharing his story – probably far more than argument or authoritative commands would have done. That's a lesson anyone advocating for vaccination would do well to remember.

There's a less wholesome lesson in Maalin's death. He hadn't been vaccinated against malaria because there was no vaccine available, but there could have been. The RTS,S malaria vaccine was first made by a collaboration between GlaxoSmithKline and the Walter Reed Army Institute of Research in 1987, but it's spent most of the decades since then at the bottom of the biotech valley of death. Development and testing have been so achingly slow that when Maalin died in 2013, it was still in phase 3 trials.[5]

At the end of 2021, funding was finally secured for the RTS,S vaccine to be rolled out across Africa.[6] We can't say for sure that it would have saved Maalin because it reduces the severity of malaria infection rather than preventing it. There will undoubtedly be people who die of malaria even after receiving RTS,S, but with malaria killing over half a million every year,[7] mostly children under five years old, there's no doubt that it would have saved millions of lives if it had been rolled out even ten years ago.

The story of vaccines is far from complete for the simple reason that the story of infectious disease is far from complete. As long as microbes assail us, we'll need vaccines to defend ourselves, and if today's vaccines aren't up to the job, advances in biology, chemistry and – critically, in the case of the malaria vaccine – funding priorities may give us vaccines tomorrow that are.

While the vaccines – and lack thereof – that defined Maalin's legacy have received relatively little media attention, the whole world has watched with bated breath while the COVID-19 pandemic drove the same issues to play out on a much shorter timescale.

As with the malaria that killed Maalin, 2020 set the entire world grappling with an infectious disease for which there was no treatment and no vaccine. The speed of the response owed a lot to platform technologies like viral vectors and mRNA vaccines having recently reached maturity, but also because, unlike malaria, COVID-19 is a priority in high-income countries. While the malaria vaccine spent decades awaiting funding, the COVID-19 vaccines were thoroughly tested in a matter of months.

As impressively fast as they were developed, COVID-19 vaccines are taking their sweet time to reach most people in low-income countries. Admittedly, not as long as vaccines usually take; there had been meningococcus conjugate vaccines around for years before one was rolled out across the Meningitis Belt, while COVID-19 vaccines were being deployed south of the Sahara within a few months of being rolled out in Europe. Combined with the funding for the malaria vaccine, there's reason to hope that the vaccination programmes that have already saved so many lives in low-income countries will continue to be strengthened in the coming years.

The fanfare around COVID-19 vaccines has provoked a not unexpected backlash. The impulse that sent protestors to wave placards outside vaccine clinics in 2021 is essentially the same as the impulse that sent a grenade with a rude message through Cotton Mather's Boston window in 1721.

Nobody ever said avoiding illness was ever going to be easy, for ourselves as individuals or for the nearly eight billion people currently in the world. All we can do is try to understand the pathogens we face so that we can protect ourselves as best we can.

Acknowledgements

Writing this book took two years plus all of my life before those two years. The two years were to research and write it. The other four decades and change were to become someone who could research and write it in two years.

Those four decades are why I owe an enormous debt of gratitude to the countless friends, family members, colleagues and one or two enemies who have helped me become that person. I wouldn't have had the last of those decades without the many doctors and nurses who treated my lymphoma, and I can't thank them enough for that time – any more than any of us who are living lives we wouldn't have without the NHS can thank the over-stretched professionals who make it work.

Moving on to the two years of research and writing, I have nothing but appreciation for my agent, Eli Keren at United, and editor, Holly Harley at Little, Brown, for believing I could write a book worth writing and for the hours they both put into making it worth reading.

A great many people have helped me along the way but I'd particularly like to thank Onome Akpogheneta and Sarah Hill, whose discerning eyes saved me from more than a few embarrassments, and the Chalk Scribblers – you know who you are – whose perspective kept me grounded.

I am enormously grateful to several experts who shared their perspectives when I contacted them out of the blue. I am indebted to James Cherry, Marion Crouchman, Robert Heyderman, Margaret Miles, Richard Moxon, Paul Offit, Stanley Plotkin, Ian Poxton, Euan Ross and Caroline Trotter.

It was equally valuable to hear the perspectives of people who endured the maladies at the centre of this book. Many thanks to Clair Michna, Lucy and 'Rani', who shared their stories with me and allowed me to use them.

I wrote much of this book in isolation due to the COVID-19 pandemic and if it wasn't for the many people who offered their friendship, often from a safe distance, I'd never have managed to stay focused enough to finish it. There are too many to name here, but I am particularly grateful to Olga Gridina and the cat of mysterious origin, both of whom checked in on me most days to keep my spirits up, and to my sister, Katharine, who made it all possible.

References

Introduction

1. Institute of Medicine (1991). *Adverse Effects of Pertussis and Rubella Vaccines: A Report of the Committee to Review the Adverse Consequences of Pertussis and Rubella Vaccines*. Washington, Institute of Medicine.
2. Baker, J. (2003). 'The pertussis vaccine controversy in Great Britain, 1974–1986'. *Vaccine* 21 (25–6): 4003–10.
3. Public Health England (2019). *Laboratory confirmed cases of pertussis in England. Annual report for 2019 supplementary data tables*. London, Crown Copyright.
4. Amirthalingam, G., Gupta, S. & Campbell, H. (2013). 'Pertussis immunisation and control in England and Wales, 1957 to 2012: a historical review'. *EuroSurveillance* 18 (38): 4003–10.
5. Deer, B. (2011). 'Pathology reports solve "new bowel disease" riddle'. *British Medical Journal* 343.
6. General Medical Council (2010). *Dr Andrew Jeremy Wakefield. Determination on Serious Professional Misconduct (SPM) and sanction*. London, GMC.
7. Deer, B. (2020). *The Doctor Who Fooled the World: Andrew Wakefield's war on vaccines*. London, Scribe UK.
8. Hall, C. (2002). 'Research puts MMR autism link in doubt'. *Daily Telegraph*, 23 August 2002.

Chapter 1

1. Werking, R. (1972). '"Reformation Is Our Only Preservation": Cotton Mather and Salem Witchcraft'. *William and Mary Quarterly* 29 (2): 281–90.
2. Damon, I. (2013). 'Poxviruses' in *Fields Virology* (eds: D. M. Knipe & P. M. Howley), pp2161–84. Philadelphia, Wolters Kluwer Health/ Lippincott Williams & Wilkins.

3. Boylston, A. (2012). 'The origins of inoculation'. *Journal of the Royal Society of Medicine* 105 (7): 309–13.
4. Ibid.
5. Brown, T. (1988). 'The African connection. Cotton Mather and the Boston smallpox epidemic of 1721–1722'. *Journal of the American Medical Association* 260: 2247–9.
6. Ibid.
7. Artenstein, A., Opal, J., Opal, S., Tramont, E., Peter, G. & Russell, P. (2005). 'History of U.S. military contributions to the study of vaccines against infectious diseases'. *Military Medicine* 170 Suppl: S3–S11.
8. Bazin, H. (2000). *The Eradication of Smallpox*. San Diego, Academic Press.
9. Ibid.
10. Ibid.
11. Ibid.
12. Debré, P. (1998). *Louis Pasteur*. Baltimore, Johns Hopkins University Press.
13. Ibid.
14. Ibid.
15. Ibid.
16. Ibid.
17. Ibid.
18. Institut Pasteur (2017). '130 years ago, the Institut Pasteur was under construction'. www.pasteur.fr (accessed 12 July 2021).
19. Bornside, G. (1982). 'Waldemar Haffkine's cholera vaccines and the Ferran-Haffkine priority dispute'. *Journal of the History of Medicine and Allied Sciences* 37(4): 399–422.
20. Hawgood, B. (2007). 'Waldemar Mordecai Haffkine, CIE (1860–1930): prophylactic vaccination against cholera and bubonic plague in British India'. *Journal of Medical Biography* 15(1): 9–19.
21. Bornside, G. (1982). 'Waldemar Haffkine's cholera vaccines and the Ferran-Haffkine priority dispute'. *Journal of the History of Medicine and Allied Sciences* 37(4): 399–422.
22. Austrian, R. (1978). 'The Jeremiah Metzger Lecture: Of gold and pneumococci: a history of pneumococcal vaccines in South Africa'. *Transactions of the American Clinical and Climatological Association* 89: 141–61.
23. Dunnill, M. (2012). 'Sir Almroth Wright, the Plato of Praed Street'. *Proceedings of the Scottish Society of the History of Medicine* Session 2010–2011 and 2011–2012: 17–29.
24. Ibid.
25. Wright, A. & Semple, D. (1897). 'Remarks on Vaccination against Typhoid Fever'. *British Medical Journal* 1: 256–9.
26. Dunnill, M. (2012). 'Sir Almroth Wright, the Plato of Praed Street'. *Proceedings of the Scottish Society of the History of Medicine* Session 2010–2011 and 2011–2012: 17–29.

27. Hawgood, B. (2007). 'Waldemar Mordecai Haffkine, CIE (1860–1930): prophylactic vaccination against cholera and bubonic plague in British India'. *Journal of Medical Biography* 15(1): 9–19.

28. Dunnill, M. (2012). 'Sir Almroth Wright, the Plato of Praed Street'. *Proceedings of the Scottish Society of the History of Medicine* Session 2010–2011 and 2011–2012: 17–29.

29. Debré, P. (1998). *Louis Pasteur*. Baltimore, Johns Hopkins University Press.

30. Blevins, S. & Bronze, M. (2010). 'Robert Koch and the "golden age" of bacteriology'. *International Journal of Infectious Diseases* 14: e744–51.

31. Lindenmann, J. (1984). 'Origin of the terms "antibody" and "antigen"'. *Scandinavian Journal of Immunology* 19: 281–5.

32. Cavaillon, J. M. & Legout, S. (2019). 'Duclaux, Chamberland, Roux, Grancher, and Metchnikoff: the five musketeers of Louis Pasteur'. *Microbes and Infection* 21: 192–201.

33. Dunnill, M. (2012). 'Sir Almroth Wright, the Plato of Praed Street'. *Proceedings of the Scottish Society of the History of Medicine* Session 2010–2011 and 2011–2012: 17–29.

Chapter 2

1. Sakula, A. (1982). 'Baroness Burdett-Coutts' garden party: the International Medical Congress, London, 1881'. *Medical History* 26: 183–90.

2. Lister, J. (1881). 'An Address on the treatment of wounds'. *Lancet* 118: 863–6.

3. Jessney, B. (2012). 'Joseph Lister (1827–1912): a pioneer of antiseptic surgery remembered a century after his death'. *Journal of Medical Biography* 20: 107–10.

4. Lane, N. (2015). 'The unseen world: reflections on Leeuwenhoek (1677) "Concerning little animals"'. *Philosophical Transactions of the Royal Society of London B: Biological Sciences* 370: 20140344.

5. Bar-On, Y., Phillips, R. & Milo, R. (2018). 'The biomass distribution on Earth'. *Proceedings of the National Academy of Sciences of the USA* 115: 6506–11.

6. Sender, R., Fuchs, S. & Milo, R. (2016). 'Revised Estimates for the Number of Human and Bacteria Cells in the Body'. *PLoS Biology* 14: e1002533.

7. Strachan, D. (1989). 'Hay fever, hygiene, and household size'. *British Medical Journal* 299: 1259–60.

8. Rook, G. (2010). '99th Dahlem conference on infection, inflammation and chronic inflammatory disorders: Darwinian medicine and the "hygiene" or "old friends" hypothesis'. *Clinical and Experimental Immunology* 160: 70–9.

9. Bloomfield, S., Rook, G., Scott, E., Shanahan, F., Stanwell-Smith, R. & Turner, P. (2016). 'Time to abandon the hygiene hypothesis: new

perspectives on allergic disease, the human microbiome, infectious disease prevention and the role of targeted hygiene'. *Perspectives in Public Health* 136: 213–24.

10. Cavaillon, J. M. & Legout, S. (2019). 'Duclaux, Chamberland, Roux, Grancher, and Metchnikoff: the five musketeers of Louis Pasteur'. *Microbes and Infection* 21: 192–201.

11. Beijerinck, M. (1898). 'Concerning a Contagium Vivum Fluidium as a Cause of the Spot-Disease of Tobacco Leaves'. *Verhandelingen der Koninklijke Akademie van Wetenschappen Te Amsterdam* 65: 1–22. [English translation published in 1942. *Phytopathology Classics* 7: 33–52.]

12. De Kruif, P. (1927). *Microbe Hunters*. London, Jonathan Cape.

13. Watson, J. (1968). *The Double Helix: a Personal Account of the Discovery of the Structure of DNA*. London, Weidenfeld & Nicolson.

14. Creager, A. & Morgan, G. (2008). 'After the double helix: Rosalind Franklin's research on Tobacco mosaic virus'. *Isis* 99: 239–72.

15. Watts, G. (2018). 'Aaron Klug'. *Lancet* 392: 2546.

Chapter 3

1. Kolmer, J. (1936). 'Vaccination Against Acute Anterior Poliomyelitis'. *American Journal of Public Health and the Nation's Health* 26: 126–35.

2. Branyan, H. (1991). 'Medical Charlatanism: The Goat Gland Wizard of Milford, Kansas'. *Journal of Popular Culture* 25: 31–7.

3. Kolmer, J. (1936). 'Vaccination Against Acute Anterior Poliomyelitis'. *American Journal of Public Health and the Nation's Health* 26: 126–35.

4. Williams, G. (2013). *Paralysed with Fear*. Basingstoke, Palgrave Macmillan.

5. Gilbert, S. & Green, C. (2021) *Vaxxers*. London, Hodder & Stoughton.

6. Dicks, M., Spencer, A.,Edwards, N., Wadell, G., Bojang, K., Gilbert, S., Hill, A. & Cottingham, M. (2012). 'A novel chimpanzee adenovirus vector with low human seroprevalence: improved systems for vector derivation and comparative immunogenicity'. *PLoS ONE* 7: e40385.

7. Folegatti, P., Bittaye, M., Flaxman, A., Lopez, F., Bellamy, D., Kupke, A.,Mair, C., Makinson, R., Sheridan, J., Rohde, C., Halwe, S., Jeong, Y., Park, Y. S., Kim, J., Song, M., Boyd, A.,Tran, N., Silman, D., Poulton, I., Datoo, M., Marshall, J., Themistocleous, Y., Lawrie, A.,Roberts, R., Berrie, E., Becker, S., Lambe, T., Hill, A., Ewer, K. & Gilbert, S. (2020). 'Safety and immunogenicity of a candidate Middle East respiratory syndrome coronavirus viral-vectored vaccine: a dose-escalation, open-label, non-randomised, uncontrolled, phase 1 trial'. *Lancet Infectious Diseases* 20: 816–26.

8. Grady, D. (2014). 'Ebola Vaccine, Ready for Test, Sat on the Shelf'. *New York Times*, 10 October 2014. www.nytimes.com (accessed 16 July 2021).

9. van Doremalen, N., Lambe, T., Spencer, A.,Belij-Rammerstorfer, S.,

Purushotham, J., Port, J., Avanzato, V., Bushmaker, T., Flaxman, A., Ulaszewska, M., Feldmann, F., Allen, E., Sharpe, H., Schulz, J., Holbrook, M., Okumura, A., Meade-White, K., Pérez-Pérez, L., Edwards, N., Wright, D., Bissett, C., Gilbride, C., Williamson, B., Rosenke, R., Long, D., Ishwarbhai, A.,Kailath, R., Rose, L., Morris, S., Powers, C., Lovaglio, J., Hanley, P., Scott, D., Saturday, G., de Wit, E., Gilbert, S. & Munster, V. (2020). 'ChAdOx1 nCoV-19 vaccine prevents SARS-CoV-2 pneumonia in rhesus macaques'. *Nature* 586: 578–82.

10. Shedlock, D., Silvestri, G. & Weiner, D. (2009). 'Monkeying around with HIV vaccines: using rhesus macaques to define "gatekeepers" for clinical trials'. *Nature Reviews Immunology* 9: 717–28.

11. Levine, M. & Chen, W. (2016). 'How are Vaccines Assessed in Clinical Trials?' in *The Vaccine Book. 2nd edition* (eds: B. R. Bloom & P. H. Lambert) pp97–119. London, Elsevier Inc.

12. Folegatti, P., Ewer, K., Aley, P., Angus, B., Becker, S., Belij-Rammerstorfer, S., Bellamy, D., Bibi, S., Bittaye, M., Clutterbuck, E., Dold, C., Faust, S., Finn, A., Flaxman, A., Hallis, B., Heath, P., Jenkin, D., Lazarus, R., Makinson, R., Minassian, A., Pollock, K., Ramasamy, M., Robinson, H., Snape, M., Tarrant, R., Voysey, M., Green, C., Douglas, A., Hill, A., Lambe, T., Gilbert S & Pollard, A (2020). Safety and immunogenicity of the ChAdOx1 nCoV-19 vaccine against SARS-CoV-2: a preliminary report of a phase 1/2, single-blind, randomised controlled trial'. *Lancet* 396: 467–78.

13. Gilbert, S. & Green, C. (2021). *Vaxxers*. London, Hodder & Stoughton.

14. Voysey, M., Clemens, S., Madhi, S., Weckx, L., Folegatti, P., Aley, P., Angus, B., Baillie, V., Barnabas, S., Bhorat, Q., Bibi, S., Briner,C., Cicconi, P., Collins, A., Colin- Jones, R., Cutland, C., Darton, T.,Dheda, K., Duncan, C., Emary, K., Ewer, K., Fairlie, L., Faust, S.,Feng, S., Ferreira, D., Finn, A., Goodman, A., Green, C., Green, C.,Heath, P., Hill, C., Hill, H., Hirsch, I., Hodgson, S., Izu, A., Jackson,S., Jenkin, D., Joe, C., Kerridge, S., Koen, A., Kwatra, G., Lazarus, R.,Lawrie, A., Lelliott, A., Libri, V., Lillie, P., Mallory, R., Mendes, A.,Milan, E., Minassian, A., McGregor, A., Morrison, H., Mujadidi, Y.,Nana, A., O'Reilly, P., Padayachee, S., Pittella, A., Plested, E., Pollock,K., Ramasamy, M., Rhead, S., Schwarzbold, A., Singh, N., Smith, A.,Song, R., Snape, M., Sprinz, E., Sutherland, R., Tarrant, R., Thomson,E., Torok, M., Toshner, M., Turner, D., Vekemans, J., Villafana, T.,Watson, M., Williams, C., Douglas, A., Hill, A., Lambe, T., Gilbert S &Pollard A (2021). 'Safety and efficacy of the ChAdOx1 nCoV- 19 vaccine(AZD1222) against SARS- CoV- 2: an interim analysis of four randomisedcontrolled trials in Brazil, South Africa, and the UK'. *Lancet* 397: 99–111.1.

15. Offit, P. (2007). *Vaccinated: One Man's Quest to Defeat the World's Deadliest Diseases*. New York, HarperCollins.

16. Medicines and Healthcare products Regulatory Agency (2021). 'Yellow Card'. yellowcard.mhra.gov.uk (accessed 28 July 2021).

17. European Medicines Agency (2021). 'COVID-19 Vaccine AstraZeneca: PRAC investigating cases of thromboembolic events – vaccine's benefits currently still outweigh risks – Update'. ema.europa.eu (accessed 26 July 2021).

18. Ross, E. (2021). Author interview. 1 June 2021.

19. Pottegård, A., Lund, L., Karlstad, Ø., Dahl, J., Andersen, M., Hallas, J., Lidegaard, Ø., Tapia, G., Gulseth, H., Ruiz, P. D, Watle, S., Mikkelsen, A., Pedersen, L., Sørensen, H., Thomsen, R. & Hviid, A. (2021). 'Arterial events, venous thromboembolism, thrombocytopenia, and bleeding after vaccination with Oxford-AstraZeneca ChAdOx1-S in Denmark and Norway: population based cohort study'. *British Medical Journal* 373: n1114.

20. Kim, A., Woo, W., Yon, D., Lee, S., Yang, J., Kim, J., Park, S., Koyanagi, A., Kim, M., Lee, S., Shin, J. & Smith, L. (2022). 'Thrombosis patterns and clinical outcome of COVID-19 vaccine-induced immune thrombotic thrombocytopenia: A Systematic Review and Meta-Analysis'. *International Journal of Infectious Diseases* 119: 130–9.

21. Lonergan, R. (2021). 'Comparison is key: the risk of thromboembolism following the AstraZeneca vaccine needs quantifying against combined hormonal contraception'. *British Medical Journal* 373: n1159.

Chapter 4

1. Editorial (1948). 'Sir Charles Sherrington and Diphtheria Antitoxin'. *Nature* 161: 266–7.

2. Kaufmann, S. (2017). 'Remembering Emil von Behring: from Tetanus Treatment to Antibody Cooperation with Phagocytes'. *mBio* 8: e00117.

3. De Kruif, P. (1927). *Microbe Hunters*. London, Jonathan Cape.

4. Linton, D. (2005). *Emil von Behring: Infectious Disease, Immunology, Serum Therapy*. Philadelphia, American Philosophical Society.

5. Grundbacher, F. (1992). 'Behring's discovery of diphtheria and tetanus antitoxins'. *Immunology Today* 13: 188–90.

6. Opinel, A. & Gachelin, G. (2011). 'French 19th century contributions to the development of treatments for diphtheria'. *Journal of the Royal Society of Medicine* 104: 173–8.

7. Linton, D. (2005). *Emil von Behring: Infectious Disease, Immunology, Serum Therapy*. Philadelphia, American Philosophical Society.

8. Hróbjartsson, A., Gøtzsche, P. & Gluud, C. (1998). 'The controlled clinical trial turns 100 years: Fibiger's trial of serum treatment of diphtheria'. *British Medical Journal* 317: 1243–5.

9. Ibid.

10. Opinel, A. & Gachelin, G. (2011). 'French 19th century contributions to the development of treatments for diphtheria'. *Journal of the Royal Society of Medicine* 104: 173–8.

11. Kaufmann, S. (2017). 'Remembering Emil von Behring: from Tetanus Treatment to Antibody Cooperation with Phagocytes'. *mBio* 8: e00117.
12. Editorial (1917). 'Obituary: Emil von Behring'. *Lancet* 189: 890.
13. Butler, D. (2016). 'Close but no Nobel: the scientists who never won'. nature.com (accessed 23 December 2020).
14. Allen, A. (2007). *Vaccine*. New York, WW Norton & Company, Inc.
15. Bazin, H. (2000). *The Eradication of Smallpox*. San Diego, Academic Press.
16. Allen, A. (2007). *Vaccine*. New York, WW Norton & Company, Inc.
17. Lewis, J. (1986). 'The prevention of diphtheria in Canada and Britain 1914–1945'. *Journal of Social History* 20: 163–76.
18. Ibid.
19. Mortimer, P. (2011). 'The diphtheria vaccine debacle of 1940 that ushered in comprehensive childhood immunization in the United Kingdom'. *Epidemiology & Infection* 139: 487–93.
20. Ibid.
21. Ibid.
22. Begg, N. & Balraj, V. (1995). 'Diphtheria: are we ready for it?' *Archives of Disease in Childhood* 73: 568–72.
23. Ibid.
24. Maximescu, P., Oprişan, A., Pop, A. & Potorac, E. (1974). 'Further Studies on Corynebacterium Species Capable of Producing Diphtheria Toxin (*C. diphtheriae*, *C. ulcerans*, *C. ovis*)'. *Journal of General Microbiology* 82: 49–56.
25. Gill, D. (1982). 'Bacterial toxins: a table of lethal amounts'. *Microbiological Reviews* 46: 86–94.
26. Zingher, A. (1923). 'The Schick test performed on more than 150,000 children in public and parochial schools in New York (Manhattan and the Bronx)'. *American Journal of Diseases of Children* 25: 392–405.
27. Hasselhorn, H. M, Nübling, M., Tiller, F. & Hofmann, F. (1998). 'Factors influencing immunity against diphtheria in adults'. *Vaccine* 16: 70–5.
28. Swart, E., van Gageldonk, P., de Melker, H., van der Klis, F., Berbers, G. & Mollema, L. (2016). 'Long-Term Protection against Diphtheria in the Netherlands after 50 Years of Vaccination: Results from a Seroepidemiological Study'. *PLoS One* 11: e0148605.
29. Hammarlund, E., Thomas, A., Poore, E., Amanna, I., Rynko, A., Mori, M., Chen, Z. & Slifka, M. (2016). 'Durability of Vaccine-Induced Immunity Against Tetanus and Diphtheria Toxins: A Cross-sectional Analysis'. *Clinical Infectious Diseases* 62: 1111–18.
30. Public Health England (2013). 'Chapter 15: Diphtheria' in *The Green Book*. pp. 109–25.
31. Sharma, N., Efstratiou, A., Mokrousov, I., Mutreja, A., Das, B. & Ramamurthy, T. (2019). 'Diphtheria'. *Nature Reviews Disease Primers* 5: 1–18.

32. Vitek, C. & Wharton, M. (1998). 'Diphtheria in the former Soviet Union: reemergence of a pandemic disease'. *Emerging Infectious Diseases* 4: 539–50.

33. Hardy, I., Dittmann, S. & Sutter, R. (1996). 'Current situation and control strategies for resurgence of diphtheria in newly independent states of the former Soviet Union'. *Lancet* 347: 1739–44.

34. WHO (2017). 'Diphtheria global annual reported cases and DTP3 coverage, 1980–2016'. who.int (accessed 23 December 2020).

35. Clarke, K., MacNeil, A., Hadler, S., Scott, C., Tiwari, T. & Cherian, T. (2019). 'Global Epidemiology of Diphtheria, 2000–2017'. *Emerging Infectious Diseases* 25: 1834–42.

36. Dureab, F., Al-Sakkaf, M., Ismail, O., Kuunibe, N., Krisam, J., Müller, O. & Jahn, A. (2019). 'Diphtheria outbreak in Yemen: the impact of conflict on a fragile health system'. *Conflict and Health* 13: 1–7.

37. Finger, F., Funk, S., White, K., Siddiqui, M., Edmunds, W. & Kucharski, A. (2019). 'Real-time analysis of the diphtheria outbreak in forcibly displaced Myanmar nationals in Bangladesh'. *BMC Medicine* 17: 1–11.

38. Public Health England (2014). 'Vaccine coverage and COVER › Epidemiological Data › Completed Primary Courses at Two Years of Age: England and Wales, 1966–1977, England only 1978 onwards'. webarchive.nationalarchives.gov.uk (accessed 29 May 2022).

39. NHS (2021). 'Childhood Vaccination Coverage Statistics – 2020–21'. digital.nhs.uk (accessed 29 May 2022).

40. UK Health Security Agency (2021). 'Notifiable diseases: historic annual totals. Annual total figures for cases of notifiable infectious diseases from 1912 to 2020'. gov.uk (accessed 29 May 2022).

Chapter 5

1. Stride, P. (2008). 'St Kilda, the neonatal tetanus tragedy of the nineteenth century and some twenty-first-century answers'. *Journal of the Royal College of Physicians of Edinburgh* 38: 70–7.

2. Ibid.

3. Collacott, R. (1981). 'Neonatal tetanus in St Kilda'. *Scottish Medical Journal* 26: 224–7.

4. Roper, M., Wassilak, S., Scobie, H., Ridpath, A. & Orenstein, W. (2018). 'Tetanus Toxoid' in *Plotkin's Vaccines, Seventh edition* (eds: S. A. Plotkin, W. A. Orenstein, P. A. Offit & M. D. Edwards) pp1052–79. Philadelphia, Elsevier, Inc.

5. Gill, D. (1982). 'Bacterial toxins: a table of lethal amounts'. *Microbiological Reviews* 46: 86–94.

6. Licona-Cassani, C., Steen, J., Zaragoza, N., Moonen, G., Moutafis, G., Hodson, M., Power, J., Nielsen, L. & Marcellin, E. (2016). 'Tetanus toxin production is triggered by the transition from amino acid consumption to peptides'. *Anaerobe* 41: 113–24.

7. van Gijn, J. (2011). 'Charles Bell (1774–1842)'. *Journal of Neurology* 258: 1189–90.

8. Stride, P. (2008). 'St Kilda, the neonatal tetanus tragedy of the nineteenth century and some twenty-first-century answers'. *Journal of the Royal College of Physicians of Edinburgh* 38: 70–7.

9. Kantha, S. (1991). 'A centennial review; the 1890 tetanus antitoxin paper of von Behring and Kitasato and the related developments'. *Keio Journal of Medicine* 40: 35–9.

10. Shampo, M. & Kyle, R. (1999). 'Shibasaburo Kitasato – Japanese bacteriologist'. *Mayo Clinic Proceedings* 74: 146.

11. Galazka, A., Birmingham, M., Kurian, M. & Gasse, F. (2004). 'Tetanus' in *The Global Epideomiology of Infectious Diseases* (eds: J. L. Murray, A. D. Lopex & C. D. Mathers) pp151–99. Geneva, WHO.

12. Pennington, H. (2019). 'The impact of infectious disease in war time: a look back at WW1'. *Future Microbiology* 14: 165–8.

13. Wever, P. & van Bergen, L. (2012). 'Prevention of tetanus during the First World War'. *Medical Humanities* 38: 78–82.

14. Ibid.

15. MacConkey, A. (1914). 'Tetanus: Its Prevention and Treatment by Means of Antitetanic Serum'. *British Medical Journal* 2: 609–14.

16. Bruce, D. (1917). 'Note on the Incidence of Tetanus among Wounded Soldiers'. *British Medical Journal* 1: 118–19.

17. Rogers, F. & Maloney, R. (1963). 'Gaston Ramon, 1886–1963'. *Archives of Environmental Health* 7: 723–5.

18. Boyd, J. (1938). 'Active immunization against tetanus'. *Journal of the Royal Army Medical Corps* 70: 289–307.

19. Boyd. J. (1946). 'Tetanus in the African and European theatres of war, 1939–1945'. *Lancet* 1: 113–19.

20. Ibid.

21. Khan, R., Vandelaer, J., Yakubu, A., Raza, A. & Zulu, F. (2015). 'Maternal and neonatal tetanus elimination: from protecting women and newborns to protecting all'. *International Journal of Women's Health* 7: 171–80.

22. Thwaites, C., Beeching, N. & Newton, C. (2015). 'Maternal and neonatal tetanus'. *Lancet* 385: 362–70.

23. Public Health England (2020). 'Chapter 30: Tetanus' in *The Green Book*. London, PHE.

24. Haarlund, E., Thomas, A., Poore, E., Amanna, I., Rynko, A., Mori, M., Chen, Z. & Slifka, M. (2016). 'Durability of Vaccine-Induced Immunity Against Tetanus and Diphtheria Toxins: A Cross-sectional Analysis'. *Clinical Infectious Diseases* 62: 1111–18.

25. Public Health England (2020). 'Chapter 30: Tetanus' in *The Green Book*. London, PHE.

26. Public Health England (2019). *Tetanus Supplementary Data Tables England 2018*. London, PHE.

27. Ibid.

28. Collins, S., Amirthalingam, G., Beeching, N., Chand, M., Godbole, G., Ramsay, M., Fry, N. & White, J. (2016). 'Current epidemiology of tetanus in England, 2001–2014'. *Epidemiology & Infection* 144: 3343–53.

29. UNICEF/WHO (2019). 'Progress Towards Global Immunization Goals – 2019. Summary presentation of key indicators. Updated July 2020'. who.int (accessed 30 December 2020).

Chapter 6

1. Volk, A. & Atkinson, J. (2013). 'Infant and child death in the human environment of evolutionary adaptation'. *Evolution and Human Behavior* 34: 182–92.

2. Baker, J. (2003). 'The pertussis vaccine controversy in Great Britain, 1974–1986'. *Vaccine* 21 (25–6): 4003–10.

3. Cherry, J. (1984). 'The epidemiology of pertussis and pertussis immunization in the United Kingdom and the United States: a comparative study'. *Current Problems in Pediatrics* 14: 1–78.

4. Oakley, C. (1962). 'Jules Jean Baptiste Vincent Bordet, 1870–1961'. *Biographical Memoirs of Fellows of the Royal Society* 8: 818–25.

5. Ibid.

6. Cavaillon, J. M., Sansonetti, P. & Goldman, M. (2019). '100th Anniversary of Jules Bordet's Nobel Prize: Tribute to a Founding Father of Immunology'. *Frontiers in Immunology* 10: 2114.

7. Kilgore, P., Salim, A., Zervos, M. & Schmitt, H. J. (2016). 'Pertussis: Microbiology, Disease, Treatment, and Prevention'. *Clinical Microbiology Reviews* 29: 449–86.

8. Ibid.

9. Melvin, J., Scheller, E., Miller, J. & Cotter, P. (2014). '*Bordetella pertussis* pathogenesis: current and future challenges'. *Nature Reviews Microbiology* 12: 274–88.

10. Kilgore, P., Salim, A., Zervos, M. & Schmitt, H. J. (2016). 'Pertussis: Microbiology, Disease, Treatment, and Prevention'. *Clinical Microbiology Reviews* 29: 449–86.

11. Ibid.

12. Ibid.

13. Glynn, J. & Moss, P. (2020). 'Systematic analysis of infectious disease outcomes by age shows lowest severity in school-age children'. *Scientific Data* 7: 329.

14. Anderson, R. & May, R. (1990). 'Immunisation and herd immunity'. *Lancet* 335: 641–5.

15. Kendrick, P. & Eldering, G. (1939). 'A study in active immunization against pertussis'. *American Journal of Epidemiology* 29B: 133–53.

16. Eldering, G. (1971). 'Symposium on pertussis immunization, in honor of Dr. Pearl L. Kendrick in her eightieth year: historical notes on pertussis immunization'. *Health Laboratory Science* 8: 200–5.

17. Shapiro-Shapin, C. (2007). '"A Whole Community Working Together": Pearl Kendrick, Grace Eldering, and the Grand Rapids Pertussis Trials, 1932–1939'. *Michigan Historical Review* 33: 59–85.

18. Eldering, G. (1971). 'Symposium on pertussis immunization, in honor of Dr. Pearl L. Kendrick in her eightieth year: historical notes on pertussis immunization'. *Health Laboratory Science* 8: 200–5.

19. Ibid.

20. Marks, H. (2007). 'The Kendrick-Eldering-(Frost) pertussis vaccine field trial'. *Journal of the Royal Society of Medicine* 100: 242–7.

21. Ibid.

22. Kendrick, P. & Eldering, G. (1939). 'A study in active immunization against pertussis'. *American Journal of Epidemiology* 29B: 133–53.

23. Doull, J., Shibley, G. & McClelland, J. (1936). 'Active Immunization Against Whooping Cough: Interim Report of the Cleveland Experience'. *American Journal of Public Health and the Nation's Health* 26: 1097–1105.

24. Marks, H. (2007). 'The Kendrick-Eldering-(Frost) pertussis vaccine field trial'. *Journal of the Royal Society of Medicine* 100: 242–7.

25. Kendrick, P. & Eldering, G. (1939). 'A study in active immunization against pertussis'. *American Journal of Epidemiology* 29B: 133–53.

26. Medical Research Council (1944). 'Clinical trial of patulin in the common cold. Report of the Patulin Clinical Trials Committee, Medical Research Council'. *Lancet* 244: 373–5.

27. Medical Research Council (1951). 'Prevention of whooping-cough by vaccination; a Medical Research Council investigation'. *British Medical Journal* 1: 1463–71.

28. Public Health England (2019). *Laboratory confirmed cases of pertussis in England. Annual report for 2019 supplementary data tables.* London, Crown Copyright.

29. van Hoek, A. J., Campbell, H., Andrews, N., Vasconcelos, M., Amirthalingam, G. & Miller, E. (2014). 'The burden of disease and health care use among pertussis cases in school-aged children and adults in England and Wales; a patient survey'. *PLoS One* 9: e11180.

30. Amirthalingam, G., Gupta, S. & Campbell, H. (2013). 'Pertussis immunisation and control in England and Wales, 1957 to 2012: a historical review'. *EuroSurveillance* 18 (38): 4003–10.

31. Cody, C., Baraff, L., Cherry, J., Marcy, S. & Manclark, C. (1981). 'Nature and rates of adverse reactions associated with DTP and DT immunizations in infants and children'. *Pediatrics* 68: 650–60.

32. Campbell, H., Amirthalingam, G., Andrews, N., Fry, N., George, R., Harrison, T. & Miller, E. (2012). 'Accelerating control of pertussis in England and Wales'. *Emerging Infectious Diseases* 18: 38–47.

33. Kanai, K. (1980). 'Japan's experience in pertussis epidemiology and vaccination in the past thirty years'. *Japanese Journal of Medical Science and Biology* 33: 107–43.

34. Sato, Y., Kimura, M. & Fukumi, H. (1984). 'Development of a pertussis component vaccine in Japan'. *Lancet* 1: 1–6.

35. Harden, V. (1988). 'Dr. Margaret Pittman oral history 1988'. history. nih.gov (accessed 14th November 2021).

36. Allen, A. (2007). *Vaccine*. New York, WW Norton & Company, Inc.

37. Sato, Y., Kimura, M. & Fukumi, H. (1984). 'Development of a pertussis component vaccine in Japan'. *Lancet* 1: 122–6.

38. Kuno-Sakai, H. & Kimura, M. (2004). 'Safety and efficacy of acellular pertussis vaccine in Japan, evaluated by 23 years of its use for routine immunization'. *Pediatrics International* 46: 650–5.

39. Sato, Y., & Sato, H. (1999). 'Development of acellular pertussis vaccines'. *Biologicals* 27: 61–9.

40. Bart, M., Harris, S., Advani, A., Arakawa, Y., Bottero, D., Bouchez, V., Cassiday, P., Chiang, C. S., Dalby, T., Fry, N., Gaillard, M., van Gent, M., Guiso, N., Hallander, H., Harvill, E., He, Q., van der Heide, H., Heuvelman, K., Hozbor, D., Kamachi, K., Karataev, G., Lan, R., Lutyńska, A., Maharjan, R., Mertsola, J., Miyamura, T., Octavia, S., Preston, A., Quail, M., Sintchenko, V., Stefanelli, P., Tondella, M., Tsang, R., Xu, Y., Yao, S. M., Zhang, S., Parkhill, J. & Mooi, F. (2014). 'Global population structure and evolution of *Bordetella pertussis* and their relationship with vaccination'. *mBio* 5: e01074.

41. Zhang, L., Prietsch, S., Axelsson, I. & Halperin, S. (2014). 'Acellular vaccines for preventing whooping cough in children'. *Cochrane Database of Systematic Reviews* 17: CD001478.

42. Campbell, H., Amirthalingam, G., Andrews, N., Fry, N., George, R., Harrison, T. & Miller, E. (2012). 'Accelerating control of pertussis in England and Wales'. *Emerging Infectious Diseases* 18: 38–47.

43. Ibid.

44. Amirthalingam, G., Gupta, S. & Campbell, H. (2013). 'Pertussis immunisation and control in England and Wales, 1957 to 2012: a historical review'. *EuroSurveillance* 18 (38): 4003–10.

45. Wendelboe, A., Van Rie, A., Salmaso, S. & Englund, J. (2005). 'Duration of immunity against pertussis after natural infection or vaccination'. *Pediatric Infectious Disease Journal* 24: S58–S61.

46. Kilgore, P., Salim, A., Zervos, M. & Schmitt, H. J. (2016). 'Pertussis: Microbiology, Disease, Treatment, and Prevention'. *Clinical Microbiology Reviews* 29: 449–86.

47. Althouse, B. & Scarpino, S. (2015). 'Asymptomatic transmission and the resurgence of *Bordetella pertussis*'. *BMC Medicine* 13: 146.

48. Public Health England (2019). *Laboratory confirmed cases of pertussis in England. Annual report for 2019 supplementary data tables.* London, Crown Copyright.

49. World Health Organization (2015). 'Pertussis vaccines: WHO position paper – August 2015'. *Weekly Epidemiological Record* 90: 433–58.

50. Public Health England (2014). 'Vaccine coverage and COVER ›
    Epidemiological Data › Completed Primary Courses at Two Years of
    Age: England and Wales, 1966–1977, England only 1978 onwards'.
    webarchive.nationalarchives.gov.uk (accessed 29 May 2022).
51. NHS (2021). 'Childhood Vaccination Coverage Statistics – 2020–21'.
    digital.nhs.uk (accessed 29 May 2022).
52. UK Health Security Agency (2021). 'Notifiable diseases: historic annual
    totals. Annual total figures for cases of notifiable infectious diseases
    from 1912 to 2020'. gov.uk (accessed 29 May 2022).

Chapter 7

1. Hall, C. (2000). 'Babies who are not vaccinated "risk death"'. *Daily
   Telegraph* 28 December 2000.
2. Bijlmer, H. (1991). 'World-wide epidemiology of *Haemophilus
   influenzae* meningitis; industrialized versus non-industrialized
   countries'. *Vaccine* 9 Suppl: S5–S9.
3. Edmond, K., Clark, A., Korczak, V., Sanderson, C., Griffiths, U. &
   Rudan, I. (2010). 'Global and regional risk of disabling sequelae from
   bacterial meningitis: a systematic review and meta-analysis'. *Lancet
   Infectious Diseases* 10: 317–28.
4. Fildes, P. (1956). 'Richard Friedrich Johannes Pfeiffer, 1858–1945'.
   Biographical Memoirs of Fellows of the Royal Society 2: 237–47.
5. Pfeiffer, R. (1893). 'Die Aetiologie der Influenza'. *Zeitschrift für
   Hygiene* 13: 357–86.
6. Fildes, P. (1956). 'Richard Friedrich Johannes Pfeiffer, 1858–1945'.
   Biographical Memoirs of Fellows of the Royal Society 2: 237–47.
7. Ibid.
8. Winslow, C., Broadhurst, J., Buchanan, R., Krumwiede Jr, C., Rogers,
   L. & Smith, G. (1920). 'The Families and Genera of the Bacteria: Final
   Report of the Committee of the Society of American Bacteriologists
   on Characterization and Classification of Bacterial Types'. *Journal of
   Bacteriology* 5: 191–229.
9. Gessner, B. & Adegbola, R. (2008). 'The impact of vaccines on
   pneumonia: key lessons from *Haemophilus influenzae* type b conjugate
   vaccines'. *Vaccine* 26 Suppl 2: B3–8.
10. Pericone, C., Overweg, K., Hermans, P. & Weiser, J. (2000).
    'Inhibitory and bactericidal effects of hydrogen peroxide production by
    Streptococcus pneumoniae on other inhabitants of the upper respiratory
    tract'. *Infection and Immunity* 68: 3990–7.
11. Lysenko, E., Ratner, A., Nelson, A. & Weiser, J. (2005). 'The role of
    innate immune responses in the outcome of interspecies competition for
    colonization of mucosal surfaces'. *PLoS Pathogens* 1: 0003–0011.
12. Kim, K. (2003). 'Pathogenesis of bacterial meningitis: from bacteraemia
    to neuronal injury'. *Nature Reviews Neuroscience* 4: 376–85.
13. Fothergill, L. & Wright, J. (1933). 'Influenza meningitis: the relation

of age incidence to the bactericidal power of blood against the causal organism'. *Journal of Immunology* 24: 273–84.

14. Schreiber, J., Basker, C. & Siber, G. (1987). 'Effect of complement depletion on anticapsular-antibody-mediated immunity to experimental infection with Haemophilus influenzae type b'. *Infection and Immunity* 55: 2830–3.

15. Anderson, P., Peter, G., Johnston Jr, R., Wetterlow, L. & Smith, D. (1972). 'Immunization of humans with polyribophosphate, the capsular antigen of *Hemophilus influenzae*, type b'. *Journal of Clinical Investigation* 51: 39–44.

16. Smith, D. & Robbins, J. (1974). 'Prevention of Haemophilus influenzae type b disease in humans'. *Preventative Medicine* 3: 446–8.

17. Peltola, H., Mäkelä, P., Elo, O., Pettay, O., Renkonen, O. V. & Sivonen, A. (1976). 'Vaccination against meningococcal group A disease in Finland 1974-75'. *Scandinavian Journal of Infectious Diseases* 8: 169–74.

18. Peltola, H., Käyhty, H., Virtanen, M. & Mäkelä, P. (1984). 'Prevention of *Hemophilus influenzae* type b bacteremic infections with the capsular polysaccharide vaccine'. *New England Journal of Medicine* 310: 1561–6.

19. Peltola, H., Käyhty, H., Sivonen, A. & Mäkelä, H. (1977). '*Haemophilus influenzae* type b capsular polysaccharide vaccine in children: a double-blind field study of 100,000 vaccinees 3 months to 5 years of age in Finland'. *Pediatrics* 60: 730–7.

20. Bijlmer, H. (1991). 'World-wide epidemiology of *Haemophilus influenzae* meningitis; industrialized versus non-industrialized countries'. *Vaccine* 9 Suppl: S5–S9.

21. Siber, G. (2001). 'Tribute to John B. Robbins, M.D.' in *Recognition of Excellence in Vaccinology and Global Immunization. Addresses by: George R. Siber, M.D. and John B. Robbins, M.D. On the Occasion of the Presentation of the Albert B. Sabin Gold Medal to John B. Robbins, M.D.* (ed: Albert B. Sabin Vaccine Institute) pp5–10. Crystal City, Albert B. Sabin Vaccine Institute.

22. Ibid.

23. Schneerson, R., Barrera, O., Sutton, A. & Robbins, J. (1980). 'Preparation, characterization, and immunogenicity of *Haemophilus influenzae* type b polysaccharide-protein conjugates'. *Journal of Experimental Medicine* 152: 361–76.

24. McNeil, D. (2019). 'Dr. John Robbins, developer of a meningitis vaccine, dies at 86'. *New York Times*, 19 December 2019.

25. Centers for Disease Control and Prevention (1991). 'Haemophilus b conjugate vaccines for prevention of Haemophilus influenzae type b disease among infants and children two months of age and older. Recommendations of the immunization practices advisory committee (ACIP)'. *Morbidity and Mortality Weekly Report Recommendations and Reports* 40: 1–7.

26. Chu, C., Schneerson, R., Robbins, J. & Rastogi, S. (1983). 'Further studies on the immunogenicity of *Haemophilus influenzae* type b and pneumococcal type 6A polysaccharide-protein conjugates'. *Infection and Immunity* 40: 245–56.

27. Joint Committee on Vaccination and Immunisation (1991). 'Haemophilus influenzae B Vaccine Implementation Group: Minutes of the third meeting held at 10:30 am on Monday 24 June 1991 in Room 63 Hannibal House'.

28. Moxon, E. (2021). Author interview. 25 January 2021.

29. Ibid.

30. Booy, R., Hodgson, S., Carpenter, L., Mayon-White, R., Slack, M., Macfarlane, J., Haworth, E., Kiddle, M., Shribman, S., Roberts, J. & Moxon, E. (1994). 'Efficacy of *Haemophilus influenzae* type b conjugate vaccine PRP-T'. *Lancet* 344: 362–6.

31. Barbour, M., Mayon-White, R., Coles, C., Crook, D. & Moxon, E. (1995). 'The impact of conjugate vaccine on carriage of *Haemophilus influenzae* type b'. *Journal of Infectious Diseases* 171: 93–8.

32. Barbour, M. (1996). 'Conjugate vaccines and the carriage of *Haemophilus influenzae* type b'. *Emerging Infectious Diseases* 2: 176–82.

33. Ladhani, S., Ramsay, M. & Slack, M. (2011). 'The impact of *Haemophilus influenzae* serotype B resurgence on the epidemiology of childhood invasive Haemophilus influenzae disease in England and Wales'. *Pediatric Infectious Disease Journal* 30: 893–5.

34. McVernon, J., Andrews, N., Slack, M. & Ramsay, M. (2003). 'Risk of vaccine failure after *Haemophilus influenzae* type b (Hib) combination vaccines with acellular pertussis'. *Lancet* 361: 1521–3.

35. Georges, S., Lepoutre, A., Dabernat, H. & Levy-Bruhl, D. (2013). 'Impact of *Haemophilus influenzae* type b vaccination on the incidence of invasive Haemophilus influenzae disease in France, 15 years after its introduction'. *Epidemiology & Infection* 141: 1787–96.

36. Bijlmer, H. (1991). 'World-wide epidemiology of *Haemophilus influenzae* meningitis; industrialized versus non-industrialized countries'. *Vaccine* 9 Suppl: S5–S9.

37. Kelly, D., Moxon, E. & Pollard, A. (2004). '*Haemophilus influenzae* type b conjugate vaccines'. *Immunology* 113: 163–74.

38. Peltola, H. (2000). 'Worldwide *Haemophilus influenzae* type b disease at the beginning of the 21st century: global analysis of the disease burden 25 years after the use of the polysaccharide vaccine and a decade after the advent of conjugates'. *Clinical Microbiology Reviews* 13: 302–17.

39. Mulholland, K., Hilton, S., Adegbola, R., Usen, S., Oparaugo, A., Omosigho, C., Weber, M., Palmer, A., Schneider, G., Jobe, K., Lahai, G., Jaffar, S., Secka, O., Lin, K., Ethevenaux, C. & Greenwood, B. (1997). 'Randomised trial of *Haemophilus influenzae* type-b tetanus

protein conjugate vaccine [corrected] for prevention of pneumonia and meningitis in Gambian infants'. *Lancet* 349: 1191–7.

40. Adegbola, R., Secka, O., Lahai, G., Lloyd-Evans, N., Njie, A., Usen, S., Oluwalana, C., Obaro, S., Weber, M., Corrah, T., Mulholland, K., McAdam, K., Greenwood, B. & Milligan, P. (2005). 'Elimination of *Haemophilus influenzae* type b (Hib) disease from The Gambia after the introduction of routine immunisation with a Hib conjugate vaccine: a prospective study'. *Lancet* 366: 144–50.

41. World Health Organization (2006). 'WHO position paper on *Haemophilus influenzae* type b conjugate vaccines'. *Weekly Epidemiological Record* 81: 445–52.

42. GAVI (2020). 'Hib Initiative: a GAVI success story'. gavi.org (accessed 31 January 2021).

43. World Health Organization (2020). '*Haemophilus influenzae* type b (Hib)'. who.int (accessed 31 January 2021).

44. Public Health England (2014). 'Vaccine coverage and COVER › Epidemiological Data › Completed Primary Courses at Two Years of Age: England and Wales, 1966–1977, England only 1978 onwards'. webarchive.nationalarchives.gov.uk (accessed 29 May 2022).

45. NHS (2021). 'Childhood Vaccination Coverage Statistics – 2020–21'. digital.nhs.uk (accessed 29 May 2022).

46. Public Health England (2015). *Laboratory reports of Haemophilus influenzae by age group and serotype (England and Wales): October to December 2014, and consolidated annual report for 2014.* London, Crown Copyright.

47. Public Health England (2016). *Laboratory reports of Haemophilus influenzae by age group and serotype (England and Wales): October to December 2015, and consolidated annual report for 2015.* London, Crown Copyright.

48. Public Health England (2015). *Laboratory reports of Haemophilus influenzae infection by serotype and year England 1990 to 2014.* London, Crown Copyright.

49. Public Health England (2019). *Laboratory reports of Haemophilus influenzae by age group and serotype (England): 2018.* London, Crown Copyright.

50. Public Health England (2022). *Laboratory reports of Haemophilus influenzae by age group and serotype, England: annual 2020 (and 2019).* London, Crown Copyright.

Chapter 8

1. Debré, P. (1998). *Louis Pasteur.* Baltimore, Johns Hopkins University Press.

2. Austrian, R. (1981). 'Pneumococcus: The First One Hundred Years'. *Reviews of Infectious Diseases* 3: 183–9.

3. Pakenham, T. (1991). *The Scramble for Africa.* London, Abacus.

4. Maynard, G. (1913). *An enquiry into the etiology, manifestations and prevention of pneumonia amongst natives on the Rand, recruited from tropical areas.* Johannesburg, South African Institute for Medical Research.

5. Packard, R. (1993). 'The invention of the "tropical worker": medical research and the quest for central African labor on the South African gold mines, 1903–36'. *Journal of African History* 34: 271–92.

6. Cobley, A. (2014). '"Lacking in respect for whitemen": "tropical Africans" on the Witwatersrand gold mines, 1903–1904'. *International Labor and Working Class History* 86: 36–54.

7. Dunnill, M. (2012). 'Sir Almroth Wright, the Plato of Praed Street'. *Proceedings of the Scottish Society of the History of Medicine* Session 2010–2011 and 2011–2012: 17–29.

8. Wright, A., Parry Morgan, W., Colebrook, L. & Dodgson, R. (1914). 'Prophylactic inoculation against pneumococcus infections and on the results which have been achieved by it'. *Lancet* 183: 87–95.

9. Dunnill, M. (2012). 'Sir Almroth Wright, the Plato of Praed Street'. *Proceedings of the Scottish Society of the History of Medicine* Session 2010–2011 and 2011–2012: 17–29.

10. Austrian, R. (1978). 'The Jeremiah Metzger Lecture: Of gold and pneumococci: a history of pneumococcal vaccines in South Africa'. *Transactions of the American Clinical and Climatological Association* 89: 141–61.

11. Dochez, A. & Gillespie, L. (1913). 'A biologic classification of pneumococci by means of immunity reactions'. *Journal of the American Medical Association* 61: 727–32.

12. Klugman, K., Dagan, R. & Whitney, C. (2018). 'Pneumococcal Conjugate Vaccine and Pneumococcal Common Protein Vaccines' in *Plotkin's Vaccines, Seventh edition* (eds: S. A. Plotkin, W. A. Orenstein, P. A. Offit & M. D. Edwards) pp773–815. Philadelphia, Elsevier, Inc.

13. Austrian, R. (1981). 'Pneumococcus: The First One Hundred Years'. *Reviews of Infectious Diseases* 3: 183–9.

14. Heidelberger, M. & Avery, O. (1924). 'The soluble specific substance of pneumococcus: second paper'. *Journal of Experimental Medicine* 40: 301–17.

15. Ibid.

16. Dubos, R. (1956). 'Oswald Theodore Avery, 1877–1955'. *Biographical Memoirs of Fellows of the Royal Society* 2: 35–48.

17. Griffith, F. (1928). 'The Significance of Pneumococcal Types'. *Journal of Hygiene* 27: 113–59.

18. Dubos, R. (1956). 'Oswald Theodore Avery, 1877–1955'. *Biographical Memoirs of Fellows of the Royal Society* 2: 35–48.

19. Avery, O., Macleod, C. & McCarty, M. (1944). 'Studies on the chemical nature of the substance inducing transformation of pneumococcal types: induction of transformation by a desoxyribonucleic acid fraction

isolated from pneumococcus Type III'. *Journal of Experimental Medicine* 79: 137–58.

20. Brooks, L. & Mias, G. (2018). '*Streptococcus pneumoniae*'s Virulence and Host Immunity: Aging, Diagnostics, and Prevention'. *Frontiers in Immunology* 9: 1366.

21. Subramanian, K., Henriques-Normark, B. & Normark, S. (2019). 'Emerging concepts in the pathogenesis of the *Streptococcus pneumoniae*: From nasopharyngeal colonizer to intracellular pathogen'. *Cellular Microbiology* 21: e13077.

22. Goering, R., Mims, C., Dockrell, H., Zuckerman, M. & Chiodini, P. (2019) *Mims' Medical Microbiology and Immunology: Sixth Edition.* Edinburgh Elsevier.

23. Henriques-Normark, B. & Tuomanen, E. (2013). 'The pneumococcus: epidemiology, microbiology, and pathogenesis'. *Cold Spring Harbor Perspectives in Medicine* 3: 1–15.

24. Ibid.

25. Osler, W. (1892). *The Principles and Practice of Medicine, Designed for the Use of Practitioners and Students of Medicine.* Edinburgh, Young J. Putland.

26. MacLeod, C., Hodges, R., Heidelberger, M. & Bernhard, W. (1945). 'Prevention of pneumococcal pneumonia by immunization with specific capsular polysaccharides'. *Journal of Experimental Medicine* 82: 445–65.

27. Ibid.

28. Klein, J. & Plotkin, S. (2007). 'Robert Austrian: 1917–2007'. *Clinical Infectious Diseases* 45: 2–3.

29. Henriques-Normark, B. & Tuomanen, E. (2013). 'The pneumococcus: epidemiology, microbiology, and pathogenesis'. *Cold Spring Harbor Perspectives in Medicine* 3: 1–15.

30. Koornhof, H., Madhi, S., Feldman, C., von Gottberg, A. & Klugman, K. (2017). 'A century of South African battles against the pneumococcus – "the captain of death"'. *Southern African Journal of Epidemiology and Infection* 24: 7–19.

31. Austrian, R. (1977). 'Prevention of pneumococcal infection by immunization with capsular polysaccharides of *Streptococcus pneumoniae*: current status of polyvalent vaccines'. *Journal of Infectious Diseases* 136 Suppl: S38–42.

32. Austrian, R. (1975). 'Maxwell Finland Lecture. Random gleanings from a life with the pneumococcus'. *Journal of Infectious Diseases* 131: 474–84.

33. Offit, P. (2007). *Vaccinated: One Man's Quest to Defeat the World's Deadliest Diseases.* New York, HarperCollins.

34. Allen, A. (2007). *Vaccine.* New York, WW Norton & Company, Inc.

35. Smit, P., Oberholzer, D., Hayden-Smith, S., Koornhof, H. & Hilleman, M. (1977). 'Protective efficacy of pneumococcal polysaccharide vaccines'. *Journal of the American Medical Association* 238: 2613–16.

36. Geno, K., Gilbert, G., Song, J., Skovsted, I., Klugman, K., Jones, C., Konradsen, H. & Nahm, M. (2015). 'Pneumococcal Capsules and Their Types: Past, Present, and Future'. *Clinical Microbiology Reviews* 28: 871–99.

37. Tomasz, A. (1997). 'Antibiotic resistance in *Streptococcus pneumoniae*'. *Clinical Infectious Diseases* 24 (Suppl 1): S85–88.

38. Brueggemann, A., Pai, R., Crook, D. & Beall, B. (2007). 'Vaccine escape recombinants emerge after pneumococcal vaccination in the United States'. *PLoS Pathogens* 3: e168.

39. Klugman, K., Dagan, R. & Whitney, C. (2018). 'Pneumococcal Conjugate Vaccine and Pneumococcal Common Protein Vaccines' in *Plotkin's Vaccines, Seventh edition* (eds: S. A. Plotkin, W. A. Orenstein, P. A. Offit & M. D. Edwards) pp773–815. Philadelphia, Elsevier, Inc.

40. Trotter, C., Waight, P., Andrews, N., Slack, M., Efstratiou, A., George, R. & Miller, E. (2010). 'Epidemiology of invasive pneumococcal disease in the pre-conjugate vaccine era: England and Wales, 1996–2006'. *Journal of Infection* 60: 200–8.

41. Miller, E., Waight, P., Efstratiou, A., Brisson, M., Johnson, A. & George, R. (2000). 'Epidemiology of invasive and other pneumococcal disease in children in England and Wales 1996–1998'. *Acta Paediatrica* 89 Suppl: S11–S16.

42. Waight, P., Andrews, N., Ladhani, S., Sheppard, C., Slack, M. & Miller, E. (2015). 'Effect of the 13-valent pneumococcal conjugate vaccine on invasive pneumococcal disease in England and Wales 4 years after its introduction: an observational cohort study'. *Lancet Infectious Diseases* 15: 535–43.

43. Ladhani, S., Collins, S., Djennad, A., Sheppard, C., Borrow, R., Fry, N., Andrews, N., Miller, E. & Ramsay, M. (2018). 'Rapid increase in non-vaccine serotypes causing invasive pneumococcal disease in England and Wales, 2000–17: a prospective national observational cohort study'. *Lancet Infectious Diseases* 18: 441–51.

44. Waight, P., Andrews, N., Ladhani, S., Sheppard, C., Slack, M. & Miller, E. (2015). 'Effect of the 13-valent pneumococcal conjugate vaccine on invasive pneumococcal disease in England and Wales 4 years after its introduction: an observational cohort study'. *Lancet Infectious Diseases* 15: 535–43.

45. Djennad, A., Ramsay, M., Pebody, R., Fry, N., Sheppard, C., Ladhani, S. & Andrews, N. (2018). 'Effectiveness of 23-Valent Polysaccharide Pneumococcal Vaccine and Changes in Invasive Pneumococcal Disease Incidence from 2000 to 2017 in Those Aged 65 and Over in England and Wales'. *EClinicalMedicine* 6: 42–50.

46. Hicks, L., Harrison, L., Flannery, B., Hadler, J., Schaffner, W., Craig, A., Jackson, D., Thomas, A., Beall, B., Lynfield, R., Reingold, A., Farley, M. & Whitney, C. (2007). 'Incidence of pneumococcal disease due to non-pneumococcal conjugate vaccine (PCV7) serotypes in the

United States during the era of widespread PCV7 vaccination, 1998–2004'. *Journal of Infectious Diseases* 196: 1346–54.

47. Ladhani, S., Collins, S., Djennad, A., Sheppard, C., Borrow, R., Fry, N., Andrews, N., Miller, E. & Ramsay, M. (2018). 'Rapid increase in non-vaccine serotypes causing invasive pneumococcal disease in England and Wales, 2000–17: a prospective national observational cohort study'. *Lancet Infectious Diseases* 18: 441–51.

48. Henriques-Normark, B., Blomberg, C., Dagerhamn, J., Bättig, P. & Normark, S. (2008). 'The rise and fall of bacterial clones: *Streptococcus pneumoniae*'. *Nat Rev Microbiol* 6: 827–37.

49. Dagan, R., Poolman, J. & Siegrist, C. A. (2010). 'Glycoconjugate vaccines and immune interference: A review'. *Vaccine* 28: 5513–23.

50. Uchida, T., Pappenheimer Jr, A. & Greany, R. (1973). 'Diphtheria toxin and related proteins. I. Isolation and properties of mutant proteins serologically related to diphtheria toxin'. *Journal of Biological Chemistry* 248: 3838–44.

51. Whitney, C., Pilishvili, T., Farley, M., Schaffner, W., Craig, A., Lynfield, R., Nyquist, A. C., Gershman, K., Vazquez, M., Bennett, N., Reingold, A., Thomas, A., Glode, M., Zell, E., Jorgensen, J., Beall, B. & Schuchat, A. (2006). 'Effectiveness of seven-valent pneumococcal conjugate vaccine against invasive pneumococcal disease: a matched case-control study'. *Lancet* 368: 1495–1502.

52. Lucero, M., Puumalainen, T., Ugpo, J., Williams, G., Käyhty, H. & Nohynek, H. (2004). 'Similar antibody concentrations in Filipino infants at age 9 months, after 1 or 3 doses of an adjuvanted, 11-valent pneumococcal diphtheria/tetanus-conjugated vaccine: a randomized controlled trial'. *Journal of Infectious Diseases* 189: 2077–84.

53. Goldblatt, D., Southern, J., Andrews, N., Burbidge, P., Partington, J., Roalfe, L., Valente Pinto, M., Thalasselis, V., Plested, E., Richardson, H., Snape, M. & Miller, E. (2018). 'Pneumococcal conjugate vaccine 13 delivered as one primary and one booster dose (1 + 1) compared with two primary doses and a booster (2 + 1) in UK infants: a multicentre, parallel group randomised controlled trial'. *Lancet Infectious Diseases* 18: 171–9.

54. Wahl, B., O'Brien, K., Greenbaum, A., Majumder, A., Liu, L., Chu, Y., Lukšić, I., Nair, H., McAllister, D., Campbell, H., Rudan, I., Black, R. & Knoll, M. (2018). 'Burden of *Streptococcus pneumoniae* and *Haemophilus influenzae* type b disease in children in the era of conjugate vaccines: global, regional, and national estimates for 2000–15'. *Lancet Glob Health* 6: e744–57.

55. Cutts, F., Zaman, S., Enwere, G., Jaffar, S., Levine, O., Okoko, J., Oluwalana, C., Vaughan, A., Obaro, S., Leach, A., McAdam, K., Biney, E., Saaka, M., Onwuchekwa, U., Yallop, F., Pierce, N., Greenwood, B. & Adegbola, R. (2005). 'Efficacy of nine-valent pneumococcal conjugate vaccine against pneumonia and invasive pneumococcal disease in The

Gambia: randomised, double-blind, placebo-controlled trial'. *Lancet* 365: 1139–46.

56. von Gottberg, A., de Gouveia, L., Tempia, S., Quan, V., Meiring, S., von Mollendorf, C., Madhi, S., Zell, E., Verani, J., O'Brien, K., Whitney, C., Klugman, K. & Cohen, C. (2014). 'Effects of vaccination on invasive pneumococcal disease in South Africa'. *New England Journal of Medicine* 371: 1889–99.

57. Johnson, H., Deloria-Knoll, M., Levine, O., Stoszek, S., Freimanis Hance, L., Reithinger, R., Muenz, L. & O'Brien, K. (2010). 'Systematic evaluation of serotypes causing invasive pneumococcal disease among children under five: the pneumococcal global serotype project'. *PLoS Medicine* 7: e1000348.

58. Wahl, B., O'Brien, K., Greenbaum, A., Majumder, A., Liu, L., Chu, Y., Lukšić, I., Nair, H., McAllister, D., Campbell, H., Rudan, I., Black, R. & Knoll, M. (2018). 'Burden of *Streptococcus pneumoniae* and *Haemophilus influenzae* type b disease in children in the era of conjugate vaccines: global, regional, and national estimates for 2000–15'. *Lancet Glob Health* 6: e744–57.

59. World Health Organization (2020). 'Pneumococcal conjugate vaccines (PCV3) immunization coverage among 1-year-olds (%)'. who.int (accessed 25 February 2021).

60. Pelders, J. & Nelson, G. (2018). 'Living conditions of mine workers from eight mines in South Africa'. *Development Southern Africa* 36: 265–82.

61. Corbett, E., Churchyard, G., Charalambos, S., Samb, B., Moloi, V., Clayton, T., Grant, A., Murray, J., Hayes, R. & De Cock, K. (2002). 'Morbidity and mortality in South African gold miners: impact of untreated disease due to human immunodeficiency virus'. *Clinical Infectious Diseases* 34: 1251–8.

62. Stuckler, D., Steele, S., Lurie, M. & Basu, S. (2013). '"Dying for gold": the effects of mineral mining on HIV, tuberculosis, silicosis, and occupational diseases in southern Africa'. *International Journal of Health Services* 43: 639–49.

Chapter 9

1. Meningitis Now (2020). 'Clair's story'. meningitisnow.org (accessed 12 March 2021).

2. Stephens, D., Greenwood, B. & Brandtzaeg, P. (2007). 'Epidemic meningitis, meningococcaemia, and *Neisseria meningitidis*'. *Lancet* 369: 2196–2210.

3. Michna, C. (2021). Author interview. 17 March 2021.

4. Read, R., Baxter, D., Chadwick, D., Faust, S., Finn, A., Gordon, S., Heath, P., Lewis, D., Pollard, A., Turner, D., Bazaz, R., Ganguli, A., Havelock, T., Neal, K., Okike, I., Morales-Aza, B., Patel, K., Snape, M., Williams, J., Gilchrist, S., Gray, S., Maiden, M., Toneatto, D.,

Wang, H., McCarthy, M., Dull. P. & Borrow, R. (2014). 'Effect of a quadrivalent meningococcal ACWY glycoconjugate or a serogroup B meningococcal vaccine on meningococcal carriage: an observer-blind, phase 3 randomised clinical trial'. *Lancet* 384: 2123–31.

5. Nadel, S. & Ninis, N. (2018). 'Invasive Meningococcal Disease in the Vaccine Era'. *Frontiers in Pediatrics* 6: 321.

6. Olbrich, K., Müller, D., Schumacher, S., Beck, E., Meszaros, K. & Koerber, F. (2018). 'Systematic Review of Invasive Meningococcal Disease: Sequelae and Quality of Life Impact on Patients and Their Caregivers'. *Infectious Diseases and Therapy* 7: 421–38.

7. Harrison, L., Granoff, D. & Pollard, A. (2018). 'Meningococcal Capsular Group A, C, W, and Y Conjugate Vaccines' in *Plotkin's Vaccines, Seventh edition* (eds: S. A. Plotkin, W. A. Orenstein, P. A. Offit & M. D. Edwards) pp619–43. Philadelphia, Elsevier, Inc.

8. Meningitis Now (2020). 'Clair's story'. meningitisnow.org (accessed 12 March 2021).

9. Ibid.

10. Tyler, K. (2010). 'Chapter 28: a history of bacterial meningitis'. *Handbook of Clinical Neurology* 95: 417–33.

11. Garrod, L. (1954). 'Mervyn Henry Gordon 1872–1953'. *Obituary Notices of Fellows of the Royal Society* 9: 153–63.

12. Gordon, M. (1918). 'Identification of the Meningococcus'. *Journal of Hygiene* 17: 290–315.

13. Greenwood, M. (1917). 'The outbreak of cerebrospinal fever at Salisbury in 1914–15'. *Proceedings of the Royal Society of Medicine* 10: 44–60.

14. Branham, S. (1953). 'Serological relationships among meningococci'. *Bacteriological Reviews* 17: 175–88.

15. Swartley, J., Marfin, A., Edupuganti, S., Liu, L. J, Cieslak, P., Perkins, B., Wenger, J. & Stephens, D. (1997). 'Capsule switching of *Neisseria meningitidis*'. *Proceedings of the National Academy of Sciences of the USA* 94: 271–6.

16. Harrison, L., Trotter, C. & Ramsay, M. (2009). 'Global epidemiology of meningococcal disease'. *Vaccine* 27 (Suppl 2): B51–63.

17. Gold, R. & Artenstein, M. (1971). 'Meningococcal infections. 2. Field trial of group C meningococcal polysaccharide vaccine in 1969-70'. *Bulletin of the World Health Organization* 45: 279–82.

18. Public Health England (2020). 'Notifiable diseases: annual totals from 1982 to 2019'. gov.uk (accessed 21 March 2021).

19. Nadel, S. & Ninis, N. (2018). 'Invasive Meningococcal Disease in the Vaccine Era'. *Frontiers in Pediatrics* 6: 321.

20. Harrison, L., Granoff, D. & Pollard, A. (2018). 'Meningococcal Capsular Group A, C, W, and Y Conjugate Vaccines' in *Plotkin's Vaccines, Seventh edition* (eds: S. A. Plotkin, W. A. Orenstein, P. A. Offit & M. D. Edwards) pp619–43. Philadelphia, Elsevier, Inc.

21. Fairley, C., Begg, N., Borrow, R., Fox, A., Jones, D. & Cartwright, K. (1996). 'Conjugate meningococcal serogroup A and C vaccine: reactogenicity and immunogenicity in United Kingdom infants'. *Journal of Infectious Diseases* 174: 1360–3.

22. Richmond, P., Borrow, R., Miller, E., Clark, S., Sadler, F., Fox, A., Begg, N., Morris, R. & Cartwright, K. (1999). 'Meningococcal serogroup C conjugate vaccine is immunogenic in infancy and primes for memory'. *Journal of Infectious Diseases* 179: 1569–72.

23. MacLennan, J., Shackley, F., Heath, P., Deeks, J., Flamank, C., Herbert, M., Griffiths, H., Hatzmann, E., Goilav, C. & Moxon, E. (2000). 'Safety, immunogenicity, and induction of immunologic memory by a serogroup C meningococcal conjugate vaccine in infants: A randomized controlled trial'. *Journal of the American Medical Association* 283: 2795–801.

24. Campbell, H., Andrews, N., Borrow, R., Trotter, C. & Miller, E. (2010). 'Updated postlicensure surveillance of the meningococcal C conjugate vaccine in England and Wales: effectiveness, validation of serological correlates of protection, and modeling predictions of the duration of herd immunity'. *Clinical and Vaccine Immunology* 17: 840–7.

25. Trotter, C., Andrews, N., Kaczmarski, E., Miller, E. & Ramsay, M. (2004). 'Effectiveness of meningococcal serogroup C conjugate vaccine 4 years after introduction'. *Lancet* 364: 365–7.

26. Ramsay, M., Andrews, N., Trotter, C., Kaczmarski, E. & Miller, E. (2003). 'Herd immunity from meningococcal serogroup C conjugate vaccination in England: database analysis'. *British Medical Journal* 326: 365–6.

27. Ladhani, S., Flood, J., Ramsay, M., Campbell, H., Gray, S., Kaczmarski, E., Mallard, R., Guiver, M., Newbold, L. & Borrow, R. (2012). 'Invasive meningococcal disease in England and Wales: implications for the introduction of new vaccines'. *Vaccine* 30: 3710–16.

28. Taha, M. K., Achtman, M., Alonso J. M., Greenwood, B., Ramsay, M., Fox, A., Gray, S. & Kaczmarski, E. (2000). 'Serogroup W135 meningococcal disease in Hajj pilgrims'. *Lancet* 356: 23–30.

29. Mayer, L., Reeves, M., Al-Hamdan, N., Sacchi, C., Taha M.-K., Ajello, G., Schmink, S., Noble, C., Tondella, M., Whitney, A., Al-Mazrou, Y., Al-Jefri, M., Mishkhis, A., Sabban, S., Caugant, D., Lingappa, J., Rosenstein, N. & Popovic, T. (2002). 'Outbreak of W135 meningococcal disease in 2000: not emergence of a new W135 strain but clonal expansion within the electophoretic type-37 complex'. *Journal of Infectious Diseases* 185: 1596–1605.

30. Taha, M. K., Giorgini, D., Ducos-Galand, M. & Alonso, J. M. (2004). 'Continuing diversification of *Neisseria meningitidis* W135 as a primary cause of meningococcal disease after emergence of the serogroup in 2000'. *Journal of Clinical Microbiology* 42: 4158–63.

31. Mustapha, M., Marsh, J. & Harrison, L. (2016). 'Global epidemiology of capsular group W meningococcal disease (1970–2015): Multifocal

emergence and persistence of hypervirulent sequence type (ST)-11 clonal complex'. *Vaccine* 34: 1515–23.

32. Ladhani, S., Beebeejaun, K., Lucidarme, J., Campbell, H., Gray, S., Kaczmarski, E., Ramsay, M. & Borrow, R. (2015). 'Increase in endemic *Neisseria meningitidis* capsular group W sequence type 11 complex associated with severe invasive disease in England and Wales'. *Clinical Infectious Diseases* 60: 578–85.

33. Public Health England (2016). 'Chapter 22: Meningococcal' in *The Green Book*. London, PHE.

34. Campbell, H., Saliba, V., Borrow, R., Ramsay, M. & Ladhani, S. (2015). 'Targeted vaccination of teenagers following continued rapid endemic expansion of a single meningococcal group W clone (sequence type 11 clonal complex), United Kingdom 2015'. *EuroSurveillance* 20: 1–5.

35. Campbell, H., Edelstein, M., Andrews, N., Borrow, R., Ramsay, M. & Ladhani, S. (2017). 'Emergency Meningococcal ACWY Vaccination Program for Teenagers to Control Group W Meningococcal Disease, England, 2015–2016'. *Emerging Infectious Diseases* 23: 1184–7.

36. Granoff, D. (2010). 'Review of meningococcal group B vaccines'. *Clinical Infectious Diseases* 50 (Suppl 2): S54–65.

37. Granoff, D. & Harrison, L. (2018). 'Meningococcal Capsular Group B Vaccines' in *Plotkin's Vaccines, Seventh edition* (eds: S. A. Plotkin, W. A. Orenstein, P. A. Offit & M. D. Edwards) pp644–62. Philadelphia, Elsevier, Inc.

38. Sierra, G., Campa, H., Varcacel, N., Garcia, I., Izquierdo, P., Sotolongo, P., Casanueva, G., Rico, C., Rodriguez, C. & Terry, M. (1991). 'Vaccine against group B *Neisseria meningitidis*: protection trial and mass vaccination results in Cuba'. *NIPH Annals* 14: 195–210.

39. Harrison, L., Shutt, K., Schmink, S., Marsh, J., Harcourt, B., Wang X, Whitney, A., Stephens, D., Cohn, A., Messonnier, N. & Mayer, L. (2010). 'Population structure and capsular switching of invasive *Neisseria meningitidis* isolates in the pre-meningococcal conjugate vaccine era – United States, 2000–2005'. *Journal of Infectious Diseases* 201: 1208–24.

40. Holst, J., Aaberge, I., Oster, P., Lennon, D., Martin, D., O'Hallahan, J., Nord, K., Nøkleby, H., Næss, L., Næss, L., Kristiansen, P., Skryten, A., Bryn, K., Aase, A., Rappuoli, R. & Rosenqvist, E. (2003). 'A "tailor made" vaccine trialled as part of public health response to group B meningococcal epidemic in New Zealand'. *EuroSurveillance* 7: 2262.

41. Galloway, Y., Stehr-Green, P., McNicholas, A. & O'Hallahan, J. (2009). 'Use of an observational cohort study to estimate the effectiveness of the New Zealand group B meningococcal vaccine in children aged under 5 years'. *International Journal of Epidemiology* 38: 413–18.

42. Rappuoli, R. (2017). '2017 Canada Gairdner International Award Laureate lecture'. Hamilton.

43. Pizza, M. (2017). 'Spotlight on ... Mariagrazia Pizza'. *FEMS Microbiology Letters* 364: 1–2.

44. Pizza, M., Scarlato, V., Masignani, V., Giuliani, M., Aricò, B.,
    Comanducci, M., Jennings, G., Baldi, L., Bartolini, E., Capecchi, B.,
    Galeotti, C., Luzzi, E., Manetti, R., Marchetti, E., Mora, M., Nuti,
    S., Ratti, G., Santini, L., Savino, S., Scarselli, M., Storni, E., Zuo, P.,
    Broeker, M., Hundt, E., Knapp, B., Blair, E., Mason, T., Tettelin, H.,
    Hood, D., Jeffries, A., Saunders, N., Granoff, D., Venter, J., Moxon, E.,
    Grandi, G. & Rappuoli, R. (2000). 'Identification of vaccine candidates
    against serogroup B meningococcus by whole-genome sequencing'.
    Science 287: 1816–20.

45. Rappuoli, R. (2017). '2017 Canada Gairdner International Award
    Laureate lecture'. Hamilton.

46. Santolaya, M., O'Ryan, M., Valenzuela, M., Prado, V., Vergara, R.,
    Muñoz, A., Toneatto, D., Graña, G., Wang, H., Clemens, R. & Dull,
    P. (2012). 'Immunogenicity and tolerability of a multicomponent
    meningococcal serogroup B (4CMenB) vaccine in healthy adolescents
    in Chile: a phase 2b/3 randomised, observer-blind, placebo-controlled
    study'. *Lancet* 379: 617–24.

47. Pollard, A., Riordan, A. & Ramsay, M. (2014). 'Group B meningococcal
    vaccine: recommendations for UK use'. *Lancet* 383: 1103–4.

48. Parikh, S., Andrews, N., Beebeejaun, K., Campbell, H., Ribeiro, S.,
    Ward, C., White, J., Borrow, R., Ramsay, M. & Ladhani, S. (2016).
    'Effectiveness and impact of a reduced infant schedule of 4CMenB
    vaccine against group B meningococcal disease in England: a national
    observational cohort study'. *Lancet* 388: 2775–82.

49. Isitt, C., Cosgrove, C., Ramsay, M. & Ladhani, S. (2020). 'Success of
    4CMenB in preventing meningococcal disease: evidence from real-world
    experience'. *Archives of Disease in Childhood* 105: 784–90.

50. Jódar, L., LaForce, F., Ceccarini, C., Aguado, T. & Granoff, D. (2003).
    'Meningococcal conjugate vaccine for Africa: a model for development
    of new vaccines for the poorest countries'. *Lancet* 361: 1902–4.

51. Greenwood, B. (1999). 'Manson Lecture. Meningococcal meningitis in
    Africa'. *Transactions of the Royal Society of Tropical Medicine and
    Hygiene* 93: 341–53.

52. Lapeyssonnie, L. (1963). 'La méningite cérébrospinale en Afrique'.
    Bulletin of the World Health Organization 28: 1–114.

53. Halperin, S., Bettinger, J., Greenwood, B., Harrison, L., Jelfs, J.,
    Ladhani, S., McIntyre, P., Ramsay, M. & Sáfadi, M. (2012). 'The
    changing and dynamic epidemiology of meningococcal disease'. *Vaccine*
    30 (Suppl 2): B26–36.

54. Jódar, L., LaForce, F., Ceccarini, C., Aguado, T. & Granoff, D. (2003).
    'Meningococcal conjugate vaccine for Africa: a model for development
    of new vaccines for the poorest countries'. *Lancet* 361: 1902–4.

55. Harrison, L., Granoff, D. & Pollard, A. (2018). 'Meningococcal
    Capsular Group A, C, W, and Y Conjugate Vaccines' in *Plotkin's
    Vaccines, Seventh edition* (eds: S. A. Plotkin, W. A. Orenstein, P. A.

Offit & M. D. Edwards) pp619–43. Philadelphia, Elsevier, Inc.

56. Jódar, L., LaForce, F., Ceccarini, C., Aguado, T. & Granoff, D. (2003). 'Meningococcal conjugate vaccine for Africa: a model for development of new vaccines for the poorest countries'. *Lancet* 361: 1902–4.

57. Djingarey, M., Barry, R., Bonkoungou, M., Tiendrebeogo, S., Sebgo, R., Kandolo, D., Lingani, C., Preziosi, M. P., Zuber, P., Perea, W., Hugonnet, S., Dellepiane de Rey Tolve, N., Tevi-Benissan, C., Clark, T., Mayer, L., Novak, R., Messonier, N., Berlier, M., Toboe, D., Nshimirimana, D., Mihigo, R., Aguado, T., Diomandé, F., Kristiansen, P., Caugant, D. & Laforce, F. (2012). 'Effectively introducing a new meningococcal A conjugate vaccine in Africa: the Burkina Faso experience'. *Vaccine* 30 (Suppl 2): B40–5.

58. Kristiansen, P., Diomandé, F., Ba, A., Sanou, I., Ouédraogo, A.-S., Ouédraogo, R., Sangaré, L., Kandolo, D., Aké, F., Saga, I., Clark, T., Misegades, L., Martin, S., Thomas, J., Tiendrebeogo, S., Hassan-King, M., Djingarey, M., Messonnier, N., Préziosi, M., Laforce, F. & Caugant, D. (2013). 'Impact of the serogroup A meningococcal conjugate vaccine, MenAfriVac, on carriage and herd immunity'. *Clinical Infectious Diseases* 56: 354–63.

59. Kristiansen, P., Ba, A., Ouédraogo, A.-S., Sanou, I., Ouédraogo, R., Sangaré, L., Diomandé, F., Kandolo, D., Saga, I., Misegades, L., Clark, T., Préziosi M. P. & Caugant, D. (2014). 'Persistent low carriage of serogroup A *Neisseria meningitidis* two years after mass vaccination with the meningococcal conjugate vaccine, MenAfriVac'. *BMC Infectious Diseases* 14: 1–11.

60. Trotter, C., Lingani, C., Fernandez, K., Cooper, L., Bita, A., Tevi-Benissan, C., Ronveaux, O., Préziosi, M. & Stuart, J. (2017). 'Impact of MenAfriVac in nine countries of the African meningitis belt, 2010–15: an analysis of surveillance data'. *Lancet Infectious Diseases* 17: 867–72.

61. Exchange Rates UK (2021). 'British pound to US dollar spot exchange rates for 2010'. exchangerates.org.uk (accessed 03 April 2021).

62. Berman, G. (2012). *The cost of international military operations.* London, UK Parliament.

63. Trotter, C. (2021). Author interview. 25 March 2021.

64. Chen, W., Neuzil, K., Boyce, C., Pasetti, M., Reymann, M., Martellet, L., Hosken, N., LaForce, F., Dhere, R., Pisal, S., Chaudhari, A., Kulkarni, P., Borrow, R., Findlow, H., Brown, V., McDonough, M., Dally, L. & Alderson, M. (2018). 'Safety and immunogenicity of a pentavalent meningococcal conjugate vaccine containing serogroups A, C, Y, W and X in healthy adults: a phase 1, single-centre, double-blind, randomised, controlled study'. *Lancet Infectious Diseases* 18: 1088–96.

65. Ibid.

66. Heyderman, R. (2021). Author interview. 8 November 2021.

67. Michna, C. (2021). Author interview. 17 March 2021.

Chapter 10

1. Frierson, J. (2010). 'The yellow fever vaccine: a history'. *Yale Journal of Biology and Medicine* 83: 77–85.

2. Thomas, R., Lorenzetti, D. & Spragins, W. (2013). 'Mortality and morbidity among military personnel and civilians during the 1930s and World War II from transmission of hepatitis during yellow fever vaccination: systematic review'. *American Journal of Public Health* 103: e16–29.

3. Findlay, G. & MacCallum, F. O. (1937). 'Note on acute hepatitis and yellow fever immunization'. *Transactions of the Royal Society of Tropical Medicine and Hygiene* 31: 297–308.

4. Fox, J., Manso, C., Penna, H. & Pará, M. (1942). 'Observations on the occurrence of icterus in Brazil following vaccination against yellow fever'. *American Journal of Epidemiology* 36: 68–116.

5. Thomas, R., Lorenzetti, D. & Spragins, W. (2013). 'Mortality and morbidity among military personnel and civilians during the 1930s and World War II from transmission of hepatitis during yellow fever vaccination: systematic review'. *American Journal of Public Health* 103: e16–29.

6. Frierson, J. (2010). 'The yellow fever vaccine: a history'. *Yale Journal of Biology and Medicine* 83: 77–85.

7. Martin, N. (2003). 'The discovery of viral hepatitis: a military perspective'. *Journal of the Royal Army Medical Corps* 149: 121–4.

8. Findlay, G., Martin, N. & Mitchell, J. (1944). 'Hepatitis after yellow fever inoculation relation to infective hepatitis II. immunology and epidemiology'. *Lancet* 244: 365–70.

9. Grist, N. (1995). 'Frederick Ogden MacCallum'. *Bulletin of the Royal College of Pathologists* 90: 6–7.

10. Martin, N. (2003). 'The discovery of viral hepatitis: a military perspective'. *Journal of the Royal Army Medical Corps* 149: 121–4.

11. Neefe, J., Gellis, S. & Stokes Jr, J. (1946). 'Homologous serum hepatitis and infectious (epidemic) hepatitis; studies in volunteers bearing on immunological and other characteristics of the etiological agents'. *American Journal of Medicine* 1: 3–22.

12. MacCallum, F. (1947). 'Homologous serum hepatitis'. *Lancet* 6480: 691–2.

13. Blumberg, B., Alter, H. & Visnich, S. (1965). 'A "New" Antigen in Leukemia Sera'. *Journal of the American Medical Association* 191: 541–6.

14. Blumberg, B., Gerstley, B., Hungerford, D., London, W. & Sutnick, A. (1967). 'A serum antigen (Australia antigen) in Down's syndrome, leukemia, and hepatitis'. *Annals of Internal Medicine* 66: 924–31.

15. Okochi, K., Murakami, S., Ninomiya, K. & Kaneko, M. (1970). 'Australia Antigen, Transfusion and Hepatitis'. *Vox Sanguinis* 18: 289–300.

16. Seeger, C., Zoulim, F. & Mason, W. (2013). 'Hepadnaviruses' in *Fields Virology* (eds: D. M. Knipe & P. M. Howley) pp2185–221. Philadelphia, Wolters Kluwer Health/Lippincott Williams & Wilkins.

17. Norman, J., Beebe, G., Hoofnagle, J. & Seeff, L. (1993). 'Mortality follow-up of the 1942 epidemic of hepatitis B in the U.S. Army'. *Hepatology* 18: 790–7.

18. Senior, J., Sutnick, A., Goeser, E., London, W., Dahlke, M. & Blumberg, B. (1974). 'Reduction of post-transfusion hepatitis by exclusion of Australia antigen from donor blood in an urban public hospital'. *American Journal of Medical Science* 267: 171–7.

19. Beasley, R., Hwang, L. Y., Lin, C. C. & Chien, C. (1981). 'Hepatocellular carcinoma and hepatitis B virus. A prospective study of 22,707 men in Taiwan'. *Lancet* 2: 1129–33.

20. Dane, D., Cameron, C. & Briggs, M. (1970). 'Virus-like particles in serum of patients with Australia-antigen-associated hepatitis'. *Lancet* 1: 695–8.

21. Nobel Media (2009). 'Baruch S. Blumberg – Interview'. nobelprize.org (accessed 26 September 2020).

22. Hilleman, M., Buynak, E., Roehm, R., Tytell, A., Bertland, A. & Lampson, G. (1975). 'Purified and inactivated human hepatitis B vaccine: progress report'. *American Journal of Medical Science* 270: 401–4.

23. Nobel Media (2009). 'Baruch S. Blumberg – Interview'. nobelprize.org (accessed 26 September 2020).

24. Altman, L. (1982). 'Dr. Wolf Szmuness is dead at 63; an epidemiologist and researcher'. *New York Times,* 8 June 1982.

25. Szmuness, W., Stevens, C., Harley, E., Zang, E., Oleszko, W., William, D., Sadovsky, R., Morrison, J. & Kellner, A. (1980). 'Hepatitis B vaccine: demonstration of efficacy in a controlled clinical trial in a high-risk population in the United States'. *New England Journal of Medicine* 303: 833–41.

26. Offit, P. (2007). *Vaccinated: One Man's Quest to Defeat the World's Deadliest Diseases.* New York, HarperCollins.

27. Whittle, H., Inskip, H., Hall, A., Mendy, M., Downes, R. & Hoare, S. (1991). 'Vaccination against hepatitis B and protection against chronic viral carriage in The Gambia'. *Lancet* 337: 747–50.

28. Whittle, H., Jaffar, S., Wansbrough, M., Mendy, M., Dumpis, U., Collinson, A. & Hall, A. (2002). 'Observational study of vaccine efficacy 14 years after trial of hepatitis B vaccination in Gambian children'. *British Medical Journal* 325: 569.

29. McAleer, W., Buynak, E., Maigetter, R., Wampler, D., Miller, W. & Hilleman, M. (1984). 'Human hepatitis B vaccine from recombinant yeast'. *Nature* 307: 178–80.

30. Hall, A., Roberston, R., Crivelli, P., Lowe, Y., Inskip, H., Snow, S. & Whittle, H. (1993). 'Cost-effectiveness of hepatitis B vaccine in The

Gambia'. *Transactions of the Royal Society of Tropical Medicine and Hygiene* 87: 333–6.

31. Chiang C. J., Yang Y. W., You S. L., Lai, M. S. & Chen, C. J. (2013). 'Thirty-year outcomes of the national hepatitis B immunization program in Taiwan'. *Journal of the American Medical Association* 310: 974–6.

32. World Health Organization (2017). *Global Hepatitis Report 2017.* Geneva, World Health Organization.

33. World Health Organization (2017). 'Hepatitis B vaccines: WHO position paper – July 2017'. *Weekly Epidemiological Record* 92: 369–92.

34. Siddiqui, M., Gay, N., Edmunds, W. & Ramsay, M. (2011). 'Economic evaluation of infant and adolescent hepatitis B vaccination in the UK'. *Vaccine* 29: 466–75.

35. Yuen, M. F., Chen, D. S., Dusheiko, G., Janssen, H., Lau, D., Locarnini, S., Peters, M. & Lai, C. L. (2018). 'Hepatitis B virus infection'. *Nature Reviews Disease Primers* 4: 18035.

36. European Centre for Disease Prevention and Control (2016). *Epidemiological assessment of hepatitis B and C among migrants in the EU/EEA.* Stockholm, ECDC.

37. Joint Committee on Vaccination and Immunisation (2014). 'Minute of the meeting on 1 October 2014'. whatdotheyknow.com (accessed 27 September 2020).

38. Dhillon, S. 'DTPa-HBV-IPV/Hib Vaccine (Infanrix hexa™): A Review of its Use as Primary and Booster Vaccination'. *Drugs* 70: 1021–58.

39. Public Health England (2017). *Immunisation against infectious disease.* London, Public Health England.

40. Das, P. (2002). 'Baruch Blumberg – hepatitis B and beyond'. *Lancet Infectious Diseases* 2: 767–71.

41. Cox, A., El-Sayed, M., Kao, J. H., Lazarus, J., Lemoine, M., Lok, A. & Zoulim, F. (2020). 'Progress towards elimination goals for viral hepatitis'. *Nature Reviews Gastroenterology & Hepatology* 17: 533–42.

42. World Health Organization (2017). 'Hepatitis B vaccines: WHO position paper – July 2017'. *Weekly Epidemiological Record* 92: 369–92.

43. Fox Chase Cancer Center (2011). 'Nobelist Baruch S. Blumberg, MD, PhD, Dies at 85'. foxchase.org (accessed 28 September 2020).

Chapter 11

1. Prestwich, J. & Prestwich, M. (1980). 'John & Maggie Prestwich'. johnprestwich.co.uk (accessed 5 September 2020).

2. Leech, J. (1852). 'A Court for King Cholera'. *Punch, or the London Charivari*, 25 September 1852.

3. Nathanson, N. & Kew, O. (2010). 'From emergence to eradication: the epidemiology of poliomyelitis deconstructed'. *American Journal of Epidemiology* 172: 1213–29.

4. Pallansch, M., Oberste, M. & Whitton, J. (2013). 'Enteroviruses: Polioviruses, Coxsackieviruses, Echoviruses, and Newer Enteroviruses'

in *Fields Virology* (eds: D. M. Knipe & P. M. Howley) pp490–530. Philadelphia, Wolters Kluwer Health/Lippincott Williams & Wilkins.

5. Goldman, A., Schmalstieg, E., Freeman Jr, D., Goldman, D. & Schmalstieg Jr, F. (2003). 'What was the cause of Franklin Delano Roosevelt's paralytic illness?' *Journal of Medical Biography* 11: 232–40.
6. Allen, A. (2007). *Vaccine*. New York, WW Norton & Company, Inc.
7. Nathanson, N. & Kew, O. (2010). 'From emergence to eradication: the epidemiology of poliomyelitis deconstructed'. *American Journal of Epidemiology* 172: 1213–29.
8. Smallman-Raynor, M. & Cliff, A. (2013). 'The geographical spread of the 1947 poliomyelitis epidemic in England and Wales: spatial wave propagation of an enigmatic epidemiological event'. *Journal of Historical Geography* 40: 36–51.
9. Ibid.
10. Tyrell, D. (1987). 'John Franklin Enders, 10 February 1897 – 8 September 1985'. *Biographical Memoirs of Fellows of the Royal Society* 33: 211–13.
11. Enders, J., Weller, T. & Robbins, F. (1949). 'Cultivation of the Lansing Strain of Poliomyelitis Virus in Cultures of Various Human Embryonic Tissues'. *Science* 109: 85–7.
12. Tyrell, D. (1987). 'John Franklin Enders, 10 February 1897 – 8 September 1985'. *Biographical Memoirs of Fellows of the Royal Society* 33: 211–13.
13. Wilson, J. (1963). *Margin of Safety*. New York, Doubleday.
14. Frierson, J. (2010). 'The yellow fever vaccine: a history'. *Yale Journal of Biology and Medicine* 83: 77–85.
15. Watts, G. (2017). 'Julius Stuart Youngner'. *Lancet* 389: 2370.
16. Oshinsky, D. (2005). *Polio: an American story*. Oxford, Oxford University Press.
17. Wadman, M. (2017). *The Vaccine Race*. London, Transworld Publishers.
18. Trevelyan, B., Smallman-Raynor, M. & Cliff, A. (2005). 'The Spatial Dynamics of Poliomyelitis in the United States: From Epidemic Emergence to Vaccine-Induced Retreat, 1910–1971'. *Annals of the Association of American Geographers* 95: 269–93.
19. Millward, G. (2019). *Vaccinating Britain*. Manchester, Manchester University Press.
20. Sabin, A. (1985). 'Oral poliovirus vaccine: history of its development and use and current challenge to eliminate poliomyelitis from the world'. *Journal of Infectious Diseases* 151: 420–36.
21. Global Health Chronicles (2016). 'Sabin, Deborah'. globalhealthchronicles.org (accessed 5 September 2020).
22. Agol, V. & Drozdov, S. (1993). 'Russian contribution to OPV'. *Biologicals* 21: 321–5.
23. Kew, O. & Pallansch, M. (2018). 'Breaking the Last Chains of Poliovirus

Transmission: Progress and Challenges in Global Polio Eradication'.
Annual Review of Virology 5: 427–51.

24. Centers for Disease Control and Prevention (1997). 'Poliomyelitis
    Prevention in the United States: Introduction of A Sequential
    Vaccination Schedule of Inactivated Poliovirus Vaccine Followed by
    Oral Poliovirus Vaccine; Recommendations of the Advisory Committee
    on Immunization Practices (ACIP)'. *Morbidity and Mortality Weekly
    Report* 46: 1–25.

25. UK Health Security Agency (2019). 'Vaccination timeline table from
    1796 to present'. gov.uk (accessed 7 August 2022).

26. Nathanson, N. & Kew, O. (2010). 'From emergence to eradication: the
    epidemiology of poliomyelitis deconstructed'. *American Journal of
    Epidemiology* 172: 1213–29.

27. Nkowane, B., Wassilak, S., Orenstein, W., Bart, K., Schonberger,
    L., Hinman, A. & Kew, O. (1987). 'Vaccine-associated paralytic
    poliomyelitis. United States: 1973 through 1984'. *Journal of the
    American Medical Association* 257: 1335–40.

28. Nathanson, N. & Kew, O. (2010). 'From emergence to eradication: the
    epidemiology of poliomyelitis deconstructed'. *American Journal of
    Epidemiology* 172: 1213–29.

29. Cruz, R. (1984). 'Cuba: mass polio vaccination program, 1962–1982'.
    Reviews of Infectious Diseases 6 Suppl: S408–12.

30. Nathanson, N. & Kew, O. (2010). 'From emergence to eradication: the
    epidemiology of poliomyelitis deconstructed'. *American Journal of
    Epidemiology* 172: 1213–29.

31. Kew, O. & Pallansch, M. (2018). 'Breaking the Last Chains of Poliovirus
    Transmission: Progress and Challenges in Global Polio Eradication'.
    Annual Review of Virology 5: 427–51.

32. Shah, S. (2011). 'CIA organised fake vaccination drive to get Osama bin
    Laden's family DNA'. *Guardian*, 11 July 2011.

33. Gostin, L. (2014). 'Global polio eradication: espionage, disinformation,
    and the politics of vaccination'. *Milbank Quarterly* 92: 413–17.

34. Racaniello, V. (2013). 'Picornaviridae: The viruses and their replication'
    in *Fields Virology* (eds: D. M. Knipe & P. M. Howley) pp454–89.
    Philadelphia, Wolters Kluwer Health/Lippincott Williams & Wilkins.

35. Public Health England (2014). 'Vaccine coverage and COVER ›
    Epidemiological Data › Completed Primary Courses at Two Years of
    Age: England and Wales, 1966–1977, England only 1978 onwards'.
    webarchive.nationalarchives.gov.uk (accessed 29 May 2022).

36. NHS (2021). 'Childhood Vaccination Coverage Statistics – 2020–21'.
    digital.nhs.uk (accessed 29 May 2022).

37. UK Health Security Agency (2021). 'Notifiable diseases: historic annual
    totals. Annual total figures for cases of notifiable infectious diseases
    from 1912 to 2020'. gov.uk (accessed 29 May 2022).

Chapter 12

1. World Health Organization (2021). *World health statistics 2021: monitoring health for the SDGs, sustainable development goals.* Geneva, WHO.

2. Liu, L., Oza, S., Hogan, D., Perin, J., Rudan, I., Lawn, J., Cousens, S., Mathers, C. & Black, R. (2015). 'Global, regional, and national causes of child mortality in 2000–13, with projections to inform post-2015 priorities: an updated systematic analysis'. *Lancet* 385: 430–40.

3. Crawford, S., Ramani, S., Tate, J., Parashar, U., Svensson, L., Hagbom, M., Franco, M., Greenberg, H., O'Ryan, M., Kang, G., Desselberger, U. & Estes, M. (2017). 'Rotavirus infection'. *Nature Reviews Disease Primers* 3: e17083.

4. Velázquez, F., Matson, D., Calva, J., Guerrero, L., Morrow, A., Carter-Campbell, S., Glass, R., Estes, M., Pickering, L. & Ruiz-Palacios, G. (1996). 'Rotavirus infection in infants as protection against subsequent infections'. *New England Journal of Medicine* 335: 1022–8.

5. Velázquez, F., Calva, J., Lourdes Guerrero, M., Mass, D., Glass, R., Pickering, L. & Ruiz-Palacios, G. (1993). 'Cohort study of rotavirus serotype patterns in symptomatic and asymptomatic infections in Mexican children'. *Pediatric Infectious Disease Journal* 12: 54–61.

6. Ray, P., Kelkar, S., Walimbe, A., Biniwale, V. & Mehendale, S. (2007). 'Rotavirus immunoglobulin levels among Indian mothers of two socio-economic groups and occurrence of rotavirus infections among their infants up to six months'. *Journal of Medical Virology* 79: 341–9.

7. Krawczyk, A., Lewis, M., Venkatesh, B. & Nair, S. (2016). 'Effect of Exclusive Breastfeeding on Rotavirus Infection among Children'. *Indian Journal of Pediatrics* 83: 220–5.

8. Velázquez, F., Matson, D., Calva, J., Guerrero, L., Morrow, A., Carter-Campbell, S., Glass, R., Estes, M., Pickering, L. & Ruiz-Palacios, G. (1996). 'Rotavirus infection in infants as protection against subsequent infections'. *New England Journal of Medicine* 335: 1022–8.

9. Ansari, S., Sattar, S., Springthorpe, V., Wells, G. & Tostowaryk, W. (1988). 'Rotavirus survival on human hands and transfer of infectious virus to animate and nonporous inanimate surfaces'. *Journal of Clinical Microbiology* 26: 1513–18.

10. Estes, M. & Greenberg, H. (2013). 'Rotaviruses' in *Fields Virology* (eds: D. M. Knipe & P. M. Howley) pp1347–95. Philadelphia, Wolters Kluwer Health/Lippincott Williams & Wilkins.

11. Anderson, E. & Weber, S. (2004). 'Rotavirus infection in adults'. *Lancet Infectious Diseases* 4: 91–9.

12. Crawford, S., Ramani, S., Tate, J., Parashar, U., Svensson, L., Hagbom, M., Franco, M., Greenberg, H., O'Ryan, M., Kang, G., Desselberger, U. & Estes, M. (2017). 'Rotavirus infection'. *Nature Reviews Disease Primers* 3: e17083.

13. De Marco, G., Bracale, I., Buccigrossi, V., Bruzzese, E., Canani, R.,

Polito, G., Ruggeri, F. & Guarino, A. (2009). 'Rotavirus induces a biphasic enterotoxic and cytotoxic response in human-derived intestinal enterocytes, which is inhibited by human immunoglobulins'. *Journal of Infectious Diseases* 200: 813–19.

14. Hagbom, M., Istrate, C., Engblom, D., Karlsson, T., Rodriguez-Diaz, J., Buesa, J., Taylor, J., Loitto, V. M., Magnusson, K. E., Ahlman, H., Lundgren, O. & Svensson, L. (2011). 'Rotavirus stimulates release of serotonin (5-HT) from human enterochromaffin cells and activates brain structures involved in nausea and vomiting'. *PLoS Pathogens* 7: e1002115.

15. Greenberg, H. & Estes, M. (2009). 'Rotaviruses: from pathogenesis to vaccination'. *Gastroenterology* 136: 1939–51.

16. Parashar, U., Hummelman, E., Bresee, J., Miller, M. & Glass, R. (2003). 'Global illness and deaths caused by rotavirus disease in children'. *Emerging Infectious Diseases* 9: 565–72.

17. Rodriguez, W., Kim, H., Brandt, C., Schwartz, R., Gardner, M., Jeffries, B., Parrott, R., Kaslow, R., Smith, J. & Kapikian, A. (1987). 'Longitudinal study of rotavirus infection and gastroenteritis in families served by a pediatric medical practice: clinical and epidemiologic observations'. *Pediatric Infectious Disease Journal* 6: 170–6.

18. Robilotti, E., Deresinski, S. & Pinsky, B. (2015). 'Norovirus'. *Clinical Microbiology Reviews* 28: 134–4.

19. Velázquez, F., Matson, D., Calva, J., Guerrero, L., Morrow, A., Carter-Campbell, S., Glass, R., Estes, M., Pickering, L. & Ruiz-Palacios, G. (1996). 'Rotavirus infection in infants as protection against subsequent infections'. *New England Journal of Medicine* 335: 1022–8.

20. Kapikian, A., Wyatt, R., Dolin, R., Thornhill, T., Kalica, A. & Chanock, R. (1972). 'Visualization by immune electron microscopy of a 27-nm particle associated with acute infectious nonbacterial gastroenteritis'. *Journal of Virology* 10: 1075–81.

21. Bishop, R., Davidson, G., Holmes, I. & Ruck, B. (1973). 'Virus particles in epithelial cells of duodenal mucosa from children with acute non-bacterial gastroenteritis'. *Lancet* 2: 1281–3.

22. Flewett, T., Bryden, A., Davies, H., Woode, G., Bridger, J. & Derrick, J. (1974). 'Relation between viruses from acute gastroenteritis of children and newborn calves'. *Lancet* 2: 61–3.

23. Marsicovetere, P., Ivatury, S., White, B. & Holubar, S. (2017). 'Intestinal Intussusception: Etiology, Diagnosis, and Treatment'. *Clinics in Colon and Rectal Surgery* 30: 30–9.

24. Konno, T., Suzuki, H., Kutsuzawa, T., Imai, A., Katsushima, N., Sakamoto, M., Kitaoka, S., Tsuboi, R. & Adachi, M. (1978). 'Human rotavirus infection in infants and young children with intussusception'. *Journal of Medical Virology* 2: 265–9.

25. Kapikian, A., Hoshino, Y., Chanock, R. & Pérez-Schael, I. (1996). 'Efficacy of a quadrivalent rhesus rotavirus-based human rotavirus

vaccine aimed at preventing severe rotavirus diarrhea in infants and young children'. *Journal of Infectious Diseases* 174 Suppl 1: S65–72.

26. Centers for Disease Control and Prevention (1999). 'Rotavirus vaccine for the prevention of rotavirus gastroenteritis among children. Recommendations of the Advisory Committee on Immunization Practices (ACIP)'. *Morbidity and Mortality Weekly Report* 48: 1–20.

27. Rennels, M., Parashar, U., Holman, R., Le, C., Chang, H. G. & Glass, R. (1998). 'Lack of an apparent association between intussusception and wild or vaccine rotavirus infection'. *Pediatric Infectious Disease Journal* 17: 924–5.

28. Ibid.

29. Centers for Disease Control and Prevention (1999). 'Intussusception among recipients of rotavirus vaccine – United States, 1998–1999'. *Morbidity and Mortality Weekly Report* 48: 577–81.

30. Centers for Disease Control and Prevention (1999). 'Withdrawal of rotavirus vaccine recommendation'. *Morbidity and Mortality Weekly Report* 48: 1007.

31. Kramarz, P., France, E., DeStefano, F., Black, S., Shinefield, H., Ward, J., Chang, E., Chen, R., Shatin, D., Hill, J., Lieu, T. & Ogren, J. (2001). 'Population-based study of rotavirus vaccination and intussusception'. *Pediatric Infectious Disease Journal* 20: 410–16.

32. Murphy, T., Gargiullo, P., Massoudi, M., Nelson, D., Jumaan, A., Okoro, C., Zanardi, L., Setia, S., Fair, E., LeBaron, C., Wharton, M. & Livengood, J. (2001). 'Intussusception among infants given an oral rotavirus vaccine'. *New England Journal of Medicine* 344: 564–72.

33. Marsicovetere, P., Ivatury, S., White, B. & Holubar, S. (2017). 'Intestinal Intussusception: Etiology, Diagnosis, and Treatment'. *Clinics in Colon and Rectal Surgery* 30: 30–9.

34. Weijer, C. (2000). 'The future of research into rotavirus vaccine'. *British Medical Journal* 321: 525–6.

35. Rennels, M. (2000). 'The rotavirus vaccine story: a clinical investigator's view'. *Pediatrics* 106: 123–5.

36. Vesikari, T., Matson, D., Dennehy, P., Van Damme, P., Santosham, M., Rodriguez, Z., Dallas, M., Heyse, J., Goveia, M., Black, S., Shinefield, H., Christie, C., Ylitalo, S., Itzler, R., Coia, M., Onorato, M., Adeyi, B., Marshall, G., Gothefors, L., Campens, D., Karvonen, A., Watt, J., O'Brien, K., DiNubile, M., Clark, H., Boslego, J., Offit, P. & Heaton, P. (2006). 'Safety and efficacy of a pentavalent human-bovine (WC3) reassortant rotavirus vaccine'. *New England Journal of Medicine* 354: 23–33.

37. Heaton, P. & Ciarlet, M. (2007). 'Vaccines: the pentavalent rotavirus vaccine: discovery to licensure and beyond'. *Clinical Infectious Diseases* 45: 1618–24.

38. Ward, R. & Bernstein, D. (2009). 'Rotarix: a rotavirus vaccine for the world'. *Clinical Infectious Diseases* 48: 222–8.

39. Bernstein, D., Smith, V., Sherwood, J., Schiff, G., Sander, D., DeFeudis, D., Spriggs, D. & Ward, R. (1998). 'Safety and immunogenicity of live, attenuated human rotavirus vaccine 89-12'. *Vaccine* 16: 381–7.

40. Bernstein, D., Sack, D., Reisinger, K., Rothstein, E. & Ward, R. (2002). 'Second-year follow-up evaluation of live, attenuated human rotavirus vaccine 89-12 in healthy infants'. *Journal of Infectious Diseases* 186: 1487–9.

41. Ruiz-Palacios, G., Pérez-Schael, I., Velàzquez, F., Abate, H., Breuer, T., Clemens, S., Cheuvart, B., Espinoza, F., Gillard, P., Innis, B., Cervantes, Y., Linhares, A., López, P., Macías-Parra, M., Ortega-Barría, E., Richardson, V., Rivera-Medina, D., Rivera, L., Salinas, B., Pavía-Ruz, N., Salmerón, J., Rüttimann, R., Tinoco, J., Rubio, P., Nuñez, E., Guerrero, M., Yarzábal, J., Damaso, S., Tornieporth, N., Sáez-Llorens X, Vergara, R., Vesikari, T., Bouckenooghe, A., Clemens, R., De Vos, B. & O'Ryan, M. (2006). 'Safety and efficacy of an attenuated vaccine against severe rotavirus gastroenteritis'. *New England Journal of Medicine* 354: 11–22.

42. Marlow, R. & Finn, A. (2013). 'Introduction of immunisation against rotavirus in the UK'. *Prescriber* 24: 6–8.

43. McGeoch, L., Finn, A. & Marlow, R. (2020). 'Impact of rotavirus vaccination on intussusception hospital admissions in England'. *Vaccine* 38: 5618–26.

44. Tate, J., Burton, A., Boschi-Pinto, C. & Parashar, U. (2016). 'Global, Regional, and National Estimates of Rotavirus Mortality in Children <5 Years of Age, 2000–2013'. *Clinical Infectious Diseases* 62 Suppl 2: S96–105.

45. Ibid.

Chapter 13

1. Dahl, R. (1986). 'Measles. A dangerous illness'. roalddahl.com (acccessed 12 April 2020).

2. Castro, P. & Benet, L. (1997). 'The mourning after'. *People*, 31 March 1997.

3. de Vries, R., Mesman, A., Geijtenbeek, T., Duprex, W. & de Swart, R. (2012). 'The pathogenesis of measles'. *Current Opinion in Virology* 2: 248–55.

4. Rota, P., Moss, W., Takeda, M., de Swart, R., Thompson, K. & Goodson, J. (2019). 'Measles'. *Nature Reviews Disease Primers* 2: 16049.

5. Fine, P., Eames, K. & Heymann, D. (2011). '"Herd immunity": a rough guide'. *Clinical Infectious Diseases* 52: 911–16.

6. Chen, R., Goldbaum, G., Wassilak, S., Markowitz, L. & Orenstein, W. (1989). 'An explosive point-source measles outbreak in a highly vaccinated population. Modes of transmission and risk factors for disease'. *American Journal of Epidemiology* 129: 173–82.

7. Ehresmann, K., Hedberg, C., Grimm, M., Norton, C., MacDonald, K. & Osterholm, M. (1995). 'An outbreak of measles at an international sporting event with airborne transmission in a domed stadium'. *Journal of Infectious Diseases* 171: 679–83.

8. Patel, M., Dumolard, L., Nedelec, Y., Sodha, S., Steulet, C., Gacic-Dobo, M., Kretsinger, K., McFarland, J., Rota, P. & Goodson, J. (2019). 'Progress Toward Regional Measles Elimination – Worldwide, 2000–2018'. *MMWR Morbidity and Mortality Weekly Report* 68: 1105–11.

9. Rota, P., Moss, W., Takeda, M., de Swart, R., Thompson, K. & Goodson, J. (2019). 'Measles'. *Nature Reviews Disease Primers* 2: 16049.

10. Beckford, A., Kaschula, R. & Stephen, C. (1985). 'Factors associated with fatal cases of measles. A retrospective autopsy study'. *South African Medical Journal* 68: 858–63.

11. Mina, M., Kula, T., Leng, Y., Li, M., de Vries, R., Knip, M., Siljander, H., Rewers, M., Choy, D., Wilson, M., Larman, H., Nelson, A., Griffin, D., de Swart, R. & Elledge, S. (2019). 'Measles virus infection diminishes preexisting antibodies that offer protection from other pathogens'. *Science* 366: 599–606.

12. Brockell, G. (2019). 'Although first measles vaccine was named after him he didn't vaccinate his son'. *Washington Post*, 16 April 2019.

13. Enders, J. & Peebles, T. (1954). 'Propagation in tissue cultures of cytopathogenic agents from patients with measles'. *Proceedings of the Society of Experimental Biology and Medicine* 86: 277–86.

14. Ibid.

15. Katz, S., Kempe, C., Black, F., Lepow, M., Krugman, S., Haggerty, R. & Enders, J. (1960). 'Studies on an attenuated measles-virus vaccine. VIII. General summary and evaluation of the results of vaccination'. *American Journal of Disease in Childhood* 100: 942–6.

16. Hendriks, J. & Blume, S. (2013). 'Measles vaccination before the measles-mumps-rubella vaccine'. *American Journal of Public Health* 103: 1393–1401.

17. Rota, P., Moss, W., Takeda, M., de Swart, R., Thompson, K. & Goodson, J. (2019). 'Measles'. *Nature Reviews Disease Primers* 2: 16049.

18. Higgins, J., Soares-Weiser, K., López-López, J., Kakourou, A., Chaplin, K., Christensen, H., Martin, N., Sterne, J. & Reingold, A. (2016). 'Association of BCG, DTP, and measles containing vaccines with childhood mortality: systematic review'. *British Medical Journal* 355: i5170.

19. Brockell, G. (2019). 'Although first measles vaccine was named after him he didn't vaccinate his son'. *Washington Post*, 16 April 2019.

20. Albrecht, P., Ennis, F., Saltzman, E. & Krugman, S. (1977). 'Persistence of maternal antibody in infants beyond 12 months: mechanism of measles vaccine failure'. *Journal of Pediatrics* 91: 715–18.

21. Miller, D. (1964). 'Frequency of Complications of Measles, 1963. Report on a National Inquiry by the Public Health Laboratory Service in Collaboration with the Society of Medical Officers of Health'. *British Medical Journal* 2: 75–8.

22. Janaszek, W., Gay, N. & Gut, W. (2003). 'Measles vaccine efficacy during an epidemic in 1998 in the highly vaccinated population of Poland'. *Vaccine* 21: 473–8.

23. Rota, P., Moss, W., Takeda, M., de Swart, R., Thompson, K. & Goodson, J. (2019). 'Measles'. *Nature Reviews Disease Primers* 2: 16049.

24. Public Health England (2014). 'Vaccine coverage and COVER › Epidemiological Data › Completed Primary Courses at Two Years of Age: England and Wales, 1966–1977, England only 1978 onwards'. webarchive.nationalarchives.gov.uk (accessed 29 May 2022).

25. UK Health Security Agency (2021). 'Notifiable diseases: historic annual totals. Annual total figures for cases of notifiable infectious diseases from 1912 to 2020'. gov.uk (accessed 29 May 2022).

26. Patel, M., Dumolard, L., Nedelec, Y., Sodha, S., Steulet, C., Gacic-Dobo, M., Kretsinger, K., McFarland, J., Rota, P. & Goodson, J. (2019). 'Progress Toward Regional Measles Elimination – Worldwide, 2000–2018'. *MMWR Morbidity and Mortality Weekly Report* 68: 1105–11.

27. Ibid.

28. Public Health England (2014). 'Vaccine coverage and COVER › Epidemiological Data › Completed Primary Courses at Two Years of Age: England and Wales, 1966–1977, England only 1978 onwards'. webarchive.nationalarchives.gov.uk (accessed 29 May 2022).

29. NHS (2021). 'Childhood Vaccination Coverage Statistics – 2020–21'. digital.nhs.uk (accessed 29 May 2022).

30. UK Health Security Agency (2021). 'Notifiable diseases: historic annual totals. Annual total figures for cases of notifiable infectious diseases from 1912 to 2020'. gov.uk (accessed 29 May 2022).

Chapter 14

1. Rubin, S., Sauder, C. & Carbone, K. (2013). 'Mumps virus' in *Fields Virology* (eds: D. M. Knipe & P. M. Howley) pp1024–41. Philadelphia, Wolters Kluwer Health/Lippincott Williams & Wilkins.

2. Biggerstaff, M., Cauchemez, S., Reed, C., Gambhir, M. & Finelli, L. (2014). 'Estimates of the reproduction number for seasonal, pandemic, and zoonotic influenza: a systematic review of the literature'. *BMC Infectious Diseases* 14: 480.

3. Edmunds, W., Gay, N., Kretzschmar, M., Pebody, R. & Wachmann, H. (2000). 'The pre-vaccination epidemiology of measles, mumps and rubella in Europe: implications for modelling studies'. *Epidemiology & Infection* 125: 635–50.

4. Rubin, S., Sauder, C. & Carbone, K. (2013). 'Mumps virus' in *Fields Virology* (eds: D. M. Knipe & P. M. Howley) pp1024–41. Philadelphia, Wolters Kluwer Health/Lippincott Williams & Wilkins.

5. Hamilton, R. (1790). 'An Account of a Distemper, by the Common People in England Vulgarly Called the Mumps'. *London Medical Journal* 11: 190–211.

6. Hviid, A., Rubin, S. & Muhlemann, K. (2008). 'Mumps'. *Lancet* 371: 932–44.

7. Rubin, S., Eckhaus, M., Rennick, L., Bamford, C. & Duprex, W. (2015). 'Molecular biology, pathogenesis and pathology of mumps virus'. *Journal of Pathology* 235: 242–52.

8. Ibid.

9. Johnson, C. & Goodpasture, E. (1935). 'An Investigation of the Etiology of Mumps'. *Journal of Experimental Medicine* 59: 1–19.

10. Woodruff, A. & Goodpasture, E. (1931). 'The Susceptibility of the Chorio-Allantoic Membrane of Chick Embryos to Infection with the Fowl-Pox Virus'. *American Journal of Pathology* 7: 209–22.

11. Goodpasture, E., Woodruff, A. & Buddingh, G. (1931). 'The Cultivation of Vaccine and Other Viruses in the Chorioallantoic Membrane of Chick Embryos'. *Science* 74: 371–2.

12. Enders, J. (1946). 'Mumps: techniques of laboratory diagnosis, tests for susceptibility, and experiments on specific prophylaxis'. *Journal of Pediatrics* 29: 129–42.

13. Conniff, R. (2013). 'A Forgotten Pioneer of Vaccines'. *New York Times*, 6 May 2013.

14. College of Physicians of Philadelphia (2020). 'Mumps: Jeryl Lynn Story'. historyofvaccines.org (accessed 11 October 2020).

15. Stokes Jr, J., Weibel, R., Buynak, E. & Hilleman, M. (1967). 'Live attenuated mumps virus vaccine. II. Early clinical studies'. *Pediatrics* 39: 363–71.

16. Collins, H. (1999). 'The Man Who Saved Your Life – Maurice R. Hilleman – Developer of Vaccines for Mumps and Pandemic Flu'. *Philadelphia Inquirer*, 30 August 1999.

17. Buynak, E. & Hilleman, M. (1966). 'Live attenuated mumps virus vaccine. 1. Vaccine development'. *Proceedings of the Society for Experimental Biology and Medicine* 123: 768–75.

18. Hilleman, M., Weibel, R., Buynak, E., Stokes Jr, J. & Whitman Jr, J. (1967). 'Live attenuated mumps-virus vaccine. IV. Protective efficacy as measured in a field evaluation'. *New England Journal of Medicine* 276: 252–8.

19. Ibid.

20. SI-BONE (2021). 'Jeryl Lynn Hilleman. Director'. investory.si-bone.com (accessed 9 December 2021).

21. Conniff, R. (2013). 'A Forgotten Pioneer of Vaccines'. *New York Times*, 6 May 2013.

22. Hilleman, M. (1992). 'Past, present, and future of measles, mumps, and rubella virus vaccines'. *Pediatrics* 90: 149–53.

23. Joint Committee on Vaccination and Immunisation (1987). 'Minutes of the meeting held on 1 May 1987'. webarchive.nationalarchives.gov.uk (accessed 9 October 2020).

24. Balraj, V. & Miller, E. (1995). 'Complications of Mumps Vaccines'. *Reviews in Medical Microbiology* 5: 219–27.

25. Fujinaga, T., Motegi, Y., Tamura, H. & Kuroume, T. (1991). 'A prefecture-wide survey of mumps meningitis associated with measles, mumps and rubella vaccine'. *Pediatric Infectious Disease Journal* 10: 204–9.

26. Miller, E., Andrews, N., Stowe, J., Grant, A., Waight, P. & Taylor, B. (2007). 'Risks of convulsion and aseptic meningitis following measles-mumps-rubella vaccination in the United Kingdom'. *American Journal of Epidemiology* 165: 704–9.

27. Hviid, A., Rubin, S. & Muhlemann, K. (2008). 'Mumps'. *Lancet* 371: 932–44.

28. Balraj, V. & Miller, E. (1995). 'Complications of Mumps Vaccines'. *Reviews in Medical Microbiology* 5: 219–27.

29. Di Pietrantonj, C., Rivetti, A., Marchione, P., Debalini, M. & Demicheli, V. (2020). 'Vaccines for measles, mumps, rubella, and varicella in children'. *Cochrane Database of Systematic Reviews* 4: CD004407.

30. Miller, E., Andrews, N., Stowe, J., Grant, A., Waight, P. & Taylor, B. (2007). 'Risks of convulsion and aseptic meningitis following measles-mumps-rubella vaccination in the United Kingdom'. *American Journal of Epidemiology* 165: 704–9.

31. Hamilton, R. (1790). 'An Account of a Distemper, by the Common People in England Vulgarly Called the Mumps'. *London Medical Journal* 11: 190–211.

32. Gordon, J. & Kilham, L. (1949). 'Ten years in the epidemiology of mumps'. *American Journal of the Medical Sciences* 218: 338–59.

33. Public Health England (2020). 'Mumps outbreaks across England'. gov. uk (accessed 9 October 2020).

34. Waugh, C., Willocks, L., Templeton, K. & Stevenson, J. (2020). 'Recurrent outbreaks of mumps in Lothian and the impact of waning immunity'. *Epidemiology & Infection* 148: 1–5.

35. Barskey, A., Schulte, C., Rosen, J., Handschur, E., Rausch-Phung, E., Doll, M., Cummings, K., Alleyne, E., High, P., Lawler, J., Apostolou, A., Blog, D., Zimmerman, C., Montana, B., Harpaz, R., Hickman, C., Rota, P., Rota, J., Bellini, W. & Gallagher, K. (2012). 'Mumps outbreak in Orthodox Jewish communities in the United States'. *New England Journal of Medicine* 367: 1704–13.

36. Sane, J., Gouma, S., Koopmans, M., de Melker, H., Swaan, C., van Binnendijk, R. & Hahne, S. (2014). 'Epidemic of mumps among

vaccinated persons, The Netherlands, 2009–2012'. *Emerging Infectious Diseases* 20: 643–8.

Chapter 15

1. Lancaster, P. (1996). 'Gregg, Sir Norman McAlister (1892–1966)'. adb. anu.edu.au (accessed 23 October 2020).
2. Gregg, N. (1941). 'Congenital cataract following German measles in the mother'. *Transactions of the Ophthalmological Society of Australia* 3: 35–46.
3. Hobman, T. (2013). 'Rubella virus' in *Fields Virology* (eds: D. M. Knipe & P. M. Howley) pp688–708. Philadelphia, Wolters Kluwer Health/ Lippincott Williams & Wilkins.
4. Ibid.
5. Ibid.
6. Veale, H. (1866). 'History of an Epidemic of Rötheln, with Observations on Its Pathology'. *Edinburgh Medical Journal* 12: 404–14.
7. Hobman, T. (2013). 'Rubella virus' in *Fields Virology* (eds: D. M. Knipe & P. M. Howley) pp688–708. Philadelphia, Wolters Kluwer Health/ Lippincott Williams & Wilkins.
8. Ibid.
9. Liang, R. & Rentmeester, C. (1965). 'The Agony of Mothers'. *Life*, 4 June 1965.
10. Hobman, T. (2013). 'Rubella virus' in *Fields Virology* (eds: D. M. Knipe & P. M. Howley) pp688–708. Philadelphia, Wolters Kluwer Health/ Lippincott Williams & Wilkins.
11. Liang, R. & Rentmeester, C. (1965). 'The Agony of Mothers'. *Life*, 4 June 1965.
12. National Communicable Disease Center (1969). 'Rubella Surveillance no. 1, 1969'. stacks.cdc.gov.
13. Cooper, L. (1985). 'The history and medical consequences of rubella'. *Reviews of Infectious Diseases* 7 Suppl 1: S2–10.
14. Chess, S., Fernandez, P. & Korn, S. (1978). 'Behavioral consequences of congenital rubella'. *Journal of Pediatrics* 93: 699–703.
15. Amaral, D. (2017). 'Examining the Causes of Autism'. *Cerebrum* 2017: 1–17.
16. Plotkin, S. (2002). 'The late sequelae of *Arrowsmith*'. *Pediatric Infectious Disease Journal* 21: 807–9.
17. Plotkin, S. (2021). Author interview. 23 August 2021.
18. Parkman, P., Buescher, E. & Artenstein, M. (1962). 'Recovery of rubella virus from army recruits'. *Proceedings of the Society for Experimental Biology and Medicine* 111: 225–30.
19. Wadman, M. (2017). *The Vaccine Race*. London, Transworld Publishers.
20. Hayflick, L. (1965). 'The Limited in Vitro Lifetime of Human Diploid Cell Strains'. *Experimental Cell Research* 37: 614–36.

21. Plotkin, S., Cornfeld, D. & Ingalls, T. (1965). 'Studies of immunization with living rubella virus. Trials in children with a strain cultured from an aborted fetus'. *American Journal of Diseases of Children* 110: 381–9.

22. Plotkin, S., Farquhar, J., Katz, M. & Ingalls, T. (1967). 'A new attenuated rubella virus grown in human fibroblasts: evidence for reduced nasopharyngeal excretion'. *American Journal of Epidemiology* 86: 468–77.

23. Buynak, E., Hilleman, M., Weibel, R. & Stokes Jr, J. (1968). 'Live attenuated rubella virus vaccines prepared in duck embryo cell culture. I. Development and clinical testing'. *Journal of the American Medical Association* 204: 195–200.

24. Plotkin, S., Farquhar, J., Katz, M. & Hertz, C. (1969). 'Further studies of an attenuated rubella strain grown in WI-38 cells'. *American Journal of Epidemiology* 89: 232–8.

25. Weibel, R., Stokes Jr, J., Buynak, E., Whitman Jr, J., Leagus, M. & Hilleman, M. (1968). 'Live attenuated rubella virus vaccines prepared in duck embryo cell culture. II. Clinical tests in families and in an institution'. *Journal of the American Medical Association* 205: 554–8.

26. Beasley, R., Detels, R., Kim, K., Gale, J., Lin T. L. & Grayston, J. (1969). 'Prevention of rubella during an epidemic on Taiwan. HPV-77 and RA 27-3 rubella vaccines administered subcutaneously and intranasally HPV-77 vaccine mixed with mumps and-or measles vaccines'. *American Journal of Diseases of Children* 118: 301–6.

27. Plotkin, S. (2021). Author interview. 23 August 2021.

28. Wadman, M. (2017). *The Vaccine Race*. London, Transworld Publishers.

29. Hilleman, M. (1992). 'Past, present, and future of measles, mumps, and rubella virus vaccines'. *Pediatrics* 90: 149–53.

30. Buynak, E., Weibel, R., Whitman Jr, J., Stokes Jr, J. & Hilleman, M. (1969). 'Combined live measles, mumps, and rubella virus vaccines'. *Journal of the American Medical Association* 207: 2259–62.

31. Stokes Jr, J., Weibel, R., Villarejos, V., Arguedas, J., Buynak, E. & Hilleman, M. (1971). 'Trivalent combined measles-mumps-rubella vaccine. Findings in clinical-laboratory studies'. *Journal of the American Medical Association* 218: 57–61.

32. Plotkin, S., Farquhar, J. & Ogra, P. (1973). 'Immunologic properties of RA27-3 rubella virus vaccine. A comparison with strains presently licensed in the United States'. *Journal of the American Medical Association* 225: 585–90.

33. Horstmann, D., Schluederberg, A., Emmons, J., Evans, B., Randolph, M. & Andiman, W. (1985). 'Persistence of vaccine-induced immune responses to rubella: comparison with natural infection'. *Reviews of Infectious Diseases* 7 Suppl 1: S80–5.

34. Wadman, M. (2017). *The Vaccine Race*. London, Transworld Publishers.

35. Weibel, R., Stokes Jr, J., Buynak, E., Whitman Jr, J., Leagus, M. & Hilleman, M. (1968). 'Live attenuated rubella virus vaccines prepared in duck embryo cell culture. II. Clinical tests in families and in an institution'. *Journal of the American Medical Association* 205: 554–8.

36. Dudgeon, J. (1985). 'Selective immunization: protection of the individual'. *Reviews of Infectious Diseases* 7 Suppl 1: S185–90.

37. Miller, E. (1991). 'Rubella in the United Kingdom'. *Epidemiology and Infection* 107: 31–42.

38. Ibid.

39. Centers for Disease Control and Prevention (2005). 'Achievements in Public Health: Elimination of Rubella and Congenital Rubella Syndrome – United States, 1969–2004'. *Morbidity and Mortality Weekly Report* 54: 279–82.

40. Noah, N. & Fowle, S. (1988). 'Immunity to rubella in women of childbearing age in the United Kingdom'. *British Medical Journal* 297: 1301–4.

41. Hobman, T. (2013). 'Rubella virus' in *Fields Virology* (eds: D. M. Knipe & P. M. Howley) pp688–708. Philadelphia, Wolters Kluwer Health/ Lippincott Williams & Wilkins.

42. Joint Committee on Vaccination and Immunisation (1987). 'Minutes of the meeting held on 1 May 1987'. webarchive.nationalarchives.gov.uk (accessed 9 October 2020).

43. Hobman, T. (2013). 'Rubella virus' in *Fields Virology* (eds: D. M. Knipe & P. M. Howley) pp688–708. Philadelphia, Wolters Kluwer Health/ Lippincott Williams & Wilkins.

44. Bukasa, A., Campbell, H., Brown, K., Bedford, H., Ramsay, M., Amirthalingam, G. & Tookey, P. (2018). 'Rubella infection in pregnancy and congenital rubella in United Kingdom, 2003 to 2016'. *EuroSurveillance* 23: 1–8.

45. Public Health England (2014). 'Vaccine coverage and COVER › Epidemiological Data › Completed Primary Courses at Two Years of Age: England and Wales, 1966–1977, England only 1978 onwards'. webarchive.nationalarchives.gov.uk (accessed 29 May 2022).

46. NHS (2021). 'Childhood Vaccination Coverage Statistics – 2020–21'. digital.nhs.uk (accessed 29 May 2022).

47. UK Health Security Agency (2021). 'Notifiable diseases: historic annual totals. Annual total figures for cases of notifiable infectious diseases from 1912 to 2020'. gov.uk (accessed 29 May 2022).

Chapter 16

1. Scotto, J. & Bailar III, J. (1969). 'Rigoni-Stern and medical statistics. A nineteenth-century approach to cancer research'. *Journal of the History of Medicine and Allied Sciences* 24: 65–75.

2. Ibid.

3. Rotkin, I. (1967). 'Epidemiology of cancer of the cervix. 3. Sexual characteristics of a cervical cancer population'. *American Journal of Public Health and the Nations Health* 57: 815–29.

4. Eddy, B. & Stewart, S. (1959). 'Characteristics of the SE polyoma virus'. *American Journal of Public Health and the Nations Health* 49: 1486–92.

5. Gissmann, L., Wolnik, L., Ikenberg, H., Koldovsky, U., Schnürch, H. & zur Hausen, H. (1983). 'Human papillomavirus types 6 and 11 DNA sequences in genital and laryngeal papillomas and in some cervical cancers'. *Proceedings of the National Academy of Sciences of the USA* 80: 560–3.

6. zur Hausen, H. (2009). 'Papillomaviruses in the causation of human cancers – a brief historical account'. *Virology* 384: 260–5.

7. Howley, P., Schiller, J. & Lowy, D. (2013). 'Papillomaviruses' in *Fields Virology* (eds: D. M. Knipe & P. M. Howley) pp1662–1703. Philadelphia, Wolters Kluwer Health/Lippincott Williams & Wilkins.

8. Australian Academy of Sciences (2008). 'Interviews with Australian Scientists: Professor Ian Frazer, Immunologist'. web.archive.org (accessed 17 September 2020).

9. Zhao, K. N., Zhang, L. & Qu, J. (2017). 'Dr. Jian Zhou: The great inventor of cervical cancer vaccine'. *Protein & Cell* 8: 79–82.

10. Frazer, I. (2019). 'The HPV Vaccine Story'. *ACS Pharmacology & Translational Science* 2: 210–12.

11. Howley, P., Schiller, J. & Lowy, D. (2013). 'Papillomaviruses' in *Fields Virology* (eds: D. M. Knipe & P. M. Howley) pp1662–1703. Philadelphia, Wolters Kluwer Health/Lippincott Williams & Wilkins.

12. Zhou, J., Sun, X., Stenzel, D. & Frazer, I. (1991). 'Expression of vaccinia recombinant HPV 16 L1 and L2 ORF proteins in epithelial cells is sufficient for assembly of HPV virion-like particles'. *Virology* 185: 251–7.

13. GAVI (2012). 'Professor Ian Frazer talks about how he invented the HPV vaccine against cervical cancer'. gavi.org (accessed 17 September 2020).

14. Frazer, I. (2019). 'The HPV Vaccine Story'. *ACS Pharmacology & Translational Science* 2: 210–12.

15. de Villiers, E. M., Fauquet, C., Broker, T., Bernard, H. U. & zur Hausen, H. (2004). 'Classification of papillomaviruses'. *Virology* 324: 17–27.

16. International Committee on the Taxonomy of Viruses (2020). 'Papillomaviridae'. talk.ictvonline.org (accessed 12 December 2021).

17. Blast! plc (2019). *Jade: The Reality Star Who Changed Britain*. Channel 4, London.

18. Newman, V. (2019). 'Inside Jade Goody's wedding days before tragic death with Mark Wright as best man'. *Daily Mirror*, 14 August 2019.

19. Asiaf, A., Ahmad, S., Mohammad, S. & Zargar, M. (2014). 'Review of the current knowledge on the epidemiology, pathogenesis, and

prevention of human papillomavirus infection'. *European Journal of Cancer Prevention* 23: 206–24.

20. Winer, R., Hughes, J., Feng, Q., O'Reilly, S., Kiviat, N., Holmes, K. & Koutsky, L. (2006). 'Condom use and the risk of genital human papillomavirus infection in young women'. *New England Journal of Medicine* 354: 2645–54.

21. Ibid.

22. de Martel, C., Plummer, M., Vignat, J. & Franceschi, S. (2017). 'Worldwide burden of cancer attributable to HPV by site, country and HPV type'. *International Journal of Cancer* 141: 664–70.

23. Asiaf, A., Ahmad, S., Mohammad, S. & Zargar, M. (2014). 'Review of the current knowledge on the epidemiology, pathogenesis, and prevention of human papillomavirus infection'. *European Journal of Cancer Prevention* 23: 206–24.

24. NHS (2021). 'Treatment. Cervical Cancer'. nhs.uk (accessed 12 December 2021).

25. Cancer Research UK (undated). 'Cervical cancer incidence statistics'. cancerresearchuk.org (accessed 17 September 2020).

26. Schiller, J., Markowitz, L., Hildesheim, A. & Lowy, D. (2018). 'Human Papillomavirus Vaccines' in *Plotkin's Vaccines, Seventh edition* (eds: S. A. Plotkin, W. A. Orenstein, P. A. Offit & M. D. Edwards) pp430–55. Philadelphia, Elsevier, Inc.

27. NHS (2019). 'HPV vaccine safety'. nhs.uk (accessed 7 August 2022).

28. Dobson, S., McNeil, S., Dionne, M., Dawar, M., Ogilvie, G., Krajden, M., Sauvageau, C., Scheifele, D., Kollmann, T., Halperin, S., Langley, J., Bettinger, J., Singer, J., Money, D., Miller, D., Naus, M., Marra, F. & Young, E. (2013). 'Immunogenicity of 2 doses of HPV vaccine in younger adolescents vs 3 doses in young women: a randomized clinical trial'. *Journal of the American Medical Association* 309: 1793–1802.

29. Fleming, N. (2007). 'Girls of 12 to have cervical cancer jab'. *Daily Telegraph*, 20 June 2007.

30. Hilton, S. & Smith, E. (2011). '"I thought cancer was one of those random things. I didn't know cancer could be caught . . . ": adolescent girls' understandings and experiences of the HPV programme in the UK'. *Vaccine* 29: 4409–15.

31. Bednarczyk, R., Davis, R., Ault, K., Orenstein, W. & Omer, S. (2012). 'Sexual activity-related outcomes after human papillomavirus vaccination of 11- to 12-year-olds'. *Pediatrics* 130: 798–805.

32. Karpf, A. (2008). 'The state wants my daughter to be vaccinated, but I want to know more'. *Guardian*, 1 March 2008.

33. Scheller, N., Pasternak, B., Mølgaard-Nielsen, D., Svanström, H. & Hviid, A. (2017) 'Quadrivalent HPV Vaccination and the Risk of Adverse Pregnancy Outcomes'. *New England Journal of Medicine* 376: 1223–33.

34. Prue, G., Grimes, D., Baker, P. & Lawler, M. (2018). 'Access to HPV

vaccination for boys in the United Kingdom'. *Medicine Access @ Point of Care*: 1–9.

35. Sandulache, V., Wilde, D., Sturgis, E., Chiao, E. & Sikora, A. (2019). 'A Hidden Epidemic of "Intermediate Risk" Oropharynx Cancer'. *Laryngoscope Investigative Otolaryngology* 4: 617–23.

36. Falcaro, M., Castañon, A., Ndlela, B., Checchi, M., Soldan, K., Lopez-Bernal, J., Elliss-Brookes, L. & Sasieni, P. (2021). 'The effects of the national HPV vaccination programme in England, UK, on cervical cancer and grade 3 cervical intraepithelial neoplasia incidence: a register-based observational study'. *Lancet* 398: 2084–92.

37. Brisson, M., Bénard, E., Drolet, M., Bogaards, J., Baussano, I., Vänskä, S., Jit, M., Boily M.-C., Smith, M., Berkhof, J., Canfell, K., Chesson, H., Burger, E., Choi, Y., De Blasio, B., De Vlas, S., Guzzetta, G., Hontelez, J., Horn, J., Jepsen, M., Kim, J., Lazzarato, F., Matthijsse, S., Mikolajczyk, R., Pavelyev, A., Pillsbury, M., Shafer, L., Tully, S., Turner, H., Usher, C. & Walsh, C. (2016). 'Population-level impact, herd immunity, and elimination after human papillomavirus vaccination: a systematic review and meta-analysis of predictions from transmission-dynamic models'. *Lancet Public Health* 1: e8–17.

Chapter 17

1. Lucy (2020). Author interview. 2 December 2020.
2. Wat, D. (2004). 'The common cold: a review of the literature'. *European Journal of Internal Medicine* 15: 79–88.
3. Ibid.
4. Magnus, P., Gunnes, N., Tveito, K., Bakken, I., Ghaderi, S., Stoltenberg, C., Hornig, M., Lipkin, W., Trogstad, L. & Haberg, S. (2015). 'Chronic fatigue syndrome/myalgic encephalomyelitis (CFS/ME) is associated with pandemic influenza infection, but not with an adjuvanted pandemic influenza vaccine'. *Vaccine* 33: 6173–7.
5. Surtees, R. & DeSousa, C. (2006). 'Influenza virus associated encephalopathy'. *Archives of Disease in Childhood* 91: 455–6.
6. Sellers, S., Hagan, R., Hayden, F. & Fischer II, W. (2017). 'The hidden burden of influenza: A review of the extra-pulmonary complications of influenza infection'. *Influenza and Other Respiratory Viruses* 11: 372–93.
7. Barry, J. (2004). 'The site of origin of the 1918 influenza pandemic and its public health implications'. *Journal of Translational Medicine* 2: 1–4.
8. Gates, F. (1918). 'A Report on Antimeningitis Vaccination and Observations on Agglutinins in the Blood of Chronic Meningococcus Carriers'. *Journal of Experimental Medicine* 28: 449–74.
9. Barry, J. (2004). 'The site of origin of the 1918 influenza pandemic and its public health implications'. *Journal of Translational Medicine* 2: 1–4.
10. Brankston, G., Gitterman, L., Hirji, Z., Lemieux, C. & Gardam,

M. (2007). 'Transmission of influenza A in human beings'. *Lancet Infectious Diseases* 7: 257–65.

11. Mukherjee, D., Cohen, B., Bovino, M., Desai, S., Whittier, S. & Larson, E. (2012). 'Survival of influenza virus on hands and fomites in community and laboratory settings'. *American Journal of Infection Control* 40: 590–4.

12. World Bank Group (2021). 'Urban population (% of total population)'. data.worldbank.org (accessed 23 December 2021).

13. Johnson, N. & Mueller, J. (2002). 'Updating the accounts: global mortality of the 1918–1920 "Spanish" influenza pandemic'. *Bulletin of the History of Medicine* 76: 105–15.

14. European Centre for Disease Prevention and Control (2020). 'Questions and answers on influenza pandemics'. ecdc.europa.eu (accessed 10 December 2020).

15. Cunha, B. (2004). 'Influenza: historical aspects of epidemics and pandemics'. *Infectious Disease Clinics of North America* 18: 141–55.

16. Horimoto, T. & Kawaoka, Y. (2001). 'Pandemic threat posed by avian influenza A viruses'. *Clinical Microbiology Reviews* 14: 129–49.

17. Scholtissek, C., Burger, H., Kistner, O. & Shortridge, K. (1985). 'The nucleoprotein as a possible major factor in determining host specificity of influenza H3N2 viruses'. *Virology* 147: 287–94.

18. Barberis, I., Myles, P., Ault, S., Bragazzi, N. & Martini, M. (2016). 'History and evolution of influenza control through vaccination: from the first monovalent vaccine to universal vaccines'. *Journal of Preventative Medicine and Hygiene* 57: E115–20.

19. Bresalier, M. (2012). 'Uses of a Pandemic: Forging the Identities of Influenza and Virus Research in Interwar Britain'. *Social History of Medicine* 25: 400–24.

20. Evans, D. (1966). 'Wilson Smith, 1897–1965'. *Biographical Memoirs of the Fellows of the Royal Society* 12: 478–87.

21. Tyrell, D. (1991). 'Christopher Howard Andrewes, 7 June 1986–31 December 1987'. *Biographical Memoirs of Fellows of the Royal Society* 37: 33–54.

22. Bresalier, M. (2013). '80 years ago today: MRC researchers discover viral cause of flu'. *Guardian*, 8 July 2013.

23. Smith, W., Andrewes, C. & Laidlaw, P. (1933). 'A virus obtained from influenza patients'. *Lancet* 222: 66–8.

24. Evans, D. (1966). 'Wilson Smith, 1897–1965'. *Biographical Memoirs of the Fellows of the Royal Society* 12: 478–87.

25. Burnet, F. (1940). 'Influenza Virus Infections of the Chick Embryo Lung'. *British Journal of Experimental Pathology* 21: 147–53.

26. Salk, J. & Suriano, P. (1949). 'Importance of antigenic composition of influenza virus vaccine in protecting against the natural disease; observations during the winter of 1947–1948'. *American Journal of Public Health and the Nation's Health* 39: 345–55.

27. Matias, G., Taylor, R., Haguinet, F., Schuck-Paim, C., Lustig, R. & Fleming, D. (2016). 'Modelling estimates of age-specific influenza-related hospitalisation and mortality in the United Kingdom'. *BMC Public Health* 16: 481.

28. Cassini, A., Colzani, E., Pini, A., Mangen, M.-J., Plass, D., McDonald, S., Maringhini, G., van Lier, A., Haagsma, J., Havelaar, A., Kramarz, P. & Kretzschmar, M. (2018). 'Impact of infectious diseases on population health using incidence-based disability-adjusted life years (DALYs): results from the Burden of Communicable Diseases in Europe study, European Union and European Economic Area countries, 2009 to 2013'. *EuroSurveillance* 23: 17-00454.

29. Tyrell, D. (1991). 'Christopher Howard Andrewes, 7 June 1986 -31 December 1987'. *Biographical Memoirs of Fellows of the Royal Society* 37: 33 -54.3.

30. World Health Organization (2020). 'Global Influenza Surveillance and Response System (GISRS)'. who.int (acccessed 10 December 2020).

31. Barberis, I., Myles, P., Ault, S., Bragazzi, N. & Martini, M. (2016). 'History and evolution of influenza control through vaccination: from the first monovalent vaccine to universal vaccines'. *Journal of Preventative Medicine and Hygiene* 57: E115–20.

32. World Health Organization (2013). *Pandemic Influenza Risk Management. WHO Interim Guidance.* Geneva, WHO.

33. Wright, P., Neuman, G. & Kawaoka, Y. (2013). 'Orthomyxoviruses' in *Fields Virology* (eds: D. M. Knipe & P. M. Howley) pp1187–1239. Philadelphia, Wolters Kluwer Health/Lippincott Williams & Wilkins.

34. Kilbourne, E. (2004). 'Mating of a Flasher'. yjhm.yale.edu (accessed 10 December 2020).

35. Kilbourne, E. & Murphy, J. (1960). 'Genetic studies of influenza viruses. I. Viral morphology and growth capacity as exchangeable genetic traits. Rapid in ovo adaptation of early passage Asian strain isolates by combination with PR8'. *Journal of Experimental Medicine* 111: 387–406.

36. Kilbourne, E., Schulman, J., Schild, G., Schloer, G., Swanson, J. & Bucher, D. (1971). 'Related studies of a recombinant influenza-virus vaccine. I. Derivation and characterization of virus and vaccine'. *Journal of Infectious Diseases* 124: 449–62.

37. Bresee, J., Fry, A., Sambhara, S. & Cox, N. (2018). 'Inactivated Influenza Vaccines' in *Plotkin's Vaccines, Seventh edition* (eds: S. A. Plotkin, W. A. Orenstein, P. A. Offit & M. D. Edwards) pp456–88. Philadelphia, Elsevier, Inc.

38. Yardley, W. (2014). 'Hunein Maassab, Who Developed FluMist Vaccine, Dies at 87'. *New York Times*, 11 March 2014.

39. Maassab, H. (1967). 'Adaptation and growth characteristics of influenza virus at 25°C'. *Nature* 213: 612–14.

40. Wright, P., Neuman, G. & Kawaoka, Y. (2013). 'Orthomyxoviruses'

in *Fields Virology* (eds: D. M. Knipe & P. M. Howley) pp1187–1239. Philadelphia, Wolters Kluwer Health/Lippincott Williams & Wilkins.

41. Davenport, F., Hennessy, A., Maassab, H., Minuse, E., Clark, L., Abrams, G. & Mitchell, J. (1977). 'Pilot studies on recombinant cold-adapted live type A and B influenza virus vaccines'. *Journal of Infectious Diseases* 136: 17–25.

42. Kendal, A., Maassab, H., Alexandrovna, G. & Ghendon, Y. (1982). 'Development of cold-adapted recombinant live, attenuated influenza A vaccines in the U.S.A. and U.S.S.R'. *Antiviral Research* 1: 339–65.

43. Rudenko, L., Yeolekar, L., Kiseleva, I. & Isakova-Sivak, I. (2016). 'Development and approval of live attenuated influenza vaccines based on Russian master donor viruses: Process challenges and success stories'. *Vaccine* 34: 5436–41.

44. Yardley, W. (2014). 'Hunein Maassab, Who Developed FluMist Vaccine, Dies at 87'. *New York Times*, 11 March 2014.

45. Ambrose, C., Levin, M. & Belshe, R. (2011). 'The relative efficacy of trivalent live attenuated and inactivated influenza vaccines in children and adults'. *Influenza and Other Respiratory Viruses* 5: 67–75.

46. Bresee, J., Fry, A., Sambhara, S. & Cox, N. (2018). 'Inactivated Influenza Vaccines' in *Plotkin's Vaccines, Seventh edition* (eds: S. A. Plotkin, W. A. Orenstein, P. A. Offit & M. D. Edwards) pp456–88. Philadelphia, Elsevier, Inc.

47. Ibid.

48. United Kingdom Health Security Authority (2022). 'Chapter 19: Influenza' in *The Green Book*. London, UKHSA.

49. Ibid.

50. Pebody, R., Djennad, A., Ellis, J., Andrews, N., Marques, D., Cottrell, S., Reynolds, A., Gunson, R., Galiano, M., Hoschler, K., Lackenby, A., Robertson, C., O'Doherty, M., Sinnathamby, M., Panagiotopoulos, N., Yonova, I., Webb, R., Moore, C., Donati, M., Sartaj, M., Shepherd, S., McMenamin, J., de Lusignan, S. & Zambon, M. (2019). 'End of season influenza vaccine effectiveness in adults and children in the United Kingdom in 2017/18'. *EuroSurveillance* 24: 1800488.

51. Ibid.

52. Thompson, M., Pierse, N., Huang, Q., Prasad, N., Duque, J., Newbern, E., Baker, M., Turner, N. & McArthur, C. (2018). 'Influenza vaccine effectiveness in preventing influenza-associated intensive care admissions and attenuating severe disease among adults in New Zealand 2012–2015'. *Vaccine* 36: 5916–25.

Chapter 18

1. Qiu, J. (2020). 'How China's "bat woman" hunted down viruses from SARS to the new coronavirus'. *Scientific American*, 1 June 2020.

2. Nextstrain (2022). 'Genomic epidemiology of SARS-CoV-2 with

subsampling focused globally since pandemic start'. nextstrain.org (accessed 20 May 2022).

3. Zhou, P., Yang, X. L., Wang, X. G., Hu, B., Zhang, L., Zhang, W., Si, H. R., Zhu, Y., Li, B., Huang, C. L., Chen, H. D., Chen, J., Luo, Y., Guo, H., Jiang, R. D., Liu, M. Q., Chen, Y., Shen, X. R., Wang, X., Zheng, X. S., Zhao, K., Chen, Q. J., Deng, F., Liu, L. L., Yan, B., Zhan, F. X., Wang, Y. Y., Xiao, G. F. & Shi, Z. L. (2020). 'A pneumonia outbreak associated with a new coronavirus of probable bat origin'. *Nature* 579: 270–3.

4. Buckley, C. & Myers, S. (2020). 'As new coronavirus spread, China's old habits delayed fight'. *New York Times*, 1 February 2020.

5. Ibid.

6. Li, H., Mendelsohn, E., Zong, C., Zhang, W., Hagan, E., Wang, N., Li, S., Yan, H., Huang, H., Zhu, G., Ross, N., Chmura, A., Terry, P., Fielder, M., Miller, M., Shi, Z. & Daszak, P. (2019). 'Human-animal interactions and bat coronavirus spillover potential among rural residents in Southern China'. *Biosafety and Health* 1: 84–90.

7. Cherry, J. & Krogstad, P. (2004). 'SARS: the first pandemic of the 21st century'. *Pediatric Research* 56: 1–5.

8. Cui, J., Li, F. & Shi, Z. L. (2019). 'Origin and evolution of pathogenic coronaviruses'. *Nature Reviews Microbiology* 17: 181–92.

9. Qiu, J. (2020). 'How China's "bat woman" hunted down viruses from SARS to the new coronavirus'. *Scientific American*, 1 June 2020.

10. Shi, Z. (2020). 'Reply to Science Magazine'. science.org (accessed 16 May 2020).

11. World Health Organization (2020). 'Naming the coronavirus disease (COVID-19) and the virus that causes it'. who.int (accessed 16 May 2022).

12. World Health Organization (2020). 'WHO Director-General's opening remarks at the media briefing on COVID-19 – 11 March 2020'. who.int (accessed 16 May 2022).

13. Cohen, J. (2020). 'Wuhan coronavirus hunter Shi Zhengli speaks out'. *Science* 369: 487–8.

14. Shi, Z. (2020). 'Reply to Science Magazine'. science.org (accessed 16 May 2020).

15. Zhou, P., Yang X. L., Wang, X. G., Hu, B., Zhang, L., Zhang, W., Si H. R., Zhu, Y., Li, B., Huang, C. L., Chen, H. D., Chen, J., Luo, Y., Guo, H., Jiang, R. D., Liu M. Q., Chen, Y., Shen, X. R., Wang X, Zheng, X. S., Zhao, K., Chen, Q. J., Deng, F., Liu, L. L., Yan, B., Zhan, F. X., Wang, Y. Y., Xiao, G. F. & Shi, Z. L. (2020). 'A pneumonia outbreak associated with a new coronavirus of probable bat origin'. *Nature* 579: 270–3.

16. Boni, M., Lemey, P., Jiang, X., Lam, T. Y., Perry, B., Castoe, T., Rambaut, A. & Robertson, D. (2020). 'Evolutionary origins of the SARS-CoV-2 sarbecovirus lineage responsible for the COVID-19 pandemic'. *Nature Microbiology* 5: 1408–17.

17. Qiu, J. (2020). 'How China's "bat woman" hunted down viruses from SARS to the new coronavirus'. *Scientific American*, 1 June 2020.

18. Liu, Y., Gayle, A., Wilder-Smith, A. & Rocklöv, J. (2020). 'The reproductive number of COVID-19 is higher compared to SARS coronavirus'. *Journal of Travel Medicine* 27: taaa021.

19. Moriyama, M., Hugentobler, W. & Iwasaki, A. (2020). 'Seasonality of Respiratory Viral Infections'. *Annual Review of Virology* 7: 83–101.

20. Buitrago-Garcia, D., Egli-Gany, D., Counotte, M., Hossmann, S., Imeri, H., Ipekci, A., Salanti, G. & Low, N. (2020). 'Occurrence and transmission potential of asymptomatic and presymptomatic SARS-CoV-2 infections: A living systematic review and meta-analysis'. *PLoS Medicine* 17: e1003346.

21. Li, J., Huang, D., Zou, B., Yang, H., Hui, W., Rui, F., Yee, N., Liu, C., Nerurkar, S., Kai, J., Teng, M., Li, X., Zeng, H., Borghi, J., Henry, L., Cheung, R. & Nguyen, M. (2020). 'Epidemiology of COVID-19: A systematic review and meta-analysis of clinical characteristics, risk factors, and outcomes'. *Journal of Medical Virology* 93: 1449–58.

22. O'Driscoll, M., Ribeiro Dos Santos, G., Wang, L., Cummings, D., Azman, A., Paireau, J., Fontanet, A., Cauchemez, S. & Salje, H. (2020). 'Age-specific mortality and immunity patterns of SARS-CoV-2'. *Nature* 590: 140–5.

23. COVID-19 Excess Mortality Collaborators (2022). 'Estimating excess mortality due to the COVID-19 pandemic: a systematic analysis of COVID-19-related mortality, 2020–21'. *Lancet* 399: 1513–36.

24. O'Driscoll, M., Ribeiro Dos Santos, G., Wang, L., Cummings, D., Azman, A., Paireau, J., Fontanet, A., Cauchemez, S. & Salje, H. (2020). 'Age-specific mortality and immunity patterns of SARS-CoV-2'. *Nature* 590: 140–5.

25. Merad, M., Blish, C., Sallusto, F. & Iwasaki, A. (2022). 'The immunology and immunopathology of COVID-19'. *Science* 375: 1122–7.

26. Thakur, B., Dubey, P., Benitez, J., Torres, J., Reddy, S., Shokar, N., Aung, K., Mukherjee, D. & Dwivedi, A. (2021). 'A systematic review and meta-analysis of geographic differences in comorbidities and associated severity and mortality among individuals with COVID-19'. *Scientific Reports* 11: 8562.

27. Almeida, J., Berry, D., Cunningham, C., Hamre, D., Hofstad, M., Mallucci, L., McIntosh, K. & Tyrrell, D. (1968). 'Coronaviruses'. *Nature* 220: 650.

28. Folegatti, P., Bittaye, M., Flaxman, A.,Lopez, F., Bellamy, D., Kupke, A.,Mair, C., Makinson, R., Sheridan, J., Rohde, C., Halwe, S., Jeong, Y., Park, Y. S., Kim, J., Song, M., Boyd, A., Tran, N., Silman, D., Poulton, I., Datoo, M., Marshall, J., Themistocleous, Y., Lawrie, A., Roberts, R., Berrie, E., Becker, S., Lambe, T., Hill, A., Ewer, K. & Gilbert, S. (2020). 'Safety and immunogenicity of a candidate Middle East respiratory syndrome coronavirus viral-vectored vaccine: a

dose-escalation, open-label, non-randomised, uncontrolled, phase 1 trial'. *Lancet Infectious Diseases* 20: 816–26.

29. Crow, D. (2021). 'How mRNA became a vaccine game-changer; It's the "messenger" molecule of the moment that made the Pfizer and Moderna jabs so effective against COVID-19 yet mRNA was ignored for decades. Can it now revolutionise medicine?' *Financial Times*, 15 May 2021.

30. Ibid.

31. Neill, U. (2021). 'A conversation with Katalin Karikó'. *Journal of Clinical Investigation* 131: e155559.

32. de Oliveira, W., de França, G., Carmo, E., Duncan, B., de Souza Kuchenbecker, R. & Schmidt, M. (2017). 'Infection-related microcephaly after the 2015 and 2016 Zika virus outbreaks in Brazil: a surveillance-based analysis'. *Lancet* 390: 861–70.

33. Pardi, N., Hogan, M., Pelc, R., Muramatsu, H., Andersen, H., DeMaso, C., Dowd, K., Sutherland, L., Scearce, R., Parks, R., Wagner, W., Granados, A., Greenhouse, J., Walker, M., Willis, E., Yu, J. S., McGee, C., Sempowski, G., Mui, B., Tam, Y., Huang, Y. J., Vanlandingham, D., Holmes, V., Balachandran, H., Sahu, S., Lifton, M., Higgs, S., Hensley, S., Madden, T., Hope, M., Karikó, K., Santra, S., Graham, B., Lewis, M., Pierson, T., Haynes, B. & Weissman, D. (2017). 'Zika virus protection by a single low-dose nucleoside-modified mRNA vaccination'. *Nature* 543: 248–51.

34. Zheng, C., Shao, W., Chen, X., Zhang, B., Wang, G. & Zhang, W. (2022). 'Real-world effectiveness of COVID-19 vaccines: a literature review and meta-analysis'. *International Journal of Infectious Diseases* 114: 252–60.

35. Jara, A., Undurraga, E., González, C., Paredes, F., Fontecilla, T., Jara, G., Pizarro, A., Acevedo, J., Leo, K., Leon, F., Sans, C., Leighton, P., Suárez, P., García-Escorza, H. & Araos, R. (2021). 'Effectiveness of an Inactivated SARS-CoV-2 Vaccine in Chile'. *New England Journal of Medicine* 385: 875–84.

36. BBC (2020). 'COVID-19 vaccine: First person receives Pfizer jab in UK'. bbc.co.uk/news (accessed 17 May 2022).

37. World Health Organization (2022). 'Tracking SARS-CoV-2 variants'. who.int (accessed 15 April 2022).

38. Finkel, Y., Mizrahi, O., Nachshon, A., Weingarten-Gabbay, S., Morgenstern, D., Yahalom-Ronen, Y., Tamir, H., Achdout, H., Stein, D., Israeli, O., Beth-Din, A., Melamed, S., Weiss, S., Israely, T., Paran, N., Schwartz, M. & Stern-Ginossar, N. (2021). 'The coding capacity of SARS-CoV-2'. *Nature* 589: 125–30.

39. Zhang, J., Xiao, T., Cai, Y., Lavine, C., Peng, H., Zhu, H., Anand, K., Tong, P., Gautam, A., Mayer, M., Walsh, R., Jr, Rits-Volloch, S., Wesemann, D., Yang, W., Seaman, M., Lu, J. & Chen, B. (2021). 'Membrane fusion and immune evasion by the spike protein of SARS-CoV-2 Delta variant'. *Science* 374: 1353–60.

40. Liu, Y. & Rocklöv, J. (2021). 'The reproductive number of the Delta variant of SARS-CoV-2 is far higher compared to the ancestral SARS-CoV-2 virus'. *Journal of Travel Medicine* 28: 124.

41. Lin, L., Liu, Y., Tang, X. & He, D. (2021). 'The Disease Severity and Clinical Outcomes of the SARS-CoV-2 Variants of Concern'. *Frontiers in Public Health* 9: 775224.

42. Cameroni, E., Bowen, J., Rosen, L., Saliba, C., Zepeda, S., Culap, K., Pinto, D., VanBlargan, L., De Marco, A., di Iulio, J., Zatta, F., Kaiser, H., Noack, J., Farhat, N., Czudnochowski, N., Havenar-Daughton, C., Sprouse, K., Dillen, J., Powell, A., Chen, A., Maher, C., Yin, L., Sun, D., Soriaga, L., Bassi, J., Silacci-Fregni, C., Gustafsson, C., Franko, N., Logue, J., Iqbal, N., Mazzitelli, I., Geffner, J., Grifantini, R., Chu, H., Gori, A., Riva, A., Giannini, O., Ceschi, A., Ferrari, P., Cippà, P., Franzetti-Pellanda, A., Garzoni, C., Halfmann, P., Kawaoka, Y., Hebner, C., Purcell, L., Piccoli, L., Pizzuto, M., Walls, A., Diamond, M., Telenti, A., Virgin, H., Lanzavecchia, A., Snell, G., Veesler, D. & Corti, D. (2022). 'Broadly neutralizing antibodies overcome SARS-CoV-2 Omicron antigenic shift'. *Nature* 602: 664–70.

43. Lopez Bernal, J., Andrews, N., Gower, C., Gallagher, E., Simmons, R., Thelwall, S., Stowe, J., Tessier, E., Groves, N., Dabrera, G., Myers, R., Campbell, C., Amirthalingam, G., Edmunds, M., Zambon, M., Brown, K., Hopkins, S., Chand, M. & Ramsay, M. (2021). 'Effectiveness of COVID-19 Vaccines against the B.1.617.2 (Delta) Variant'. *New England Journal of Medicine* 385: 585–94.

44. Lauring, A., Tenforde, M., Chappell, J., Gaglani, M., Ginde, A., McNeal, T., Ghamande, S., Douin, D., Talbot, H., Casey, J., Mohr, N., Zepeski, A., Shapiro, N., Gibbs, K., Files, D., Hager, D., Shehu, A., Prekker, M., Erickson, H., Exline, M., Gong, M., Mohamed, A., Johnson, N., Srinivasan, V., Steingrub, J., Peltan, I., Brown, S., Martin, E., Monto, A., Khan, A., Hough, C., Busse, L., Ten Lohuis, C., Duggal, A., Wilson, J., Gordon, A., Qadir, N., Chang, S., Mallow, C., Rivas, C., Babcock, H., Kwon, J., Halasa, N., Grijalva, C., Rice, T., Stubblefield, W., Baughman, A., Womack, K., Rhoads, J., Lindsell, C., Hart, K., Zhu, Y., Adams, K., Schrag, S., Olson, S., Kobayashi, M., Verani, J., Patel, M. & Self, W. (2022). 'Clinical severity of, and effectiveness of mRNA vaccines against, COVID-19 from omicron, delta, and alpha SARS-CoV-2 variants in the United States: prospective observational study'. *British Medical Journal* 376: e069761.

45. Watson, O., Barnsley, G., Toor, J., Hogan, A., Winskill, P. & Ghani, A. (2022). 'Global impact of the first year of COVID-19 vaccination: a mathematical modelling study'. *Lancet Infectious Diseases* Online ahead of print: S1473-3099(1422)00320-00326.

46. Karim, S. & Karim, Q. (2021). 'Omicron SARS-CoV-2 variant: a new chapter in the COVID-19 pandemic'. *Lancet* 398: 2126–8.

47. Iacobucci, G. (2022). 'COVID-19: UK adds sore throat, headache,

fatigue, and six other symptoms to official list'. *British Medical Journal* 377: o892.

48. Karim, S. & Karim, Q. (2021). 'Omicron SARS-CoV-2 variant: a new chapter in the COVID-19 pandemic'. *Lancet* 398: 2126–8.

49. Willett, B., Grove, J., MacLean, O., Wilkie, C., De Lorenzo, G., Furnon, W., Cantoni, D., Scott, S., Logan, N., Ashraf, S., Manali, M., Szemiel, A., Cowton, V., Vink, E., Harvey, W., Davis, C., Asamaphan, P., Smollett, K., Tong, L., Orton, R., Hughes, J., Holland, P., Silva, V., Pascall, D., Puxty, K., da Silva Filipe, A., Yebra, G., Shaaban, S., Holden, M., Pinto, R., Gunson, R., Templeton, K., Murcia, P., Patel, A., Klenerman, P., Dunachie, S., Haughney, J., Robertson, D., Palmarini, M., Ray, S. & Thomson, E. (2022). 'SARS-CoV-2 Omicron is an immune escape variant with an altered cell entry pathway'. *Nature Microbiology* Online: Ahead of print.

50. Ito, K., Piantham, C. & Nishiura, H. (2022). 'Relative instantaneous reproduction number of Omicron SARS-CoV-2 variant with respect to the Delta variant in Denmark'. *Journal of Medical Virology* 94: 2265–8.

51. Zhao, H., Lu, L., Peng, Z., Chen, L. L., Meng, X., Zhang, C., Ip, J., Chan, W. M., Chu, A. H., Chan, K. H., Jin, D. Y., Chen, H., Yuen, K. Y. & To, K. W. (2022). 'SARS-CoV-2 Omicron variant shows less efficient replication and fusion activity when compared with Delta variant in TMPRSS2-expressed cells'. *Emerging Microbes & Infections* 11: 277–83.

52. Danza, P., Koo, T., Haddix, M., Fisher, R., Traub, E., OYong, K. & Balter, S. (2022). 'SARS-CoV-2 Infection and Hospitalization Among Adults Aged ≥18 Years, by Vaccination Status, Before and During SARS-CoV-2 B.1.1.529 (Omicron) Variant Predominance – Los Angeles County, California, November 7, 2021–January 8, 2022'. *Morbidity and Mortality Weekly Report* 71: 177–81.

53. Johnson, A., Amin, A., Ali, A., Hoots, B., Cadwell, B., Arora, S., Avoundjian, T., Awofeso, A., Barnes, J., Bayoumi, N., Busen, K., Chang, C., Cima, M., Crockett, M., Cronquist, A., Davidson, S., Davis, E., Delgadillo, J., Dorabawila, V., Drenzek, C., Eisenstein, L., Fast, H., Gent, A., Hand, J., Hoefer, D., Holtzman, C., Jara, A., Jones, A., Kamal-Ahmed, I., Kangas, S., Kanishka, F., Kaur, R., Khan, S., King, J., Kirkendall, S., Klioueva, A., Kocharian, A., Kwon, F., Logan, J., Lyons, B., Lyons, S., May, A., McCormick, D., Mendoza, E., Milroy, L., O'Donnell, A., Pike, M., Pogosjans, S., Saupe, A., Sell, J., Smith, E., Sosin, D., Stanislawski, E., Steele, M., Stephenson, M., Stout, A., Strand, K., Tilakaratne, B., Turner, K., Vest, H., Warner, S., Wiedeman, C., Zaldivar, A., Silk, B. & Scobie, H. (2022). 'COVID-19 Incidence and Death Rates Among Unvaccinated and Fully Vaccinated Adults with and Without Booster Doses During Periods of Delta and Omicron Variant Emergence – 25 U.S. Jurisdictions, April 4–December 25, 2021'. *Morbidity and Mortality Weekly Report* 71: 132–8.

54. Centre for Health Protection of the Department of Health (2022). 'Provisional Data Analysis on COVID-19 Reported Death Cases (from 31 Dec 2021 up till 18 May 2022 00:00)'. covidvaccine.gov.hk (accessed 20 May 2022).

55. Danza, P., Koo, T., Haddix, M., Fisher, R., Traub, E., OYong, K. & Balter, S. (2022). 'SARS-CoV-2 Infection and Hospitalization Among Adults Aged ≥18 Years, by Vaccination Status, Before and During SARS-CoV-2 B.1.1.529 (Omicron) Variant Predominance – Los Angeles County, California, November 7, 2021–January 8, 2022'. *Morbidity and Mortality Weekly Report* 71: 177–81.

56. Johnson, A., Amin, A., Ali, A., Hoots, B., Cadwell, B., Arora, S., Avoundjian, T., Awofeso, A., Barnes, J., Bayoumi, N., Busen, K., Chang, C., Cima, M., Crockett, M., Cronquist, A., Davidson, S., Davis, E., Delgadillo, J., Dorabawila, V., Drenzek, C., Eisenstein, L., Fast, H., Gent, A., Hand, J., Hoefer, D., Holtzman, C., Jara, A., Jones, A., Kamal-Ahmed, I., Kangas, S., Kanishka, F., Kaur, R., Khan, S., King, J., Kirkendall, S., Klioueva, A., Kocharian, A., Kwon, F., Logan, J., Lyons, B., Lyons, S., May, A., McCormick, D., Mendoza, E., Milroy, L., O'Donnell, A., Pike, M., Pogosjans, S., Saupe, A., Sell, J., Smith, E., Sosin, D., Stanislawski, E., Steele, M., Stephenson, M., Stout, A., Strand, K., Tilakaratne, B., Turner, K., Vest, H., Warner, S., Wiedeman, C., Zaldivar, A., Silk, B. & Scobie, H. (2022). 'COVID-19 Incidence and Death Rates Among Unvaccinated and Fully Vaccinated Adults with and Without Booster Doses During Periods of Delta and Omicron Variant Emergence – 25 U.S. Jurisdictions, April 4–December 25, 2021'. *Morbidity and Mortality Weekly Report* 71: 132–8.

57. Danza, P., Koo, T., Haddix, M., Fisher, R., Traub, E., OYong, K. & Balter, S. (2022). 'SARS-CoV-2 Infection and Hospitalization Among Adults Aged ≥18 Years, by Vaccination Status, Before and During SARS-CoV-2 B.1.1.529 (Omicron) Variant Predominance – Los Angeles County, California, November 7, 2021–January 8, 2022'. *Morbidity and Mortality Weekly Report* 71: 177–81.

58. Johnson, A., Amin, A., Ali, A., Hoots, B., Cadwell, B., Arora, S., Avoundjian, T., Awofeso, A., Barnes, J., Bayoumi, N., Busen, K., Chang, C., Cima, M., Crockett, M., Cronquist, A., Davidson, S., Davis, E., Delgadillo, J., Dorabawila, V., Drenzek, C., Eisenstein, L., Fast, H., Gent, A., Hand, J., Hoefer, D., Holtzman, C., Jara, A., Jones, A., Kamal-Ahmed, I., Kangas, S., Kanishka, F., Kaur, R., Khan, S., King, J., Kirkendall, S., Klioueva, A., Kocharian, A., Kwon, F., Logan, J., Lyons, B., Lyons, S., May, A., McCormick, D., Mendoza, E., Milroy, L., O'Donnell, A., Pike, M., Pogosjans, S., Saupe, A., Sell, J., Smith, E., Sosin, D., Stanislawski, E., Steele, M., Stephenson, M., Stout, A., Strand, K., Tilakaratne, B., Turner, K., Vest, H., Warner, S., Wiedeman, C., Zaldivar, A., Silk, B. & Scobie, H. (2022). 'COVID-19 Incidence and Death Rates Among Unvaccinated and Fully Vaccinated Adults

with and Without Booster Doses During Periods of Delta and Omicron Variant Emergence – 25 U.S. Jurisdictions, April 4–December 25, 2021'. *Morbidity and Mortality Weekly Report* 71: 132–8.

59. Matias, G., Taylor, R., Haguinet, F., Schuck-Paim, C., Lustig, R. & Fleming, D. (2016). 'Modelling estimates of age-specific influenza-related hospitalisation and mortality in the United Kingdom'. *BMC Public Health* 16: 481.

60. UK Health Security Agency (2022). 'Coronavirus in the UK dashboard: Deaths in United Kingdom'. coronavirus.data.gov.uk (accessed 2 May 2022).

61. Porter, K (@katemeredithp). (2020). [Tweet] 'Oh that's funny … it absolutely came from Amy. She named the group that because of her favorite trucker hat she wore when she got tested'. twitter.com (accessed 17 May 2022).

62. Nalbandian, A., Sehgal, K., Gupta, A., Madhavan, M., McGroder, C., Stevens, J., Cook, J., Nordvig, A., Shalev, D., Sehrawat, T., Ahluwalia, N., Bikdeli, B., Dietz, D., Der-Nigoghossian, C., Liyanage-Don, N., Rosner, G., Bernstein, E., Mohan, S., Beckley, A., Seres, D., Choueiri, T., Uriel, N., Ausiello, J., Accili, D., Freedberg, D., Baldwin, M., Schwartz, A., Brodie, D., Garcia, C., Elkind, M., Connors, J., Bilezikian, J., Landry, D. & Wan, E. (2021). 'Post-acute COVID-19 syndrome'. *Nature Medicine* 27: 601–15.

63. Groff, D., Sun, A., Ssentongo, A., Ba, D., Parsons, N., Poudel, G., Lekoubou, A., Oh, J., Ericson, J., Ssentongo, P. & Chinchilli, V. (2021). 'Short-term and Long-term Rates of Postacute Sequelae of SARS-CoV-2 Infection: A Systematic Review'. *JAMA Network Open* 4: e2128568.

64. Office for National Statistics (2022). 'Self-reported long COVID after infection with the Omicron variant in the UK: 6 May 2022'. ons.gov.uk (accessed 19 May 2022).

65. Office for National Statistics (2022). 'Prevalence of ongoing symptoms following coronavirus (COVID-19) infection in the UK: 6 May 2022'. ons.gov.uk (accessed 19 May 2022).

66. Masters, P. & Perlman, S. (2013). 'Coronaviridae' in *Fields Virology* (eds: D. M. Knipe & P. M. Howley) pp825–58. Philadelphia, Wolters Kluwer Health/Lippincott Williams & Wilkins.

67. Bar-On, Y., Goldberg, Y., Mandel, M., Bodenheimer, O., Freedman, L., Kalkstein, N., Mizrahi, B., Alroy-Preis, S., Ash, N., Milo, R. & Huppert, A. (2021). 'Protection of BNT162b2 Vaccine Booster against COVID-19 in Israel'. *New England Journal of Medicine* 385: 1393–1400.

68. Willett, B., Grove, J., MacLean, O., Wilkie, C., De Lorenzo, G., Furnon, W., Cantoni, D., Scott, S., Logan, N., Ashraf, S., Manali, M., Szemiel, A., Cowton, V., Vink, E., Harvey, W., Davis, C., Asamaphan, P., Smollett, K., Tong, L., Orton, R., Hughes, J., Holland, P., Silva, V., Pascall, D., Puxty, K., da Silva Filipe, A., Yebra, G., Shaaban, S.,

Holden, M., Pinto, R., Gunson, R., Templeton, K., Murcia, P., Patel, A., Klenerman, P., Dunachie, S., Haughney, J., Robertson, D., Palmarini, M., Ray, S. & Thomson, E. (2022). 'SARS-CoV-2 Omicron is an immune escape variant with an altered cell entry pathway'. *Nature Microbiology* Online: Ahead of print.

69. Sun Community News (2021). 'Meadowbrook Healthcare honors COVID-19 vaccine creator'. suncommunitynews.com (acessed 19 May 2022).

70. Neill, U. (2021). 'A conversation with Katalin Karikó'. *Journal of Clinical Investigation* 131: e155559.

Chapter 19

1. Topley, W. & Wilson, G. (1923). 'The Spread of Bacterial Infection. The Problem of Herd-Immunity'. *Journal of Hygiene (London)* 21: 243–9.

2. Drury, A. (1944). 'Prof. W.W.C. Topley, F.R.S'. *Nature* 3877: 215–16.

3. Hobman, T. (2013). 'Rubella virus' in *Fields Virology* (eds: D. M. Knipe & P. M. Howley) pp688–708. Philadelphia, Wolters Kluwer Health/ Lippincott Williams & Wilkins.

4. Anderson, R. & May, R. (1985). 'Vaccination and herd immunity to infectious diseases'. *Nature* 318: 323–9.

5. Szusz, E., Garrison, L. & Bauch, C. (2010). 'A review of data needed to parameterize a dynamic model of measles in developing countries'. *BMC Research Notes* 3: 75.

6. Hobman, T. (2013). 'Rubella virus' in *Fields Virology* (eds: D. M. Knipe & P. M. Howley) pp688–708. Philadelphia, Wolters Kluwer Health/ Lippincott Williams & Wilkins.

7. Janaszek, W., Gay, N. & Gut, W. (2003). 'Measles vaccine efficacy during an epidemic in 1998 in the highly vaccinated population of Poland'. *Vaccine* 21: 473–8.

8. Sobh, A. & Bonilla, F. (2016). 'Vaccination in primary immunodeficiency disorders'. *Journal of Allergy and Clinical Immunology: In Practice* 4: 1066–75.

9. Simons, F. (2010). 'Anaphylaxis'. *Journal of Allergy and Clinical Immunology* 125 Suppl: S161–81.

10. Kelso, J., Jones, R. & Yunginger, J. (1993). 'Anaphylaxis to measles, mumps, and rubella vaccine mediated by IgE to gelatin'. *Journal of Allergy and Clinical Immunology* 91: 867–72.

11. Bohlke, K., Davis, R., Marcy, S., Braun, M., DeStefano, F., Black, S., Mullooly, J. & Thompson, R. (2003). 'Risk of anaphylaxis after vaccination of children and adolescents'. *Pediatrics* 112: 815–20.

12. NIAID (2010). 'Community Immunity ("Herd" Immunity)'. Flickr (Creative Commons). flickr.com (accessed 30 June 2022).

Chapter 20

1. Byers, R. & Moll, F. (1948). 'Encephalopathies following prophylactic pertussis vaccine'. *Pediatrics* 1: 437–57.
2. Ibid.
3. Gordon, N. (1998). 'History of the BPNA'. bpna.org.uk (accessed 30 April 2021).
4. Amirthalingam, G., Gupta, S. & Campbell, H. (2013). 'Pertussis immunisation and control in England and Wales, 1957 to 2012: a historical review'. *EuroSurveillance* 18 (38): 4003–10.
5. Deer, B. (1998). 'The vanishing victims'. *The Sunday Times*, 1 November 1998.
6. Ibid.
7. Hedley-Whyte, J. & Milamed, D. (2019). 'International Contributions toward the Conquest of Polio'. *Ulster Medical Journal* 88: 47–54.
8. Dick, G. (1974). 'Reactions to routine immunization in childhood'. *Proceedings of the Royal Society of Medicine* 67: 371–2.
9. Dick, G. (1975). 'Whooping-cough vaccine'. *British Medical Journal* 4: 161.
10. Medical Research Council (1951). 'Prevention of whooping-cough by vaccination; a Medical Research Council investigation'. *British Medical Journal* 1: 1463–71.
11. Medical Research Council (1956). 'Vaccination against whooping-cough; relation between protection in children and results of laboratory tests; a report to the Whooping-cough Immunization Committee of the Medical Research Council and to the medical officers of health for Cardiff, Leeds, Leyton, Manchester, Middlesex, Oxford, Poole, Tottenham, Walthamstow, and Wembley'. *British Medical Journal* 2: 454–62.
12. Baker, J. (2003). 'The pertussis vaccine controversy in Great Britain, 1974–1986'. *Vaccine* 21 (25–6): 4003–10.
13. Amirthalingam, G., Gupta, S. & Campbell, H. (2013). 'Pertussis immunisation and control in England and Wales, 1957 to 2012: a historical review'. *EuroSurveillance* 18 (38): 4003–10.
14. Alderslade, R., Bellman, M., Rawson, N., Ross, E. & Miller, D. (1981). 'The National Child Encephalopathy Study' in *Whooping Cough* (eds: J. Badenoch & A. Goldberg) pp79–169. London, Crown Copyright.
15. Ibid.
16. Pollock, T. & Morris, J. (1983). 'A 7-year survey of disorders attributed to vaccination in North West Thames region'. *Lancet* 1: 753–7.
17. Melchior, J. (1977). 'Infantile spasms and early immunization against whooping cough. Danish survey from 1970 to 1975'. *Archives of Disease in Childhood* 52: 134–7.
18. Institute of Medicine (1991). *Adverse Effects of Pertussis and Rubella Vaccines: A Report of the Committee to Review the Adverse Consequences of Pertussis and Rubella Vaccines.* Washington, Institute of Medicine.

19. Alderslade, R., Bellman, M., Rawson, N., Ross, E. & Miller, D. (1981). 'The National Child Encephalopathy Study' in *Whooping Cough* (eds: J. Badenoch & A. Goldberg) pp79–169. London, Crown Copyright.

20. Kulenkampff, M., Schwartzman, J. & Wilson, J. (1974). 'Neurological complications of pertussis inoculation'. *Archives of Disease in Childhood* 49: 46–9.

21. Offit, P. (2011). *Deadly Choices: How the Anti-Vaccine Movement Threatens Us All*. New York, Basic Books.

22. Kulenkampff, M., Schwartzman, J. & Wilson, J. (1974). 'Neurological complications of pertussis inoculation'. *Archives of Disease in Childhood* 49: 46–9.

23. Deer, B. (2020). *The Doctor Who Fooled the World: Andrew Wakefield's war on vaccines*. London, Scribe UK.

24. Ross, E. (2021). Author interview. 1 June 2021.

25. Cody, C., Baraff, L., Cherry, J., Marcy, S. & Manclark, C. (1981). 'Nature and rates of adverse reactions associated with DTP and DT immunizations in infants and children'. *Pediatrics* 68: 650–60.

26. Leung, A., Hon, K. & Leung, T. (2018). 'Febrile seizures: an overview'. *Drugs in Context* 7: 212536.

27. Baumer, J., David, T., Valentine, S., Roberts, J. & Hughes, B. (1981). 'Many parents think their child is dying when having a first febrile convulsion'. *Developmental Medicine & Child Neurology* 23: 462–4.

28. Ross, E. (2021). Author interview. 1 June 2021.

29. Institute of Medicine (1991). *Adverse Effects of Pertussis and Rubella Vaccines: A Report of the Committee to Review the Adverse Consequences of Pertussis and Rubella Vaccines*. Washington, Institute of Medicine.

30. Verity, C., Greenwood, R. & Golding, J. (1998). 'Long-term intellectual and behavioral outcomes of children with febrile convulsions'. *New England Journal of Medicine* 338: 1723–8.

31. Institute of Medicine (1991). *Adverse Effects of Pertussis and Rubella Vaccines: A Report of the Committee to Review the Adverse Consequences of Pertussis and Rubella Vaccines*. Washington, Institute of Medicine.

32. Pollock, T. & Morris, J. (1983). 'A 7-year survey of disorders attributed to vaccination in North West Thames region'. *Lancet* 1: 753–7.

33. Melchior, J. (1977). 'Infantile spasms and early immunization against whooping cough. Danish survey from 1970 to 1975'. *Archives of Disease in Childhood* 52: 134–7.

34. Kilgore, P., Salim, A., Zervos, M. & Schmitt, H. J. (2016). 'Pertussis: Microbiology, Disease, Treatment, and Prevention'. *Clinical Microbiology Reviews* 29: 449–86.

35. Hodder, S. & Mortimer Jr, E. (1992). 'Epidemiology of pertussis and reactions to pertussis vaccine'. *Epidemiologic Reviews* 14: 243–67.

36. Ross, E. (2021). Author interview. 1 June 2021.

37. Dravet, C., Bureau, M., Dalla Bernardina, B. & Guerrini, R. (2011). 'Severe myoclonic epilepsy in infancy (Dravet syndrome) 30 years later'. *Epilepsia* 52 Suppl 2: 1–2.
38. Berkovic, S., Harkin, L., McMahon, J., Pelekanos, J., Zuberi, S., Wirrell, E., Gill, D., Iona, X, Mulley, J. & Scheffer, I. (2006). 'De-novo mutations of the sodium channel gene SCN1A in alleged vaccine encephalopathy: a retrospective study'. *Lancet Neurology* 5: 488–92.
39. Dravet, C., Bureau, M., Dalla Bernardina, B. & Guerrini, R. (2011). 'Severe myoclonic epilepsy in infancy (Dravet syndrome) 30 years later'. *Epilepsia* 52 Suppl 2: 1–2.
40. Reyes, I., Hsieh, D., Laux, L. & Wilfong, A. (2011). 'Alleged cases of vaccine encephalopathy rediagnosed years later as Dravet syndrome'. *Pediatrics* 128: e699–702.
41. Sturkenboom, M. (2015). 'The narcolepsy-pandemic influenza story: can the truth ever be unraveled?' *Vaccine* 33 Suppl 2: B6–13.
42. Cohet, C., van der Most, R., Bauchau, V., Bekkat-Berkani, R., Doherty, T., Schuind, A., Tavares Da Silva, F., Rappuoli, R., Garçon, N. & Innis, B. (2019). 'Safety of AS03-adjuvanted influenza vaccines: A review of the evidence'. *Vaccine* 37: 3006–21.
43. Scammell, T. (2015). 'Narcolepsy'. *New England Journal of Medicine* 373: 2654–62.
44. Sarkanen, T., Alakuijala, A., Dauvilliers, Y. & Partinen, M. (2018). 'Incidence of narcolepsy after H1N1 influenza and vaccinations: Systematic review and meta-analysis'. *Sleep Medicine Reviews* 38: 177–86.
45. Scammell, T. (2015). 'Narcolepsy'. *New England Journal of Medicine* 373: 2654–62.
46. Sturkenboom, M. (2015). 'The narcolepsy-pandemic influenza story: can the truth ever be unraveled?' *Vaccine* 33 Suppl 2: B6–13.
47. European Centre for Disease Prevention and Control (2018). *Seasonal influenza vaccination and antiviral use in EU/EEA Member States – Overview of vaccine recommendations for 2017–2018 and vaccination coverage rates for 2015–2016 and 2016–2017 influenza seasons.* Stockholm, ECDC.

Chapter 21
1. Laurance, J. (2011). 'Health: not immune to how research can hurt'. *Independent*, 22 October 2011.
2. Wakefield, A. (2015). 'CDC Whistleblower, Autism & Mandatory Vaccination. Leadership & Longevity 2015 Conference'. The Wellness Way, Green Bay.
3. Wakefield, A., Murch, S., Anthony, A., Linnell, J., Casson, D., Malik, M., Berelowitz, M., Dhillon, A., Thomson, M., Harvey, P., Valentine, A., Davies, S. & Walker-Smith, J. (1998). 'Ileal-lymphoid-nodular hyperplasia, non-specific colitis, and pervasive developmental disorder in children'. *Lancet* 351: 637–41.

4. Wakefield, A., Anthony, A., Murch, S., Thomson, M., Montgomery, S., Davies, S., O'Leary, J., Berelowitz, M. & Walker-Smith, J. (2000). 'Enterocolitis in children with developmental disorders'. *American Journal of Gastroenterology* 95: 2285–95.

5. Uhlmann, V., Martin, C., Sheils, O., Pilkington, L., Silva, I., Killalea, A., Murch, S., Walker-Smith, J., Thomson, M., Wakefield, A. & O'Leary, J. (2002). 'Potential viral pathogenic mechanism for new variant inflammatory bowel disease'. *Molecular Pathologist* 55: 84–90.

6. Wakefield, A., Anthony, A., Murch, S., Thomson, M., Montgomery, S., Davies, S., O'Leary, J., Berelowitz, M. & Walker-Smith, J. (2000). 'Enterocolitis in children with developmental disorders'. *American Journal of Gastroenterology* 95: 2285–95.

7. Taylor, B., Miller, E., Farrington, C., Petropoulos, M. C, Favot-Mayaud, I., Li, J. & Waight, P. (1999). 'Autism and measles, mumps, and rubella vaccine: no epidemiological evidence for a causal association'. *Lancet* 353: 2026–9.

8. Friederichs, V., Cameron, J. & Robertson, C. (2006). 'Impact of adverse publicity on MMR vaccine uptake: a population based analysis of vaccine uptake records for one million children, born 1987–2004'. *Archives of Disease in Childhood* 91: 465–8.

9. Lyall, K., Croen, L., Daniels, J., Fallin, M., Ladd-Acosta, C., Lee, B., Park, B., Snyder, N., Schendel, D., Volk, H., Windham, G. & Newschaffer, C. (2016). 'The Changing Epidemiology of Autism Spectrum Disorders'. *Annual Review of Public Health* 38: 81–102.

10. Ibid.

11. Wakefield, A., Murch, S., Anthony, A., Linnell, J., Casson, D., Malik, M., Berelowitz, M., Dhillon, A., Thomson, M., Harvey, P., Valentine, A., Davies, S. & Walker-Smith, J. (1998). 'Ileal-lymphoid-nodular hyperplasia, non-specific colitis, and pervasive developmental disorder in children'. *Lancet* 351: 637–41.

12. Lyall, K., Croen, L., Daniels, J., Fallin, M., Ladd-Acosta, C., Lee, B., Park, B., Snyder, N., Schendel, D., Volk, H., Windham, G. & Newschaffer, C. (2016). 'The Changing Epidemiology of Autism Spectrum Disorders'. *Annual Review of Public Health* 38: 81–102.

13. Murray, I. (1998). 'Measles vaccine's link with autism studied'. *Times*, 27 February 1998.

14. Wakefield, A., Murch, S., Anthony, A., Linnell, J., Casson, D., Malik, M., Berelowitz, M., Dhillon, A., Thomson, M., Harvey, P., Valentine, A., Davies, S. & Walker-Smith, J. (1998). 'Ileal-lymphoid-nodular hyperplasia, non-specific colitis, and pervasive developmental disorder in children'. *Lancet* 351: 637–41.

15. Afzal, M., Minor, P., Begley, J., Bentley, M., Armitage, E., Ghosh, S. & Ferguson, A. (1998). 'Absence of measles-virus genome in inflammatory bowel disease'. *Lancet* 351: 646–7.

16. Murray, I. (1998). 'Measles vaccine's link with autism studied'. *Times*, 27 February 1998.

17. Ibid.

18. Laurance, J. (2010). 'I was there when Wakefield dropped his bombshell'. *Independent*, 29 January 2010.

19. Hope, J. (1998). 'Ban three-in-one jab urge doctors after new fears'. *Daily Mail*, 27 February 1998.

20. Boseley, S. (1998). 'Undetected bowel illness led to baby's misery'. *Guardian*, 27 February 1998.

21. Deer, B (2011) 'How the vaccine crisis was meant to make money'. BMJ 342:c5258 doi:10.1136/bmj.c5258

22. Deer, B. (2011). 'How the Case Against the MMR Vaccine Was Fixed'. *British Medical Journal* 342: c6260.

23. Deer, B. (2020). *The Doctor Who Fooled the World: Andrew Wakefield's war on vaccines*. London, Scribe UK.

24. Global Health Chronicles (2016). 'Sabin, Deborah'. globalhealthchronicles.org (accessed 5 September 2020).

25. General Medical Council (2010). 'Fitness to Practice Panel Hearing 28 January 2010'. London, General Medical Council.

26. *Thrivetime Show*. (2020). 'Dr. Andy Wakefield. Discovering the terrifying truth about COVID-19 RNA-modifying luciferase 06060 vaccines'. *Thrivetime Show*, series 5, episode 769, 16 December 2020.

27. Griffin, D. (2013). 'Measles Virus' in *Fields Virology* (eds: D. M. Knipe & P. M. Howley) pp1042–69. Philadelphia, Wolters Kluwer Health/ Lippincott Williams & Wilkins.

28. Buchanan, R. & Bonthius, D. (2012). 'Measles virus and associated central nervous system sequelae'. *Seminars in Pediatric Neurology* 19: 107–14.

29. Wakefield, A., Pittilo, R., Sim, R., Cosby, S., Stephenson, J., Dhillon, A. & Pounder, R. (1993). 'Evidence of persistent measles virus infection in Crohn's disease'. *Journal of Medical Virology* 39: 345–53.

30. Deer, B. (2020). *The Doctor Who Fooled the World: Andrew Wakefield's war on vaccines*. London, Scribe UK.

31. Uhlmann, V., Martin, C., Sheils, O., Pilkington, L., Silva, I., Killalea, A., Murch, S., Walker-Smith, J., Thomson, M., Wakefield, A. & O'Leary, J. (2002). 'Potential viral pathogenic mechanism for new variant inflammatory bowel disease'. *Molecular Pathologist* 55: 84–90.

32. Bustin, S. (2004). *A-Z of Quantitative PCR*. La Jolla, International University Line.

33. Bustin, S. (2008). 'RT-qPCR and molecular diagnostics: no evidence for measles virus in the GI tract of autistic children'. *European Pharmaceutical Review* 1: 11–17.

34. Hornig, M., Briese, T., Buie, T., Bauman, M., Lauwers, G., Siemetzki, U., Hummel, K., Rota, P., Bellini, W., O'Leary, J., Sheils, O., Alden, E., Pickering, L. & Lipkin, W. (2008). 'Lack of association between measles

virus vaccine and autism with enteropathy: a case-control study'. *PLoS ONE* 3: e3140.

35. Bustin, S. (2008). 'Fading claims of MMR link to autism'. *Guardian*, 9 December 2008.

36. Autism Society San Francisco Bay Area (2015). *A Report on the Increasing Autism Rates in California*. Autism Society San Francisco Bay Area, San Francisco.

37. Hendriks, J. & Blume, S. (2013). 'Measles vaccination before the measles-mumps-rubella vaccine'. *American Journal of Public Health* 103: 1393–1401.

38. Taylor, B., Miller, E., Farrington, C., Petropoulos, M. C, Favot-Mayaud, I., Li, J. & Waight, P. (1999). 'Autism and measles, mumps, and rubella vaccine: no epidemiological evidence for a causal association'. *Lancet* 353: 2026–9.

39. Taylor, B., Jick, H. & Maclaughlin, D. (2013). 'Prevalence and incidence rates of autism in the UK: time trend from 2004–2010 in children aged 8 years'. *British Medical Journal Open* 3: e003219.

40. Nuffield Trust (2021). 'Vaccination coverage for children and mothers'. nuffieldtrust.org.uk (accessed 31 January 2021).

41. Honda, H., Shimizu, Y. & Rutter, M. (2005). 'No effect of MMR withdrawal on the incidence of autism: a total population study'. *Journal of Child Psychology and Psychiatry* 46: 572–9.

42. Sandin, S., Lichtenstein, P., Kuja-Halkola, R., Larsson, H., Hultman, C. & Reichenberg, A. (2014). 'The familial risk of autism'. *Journal of the American Medical Association* 311: 1770–7.

43. Iossifov, I., O'Roak, B., Sanders, S., Ronemus, M., Krumm, N., Levy, D., Stessman, H., Witherspoon, K., Vives, L., Patterson, K., Smith, J., Paeper, B., Nickerson, D., Dea, J., Dong, S., Gonzalez, L., Mandell, J., Mane, S. M., Murtha, M., Sullivan, C., Walker, M., Waqar, Z., Wei, L., Willsey, A., Yamrom, B., Lee, Y.-H., Grabowska, E., Dalkic, E., Wang, Z., Marks, S., Andrews, P., Leotta, A., Kendall, J., Hakker, I., Rosenbaum, J., Ma, B., Rodgers, L., Troge, J., Narzisi, G., Yoon, S., Schatz, M., Ye, K., McCombie, W., Shendure, J., Eichler, E., State, M. & Wigler, M. (2014). 'The contribution of de novo coding mutations to autism spectrum disorder'. *Nature* 515: 216–21.

44. Flores-Pajot, M. C., Ofner, M., Do, M., Lavigne, E. & Villeneuve, P. (2016). 'Childhood autism spectrum disorders and exposure to nitrogen dioxide, and particulate matter air pollution: A review and meta-analysis'. *Environmental Research* 151: 763–76.

45. Parner, E., Baron-Cohen, S., Lauritsen, M., Jørgensen, M., Schieve, L., Yeargin-Allsopp, M. & Obel, C. (2012). 'Parental age and autism spectrum disorders'. *Annals of Epidemiology* 22: 143–50.

46. Autism Society San Francisco Bay Area (2015). *A Report on the Increasing Autism Rates in California*. Autism Society San Francisco Bay Area, San Francisco.

Chapter 22

1. Harmsen, I., Mollema, L., Ruiter, R., Paulussen, T., de Melker, H. & Kok, G. (2013). 'Why parents refuse childhood vaccination: a qualitative study using online focus groups'. *BMC Public Health* 13: 1183.

2. Glenny, A., Pope, C., Waddington, H. & Wallace, U. (1926). 'The antigenic value of the toxin-antitoxin precipitate of Ramon'. *The Journal of Pathology and Bacteriology* 29: 31–40.

3. Di Pasquale, A., Preiss, S., Tavares Da Silva, F. & Garçon, N. (2015). 'Vaccine Adjuvants: from 1920 to 2015 and Beyond'. *Vaccines* 3: 320–43.

4. Garçon, N. & Friede, M. (2018), 'Evolution of Adjuvants Across the Centuries' in *Plotkin's Vaccines, Seventh edition* (eds: S. A. Plotkin, W. A. Orenstein, P. A. Offit & M. D. Edwards) pp61–74. Philadelphia, Elsevier, Inc.

5. Morefield, G., Sokolovska, A., Jiang, D., HogenEsch, H., Robinson, J. & Hem, S. (2005). 'Role of aluminum-containing adjuvants in antigen internalization by dendritic cells in vitro'. *Vaccine* 23: 1588–95.

6. Goullé, J. P. & Grangeot-Keros, L. (2020). 'Aluminum and vaccines: Current state of knowledge'. *Médecine et Maladies Infectieuses* 50: 16–21.

7. European Food Safety Authority (2008). 'Scientific opinion of the panel on food additives, flavourings, processing aids and food contact materials on a request from European Commission on safety of aluminium from dietary intake'. *EFSA Journal* 754: 1–34.

8. European Chemicals Agency (2018). *Regulation (EU) No 528/2012 concerning the making available on the market and use of biocidal products. Assessment Report. Cholecalciferol.* Helsinki, ECHA.

9. National Center for Biotechnology Information (2021). 'PubChem Compound Summary for CID 1548943, Capsaicin'. pubchem.ncbi.nlm.nih.gov (accessed 13 May 2021).

10. Altmann, P., Cunningham, J., Dhanesha, U., Ballard, M., Thompson, J. & Marsh, F. (1999). 'Disturbance of cerebral function in people exposed to drinking water contaminated with aluminium sulphate: retrospective study of the Camelford water incident'. *British Medical Journal* 319: 807–11.

11. Food Standards Agency (2004). *2000 total diet study of 12 elements – aluminium, arsenic, cadmium, chromium, copper, lead, manganese, mercury, nickel, selenium, tin and zinc.* London, FSA.

12. Krachler, M., Prohaska, T., Koellensperger, G., Rossipal, E. & Stingeder, G. (2000). 'Concentrations of selected trace elements in human milk and in infant formulas determined by magnetic sector field inductively coupled plasma-mass spectrometry'. *Biological Trace Element Research* 76: 97–112.

13. Ameratunga, R., Gillis, D., Gold, M., Linneberg, A. & Elwood, J. (2017). 'Evidence Refuting the Existence of Autoimmune/Autoinflammatory Syndrome Induced by Adjuvants (ASIA)'. *Journal of Allergy Clinical Immunology: in Practice* 5: 1551–5.

14. Linneberg, A., Jacobsen, R., Jespersen, L. & Abildstrøm, S. (2011). 'Association of subcutaneous allergen-specific immunotherapy with incidence of autoimmune disease, ischemic heart disease, and mortality'. *Journal of Allergy and Clinical Immunology* 129: 413–19.

15. Karwowski, M., Stamoulis, C., Wenren, L., Faboyede, G., Quinn, N., Gura, K., Bellinger, D. & Woolf, A. (2018). 'Blood and Hair Aluminum Levels, Vaccine History, and Early Infant Development: A Cross-Sectional Study'. *Academic Pediatrics* 18: 161–5.

16. Collier, L., Polakoff, S. & Mortimer, J. (1979). 'Reactions and antibody responses to reinforcing doses of adsorbed and plain tetanus vaccines'. *Lancet* 8131: 1364–8.

17. Feery, B., Finger, W., Kortus, Z. & Jones, G. (1985). 'The incidence and type of reactions to plain and adsorbed DTP vaccines'. *Australian Paediatric Journal* 21: 91–5.

Chapter 23

1. Singh, J. (2009). Comment: 'Old article/responses but still pertinent'. Under 'Thiomersal doesn't cause developmental disorders'. *British Medical Journal* 329: 588.

2. Pratt, R., Ball, L., Ball, R. & Sikker Jr, W. (2001). *Thimerosal [54-64-8] Nomination to the National Toxicology Program Silver Spring*, Food and Drug Administration.

3. Jamieson, W. & Powell, H. (1931). 'Merthiolate as a preservative for biological products'. *American Journal of Epidemiology* 14: 218–24.

4. Offit, P. (2007). 'Thimerosal and vaccines – a cautionary tale'. *New England Journal of Medicine* 357: 1278–9.

5. Ibid.

6. Pichichero, M., Cernichiari, E., Lopreiato, J. & Treanor, J. (2002). 'Mercury concentrations and metabolism in infants receiving vaccines containing thiomersal: a descriptive study'. *Lancet* 360: 1737–41.

7. Centers for Disease Control and Prevention (1999). 'Notice to Readers: Thimerosal in Vaccines: A Joint Statement of the American Academy of Pediatrics and the Public Health Service'. *Morbidity and Mortality Weekly Report* 48: 563–5.

8. European Medicines Agency (1999). *EMEA public statement on thiomersal containing medicinal products*. London, EMEA.

9. Plotkin, S. (2000). 'Preventing harm from thimerosal in vaccines'. *JAMA* 283: 2104–5.

10. Bernard, S., Enayati, A., Redwood, L., Roger, H. & Binstock, T. (2001). 'Autism: a novel form of mercury poisoning'. *Medical Hypotheses* 56: 462–71.

11. Gadad, B., Li, W., Yazdani, U., Grady, S., Johnson, T., Hammond, J., Gunn, H., Curtis, B., English, C., Yutuc, V., Ferrier, C., Sackett, G., Marti, C., Young, K., Hewitson, L. & German, D. (2015). 'Administration of thimerosal-containing vaccines to infant rhesus

macaques does not result in autism-like behavior or neuropathology'. *Proceedings of the National Academy of Sciences of the USA* 112: 12498–503.

12. Hviid, A., Stellfeld, M., Wohlfahrt, J. & Melbye, M. (2003). 'Association between thimerosal-containing vaccine and autism'. *Journal of the American Medical Association* 290: 1763–6.

13. Madsen, K., Lauritsen, M., Pedersen, C., Thorsen, P., Plesner, A. M., Andersen, P. & Mortensen, P. (2003). 'Thimerosal and the occurrence of autism: negative ecological evidence from Danish population-based data'. *Pediatrics* 112: 604–6.

14. Heron, J. & Golding, J. (2004). 'Thimerosal exposure in infants and developmental disorders: a prospective cohort study in the United Kingdom does not support a causal association'. *Pediatrics* 114: 577–83.

15. Andrews, N., Miller, E., Grant, A., Stowe, J., Osborne, V. & Taylor, B. (2004). 'Thimerosal exposure in infants and developmental disorders: a retrospective cohort study in the United Kingdom does not support a causal association'. *Pediatrics* 114: 584–91.

16. Verstraeten, T., Davis, R., DeStefano, F., Lieu, T., Rhodes, P., Black, S. B., Shinefield, H. & Chen, R. (2003). 'Safety of thimerosal-containing vaccines: a two-phased study of computerized health maintenance organization databases'. *Pediatrics* 112: 1039–48.

17. Schechter, R. & Grether, J. (2008). 'Continuing increases in autism reported to California's developmental services system: mercury in retrograde'. *Archives Of General Psychiatry* 65: 19–24.

18. Fombonne, E., Zakarian, R., Bennett, A., Meng, L. & McLean-Heywood, D. (2006). 'Pervasive developmental disorders in Montreal, Quebec, Canada: prevalence and links with immunizations'. *Pediatrics* 118: e139–50.

19. Dally, A. (1997). 'The rise and fall of pink disease'. *Social History of Medicine* 10: 291–304.

20. Ibid.

21. Autism Society San Francisco Bay Area (2015). *A Report on the Increasing Autism Rates in California*. Autism Society San Francisco Bay Area, San Francisco.

22. Centers for Disease Control and Prevention (2013). *Understanding Thimerosal, Mercury, and Vaccine Safety*. Atlanta, CDC.

23. Wecker, L., Miller, S., Cochran, S., Dugger, D. & Johnson, W. (1985). 'Trace element concentrations in hair from autistic children'. *Journal of Mental Deficiency Research* 29 (Pt 1): 15–22.

24. Lyall, K., Croen, L., Daniels, J., Fallin, M., Ladd-Acosta, C., Lee, B., Park, B., Snyder, N., Schendel, D., Volk, H., Windham, G. & Newschaffer, C. (2016). 'The Changing Epidemiology of Autism Spectrum Disorders'. *Annual Review of Public Health* 38: 81–102.

25. Autism Society San Francisco Bay Area (2015). *A Report on the Increasing Autism Rates in California*. Autism Society San Francisco Bay Area, San Francisco.

Chapter 24

1. Telford, R. & Rogers, A. (2003). 'What influences elderly peoples' decisions about whether to accept the influenza vaccination? A qualitative study'. *Health Education Research* 18: 743–53.

2. Demicheli, V., Jefferson, T., Ferroni, E., Rivetti, A. & Di Pietrantonj, C. (2018). 'Vaccines for preventing influenza in healthy adults'. *Cochrane Database of Systematic Reviews* 2: CD001269.

3. Matias, G., Taylor, R., Haguinet, F., Schuck-Paim, C., Lustig, R. & Fleming, D. (2016). 'Modelling estimates of age-specific influenza-related hospitalisation and mortality in the United Kingdom'. *BMC Public Health* 16: 481.

4. Paterson, P., Chantler, T. & Larson, H. (2018). 'Reasons for non-vaccination: Parental vaccine hesitancy and the childhood influenza vaccination school pilot programme in England'. *Vaccine* 36: 5397–5401.

5. Jefferson, T., Rivetti, A., Di Pietrantonj, C. & Demicheli, V. (2018). 'Vaccines for preventing influenza in healthy children'. *Cochrane Database of Systematic Reviews* 2: CD004879.

6. Moriyama, M., Hugentobler, W. & Iwasaki, A. (2020). 'Seasonality of Respiratory Viral Infections'. *Annual Review of Virology* 7: 83–101.

7. Ibid.

8. Fisman, D. (2012). 'Seasonality of viral infections: mechanisms and unknowns'. *Clinical Microbiology and Infection* 18: 946–54.

9. Wat, D. (2004). 'The common cold: a review of the literature'. *European Journal of Internal Medicine* 15: 79–88.

10. Pebody, R., Djennad, A., Ellis, J., Andrews, N., Marques, D., Cottrell, S., Reynolds, A., Gunson, R., Galiano, M., Hoschler, K., Lackenby, A., Robertson, C., O'Doherty, M., Sinnathamby, M., Panagiotopoulos, N., Yonova, I., Webb, R., Moore, C., Donati, M., Sartaj, M., Shepherd, S., McMenamin, J., de Lusignan, S. & Zambon, M. (2019). 'End of season influenza vaccine effectiveness in adults and children in the United Kingdom in 2017/18'. *EuroSurveillance* 24: 1800488.

11. Public Health England (2020). *Surveillance of Influenza and Other Respiratory Viruses in the UK: Winter 2019 to 2020*. London, PHE.

12. Pebody, R., Warburton, F., Ellis, J., Andrews, N., Potts, A., Cottrell, S., Reynolds, A., Gunson, R., Thompson, C., Galiano, M., Robertson, C., Gallagher, N., Sinnathamby, M., Yonova, I., Correa, A., Moore, C., Sartaj, M., de Lusignan, S., McMenamin, J. & Zambon, M. (2017). 'End-of-season influenza vaccine effectiveness in adults and children, United Kingdom, 2016/17'. *EuroSurveillance* 22: 17–306.

13. Pebody, R., Warburton, F., Ellis, J., Andrews, N., Potts, A., Cottrell, S., Johnston, J., Reynolds, A., Gunson, R., Thompson, C., Galiano, M., Robertson, C., Byford, R., Gallagher, N., Sinnathamby, M., Yonova, I., Pathirannehelage, S., Donati, M., Moore, C., de Lusignan, S., McMenamin, J. & Zambon, M. (2016). 'Effectiveness of seasonal influenza vaccine for adults and children in preventing

laboratory-confirmed influenza in primary care in the United Kingdom: 2015/16 end-of-season results'. *EuroSurveillance* 21: 30348.

14. Pebody, R., Green, H., Andrews, N., Boddington, N., Zhao, H., Yonova, I., Ellis, J., Steinberger, S., Donati, M., Elliot, A., Hughes, H., Pathirannehelage, S., Mullett, D., Smith, G., de Lusignan, S. & Zambon, M. (2015). 'Uptake and impact of vaccinating school age children against influenza during a season with circulation of drifted influenza A and B strains, England, 2014/15'. *EuroSurveillance* 20: 30029.

Chapter 25

1. Hilton, S., Petticrew, M. & Hunt, K. (2006). '"Combined vaccines are like a sudden onslaught to the body's immune system": parental concerns about vaccine "overload" and "immune-vulnerability"'. *Vaccine* 24: 4321–7.

2. Shearer, W., Rosenblatt, H., Gelman, R., Oyomopito, R., Plaeger, S., Stiehm, E., Wara, D., Douglas, S., Luzuriaga, K., McFarland, E., Yogev, R., Rathore, M., Levy, W., Graham, B. & Spector, S. (2003). 'Lymphocyte subsets in healthy children from birth through 18 years of age: the pediatric AIDS clinical trials group P1009 study'. *Journal of Allergy and Clinical Immunology* 112: 973–80.

3. Simon, A., Hollander, G. & McMichael, A. (2015). 'Evolution of the immune system in humans from infancy to old age'. *Proceedings of the Royal Society B: Biological Sciences* 282: 20143085.

4. Offit, P., Quarles, J., Gerber, M., Hackett, C., Marcuse, E., Kollman, T., Gellin, B. & Landry, S. (2002). 'Addressing parents' concerns: do multiple vaccines overwhelm or weaken the infant's immune system?' *Pediatrics* 109: 124–9.

5. Joint Committee on Vaccination and Immunisation (2004). 'Minutes of the meeting held on 6 February 2004'. JCVI.

6. Hviid, A., Wohlfahrt, J., Stellfeld, M. & Melbye, M. (2005). 'Childhood vaccination and nontargeted infectious disease hospitalization'. *Journal of the American Medical Association* 294: 699–705.

7. Glanz, J., Newcomer, S., Daley, M., DeStefano, F., Groom, H., Jackson, M., Lewin, B., McCarthy, N., McClure, D., Narwaney, K., Nordin, J. & Zerbo, O. (2018). 'Association Between Estimated Cumulative Vaccine Antigen Exposure Through the First 23 Months of Life and Non-Vaccine-Targeted Infections From 24 Through 47 Months of Age'. *Journal of the American Medical Association* 319: 906–13.

8. Iqbal, S., Barile, J., Thompson, W. & DeStefano, F. (2013). 'Number of antigens in early childhood vaccines and neuropsychological outcomes at age 7–10 years'. *Pharmacoepidemiology and Drug Safety* 22: 1263–70.

9. Smith, M. & Woods, C. (2010). 'On-time vaccine receipt in the first year does not adversely affect neuropsychological outcomes'. *Pediatrics* 125: 1134–41.

Epilogue

1. Anyiam-Osigwe, T. (2021). 'The Long View: The world's last smallpox patient'. gavi.org (acessed 16 July 2021).
2. Global Polio Eradication Initiative (2018). 'Remembering Ali Maalin'. polioeradication.org (accessed 6 February 2022).
3. World Health Organization (2022). 'Disease Outbreak News; Wild poliovirus type 1 (WPV1) – Malawi'. who.int (accessed 18 March 2022).
4. World Health Organization (2022). 'Mozambique confirms wild poliovirus case'. who.int (accessed 24 July 2022).
5. Laurens, M. (2020). 'RTS,S/AS01 vaccine (Mosquirix™): an overview'. *Human Vaccines and Immunotherapeutics* 16: 480–9.
6. World Health Organization (2021). 'WHO welcomes historic decision by Gavi to fund the first malaria vaccine'. who.int (accessed 6 February 2022).
7. World Health Organization (2021). *World Malaria Report 2021*. Geneva, World Health Organization.

Index